Handbook of Prescribing Medications for Geriatric Patients

Handbook of Prescribing Medications for Geriatric Patients

Judith C. Ahronheim, M.D.
Associate Professor of Geriatrics and Adult Development, and Medicine, Mount Sinai School of Medicine of the City University of New York; Attending Physician, Departments of Geriatrics and Adult Development, and Medicine, The Mount Sinai Medical Center, New York

Little, Brown and Company
Boston/ Toronto/ London

Library of Congress Catalog Card No. 91-75465

ISBN 0-316-02042-7

Printed in the United States of America

RRD-VA

To Sylvia Edith Ahronheim, M.D., mother of seven.
She taught us, among other things, not to take drugs.

Contents

Preface

Chronological age does not correlate well with biological age. At the age of 65, one may qualify for certain governmental benefits—notably Medicare and Social Security—but this is a historical phenomenon that is a tradition and cultural mandate rather than a marker of biological age. In *Handbook of Prescribing Medications for Geriatric Patients*, the *geriatric* or *elderly* patient is defined as *an individual whose biological age is advanced.* By definition, such an individual has one or more diseases, one or more silent lesions in various organ systems, and a life expectancy of approximately 10 years. In addition, there are physiological changes that affect response to or handling of medications, and because of these dosing recommendations may need to be modified. This biologically advanced age begins, on the average, after 75, but there is wide variation; some people in their sixties are quite frail and a few in their eighties or older are quite robust and able to withstand serious physiological stresses.

In this book, prescribing guidelines are conservative. They are based on the current understanding of physiological changes that are likely to be present in late life and on the possibility of silent pathology. Diseases that affect drug response and drug handling may be superimposed on these factors, requiring that the choice of medication be reassessed and the dosage modified further.

Sections of this book that describe adverse effects and drug interactions are written to highlight situations that are either very common or particularly important for the geriatric patient. These sections are detailed but are not intended to be an exhaustive summary of all situations that may arise. For complete prescribing information, the reader is advised to consult standard reference material, such as the *Physicians' Desk Reference.* Recommended readings for further information are suggested in a bibliography at the end of each chapter.

J.C.A.

Acknowledgments

A number of colleagues reviewed specific sections of the manuscript and provided expertise in their subspecialty areas, for which I am very grateful. Their astute comments have been incorporated into the text. I would like to warmly acknowledge the following physician-scholars (in alphabetical order), who gave their assistance:

From Mount Sinai School of Medicine—Philip Kanof, psychopharmacology; Diane Meier, osteoporosis; Perry Starer, urinary incontinence.

From New York University School of Medicine—Istvan Boksay, psychiatry and psychopharmacology; Michael Cohen, ophthalmology; Michael J. Faust, gastroenterology; Marty Finkelstein, infectious diseases and immunology; Govindan Gopinathan, neurology; Bernard Kaminetsky, hypertension and electrolytes; Thomas G. Kantor, rheumatology and pain control; Clement Marks, pulmonary; Mark Nachamie, cardiology; Miguel Sanchez, dermatology; Norman Sussman, psychiatry and sleep disorders; Jir Tsai, endocrinology; Stanford Wessler, anticoagulation.

From University of Chicago, Pritzker School of Medicine—Margaret Winker, geriatric clinical pharmacology.

I have also received moral and practical support from some exceptional people: Susan Pioli from Little, Brown, who is not only a fine editor but also a lovely human being, and Gerald Blandford, M.D., my own esteemed geriatrician, who was often consulted for scholarly advice but has been especially appreciated for being a wonderful and patient husband.

Handbook of Prescribing Medications for Geriatric Patients

Drug Use in the Elderly

Because biologic and chronologic age are not well matched, one cannot make sweeping generalizations about geriatric patients. However, two important pharmacologic observations have been made regarding older individuals: (1) they experience an increased incidence of adverse drug effects, and (2) there is an increased likelihood that the patient will respond atypically to a given drug. An atypical response may be manifested as an enhanced effect, a diminished effect, or an unexpected adverse effect. These problems are due partly to age-related pharmacokinetic and pharmacodynamic changes and can be mitigated by appropriate dosing and anticipation of the patient's vulnerabilities, which can aid selection of the proper drug. However, the physician must also be aware of nonpharmacologic problems that may put the patient at risk. Some of these problems, seemingly mundane, can thwart the best intentions of the most highly skilled prescriber.

PHARMACOKINETIC AND PHARMACODYNAMIC CHANGES

Physiologic and pathologic alterations occur in geriatric patients with such frequency that drug selection and dosage is often quite different than it is for younger adults. **Pharmacokinetic** factors are those having to do with drug disposition—namely, absorption, distribution, metabolism, and excretion. In the elderly, pharmacokinetic changes are brought about by certain physiological age changes as well as overt and subclinical disease in various organ systems. **Pharmacodynamic** factors are those influencing actual sensitivity to a particular concentration of the drug at the tissue level—these factors determine the degree of therapeutic response and whether or not an adverse effect will occur. Pharmacodynamic factors that may be altered with age are the quality and quantity of tissue receptors for a particular drug, and the presence of disease or age-related physiologic changes in the target organ or a distant organ.

This distinction can be illustrated by the drug digoxin. Digoxin is cleared by the kidney and is generally given to geriatric patients at half the usual adult dose in order to compensate for age-related diminution in glomerular filtration rate (GFR), a pharmacokinetic change. The presence of disease in the target organ (the heart) could result in an enhanced effect of digoxin, even in appropriate doses, leading to a toxic arrhythmia, a pharmacodynamic change. If overt or subclinical disease exists in a distant organ, for example the brain, central nervous system toxicity could occur, even in the absence of other signs of digitalis toxicity. The common co-occurrence of disease in distant organs is an important factor in management of elderly patients.

In contrast, diminished sensitivity to drugs could occur with age. Beta-receptor sensitivity may decline, and some investigators argue that a subgroup of geriatric patients exhibit a diminished response to the beta-receptor antagonists.

Functional alterations may obscure the acutal pharmacodynamic response in some cases. For example, although geriatric patients

1

tend to exhibit an enhanced sensitivity to the anticonvulsant phenytoin, demonstrating cognitive disturbances or sedation at lower than
expected drug levels, subtle changes might be unnoticed or disre-
garded. A sedentary or physically impaired patient might not notice
the lack of fine motor control and the impaired coordination produced by therapeutic levels of the drug as readily as a younger or
more robust adult whose physical demands might make such
changes readily apparent. Likewise, older patients or their caregivers might have diminished expectations of physical or intellectual capacities and might pay less attention to small decrements in
these abilities than if they were to occur in a younger or more active
person.

Pharmacokinetic and pharmacodynamic alterations and their implications are summarized in Tables 1-1 and 1-2.

Although much has been written about age-related alterations in
drug disposition, there is disagreement as to the extent and inevitability of these changes. Studies focusing on aged individuals suffer
from several problems. Cross-sectional studies comparing young
and old subjects sometimes compare young, healthy individuals
with aged subjects gathered from hospitals or nursing homes. If the
aged subjects are "healthy" they may nonetheless have subclinical
disease, which can alter outcomes in studies that seek to determine
a drug's disposition and effects. However, aged subjects that are
truly healthy may represent an elite minority so that the study's results may not be applicable to the general elderly population. Longitudinal studies are almost impossible to complete and data is sparse,
but recent findings indicate that the geriatric population is, indeed,
heterogeneous.

In addition to these pitfalls, it is not known how generalizations
about aging physiology, even if they are true, can be applied to
drug disposition, since most drugs have not been subjected to exhaustive age-specific testing and few conclusions can be reached
based on pharmacokinetic data. Even less is known about pharmacodynamic changes because the study of age-related tissue receptor
density, activity, and sensitivity is in its infancy. We must therefore
rely on clinical observations to a large extent when drawing conclusions about efficacy and potential toxicity of various agents in
use.

Table 1-1. Pharmacokinetic Changes in the Elderly

Change	Example of Drug Affected
Alpha$_1$ A glycoprotein	Lidocaine
Fat:lean ratio (F > M)	Diazepam; alcohol
GFR, tubular secretion	Digoxin; penicillin
Hepatic blood flow	Propranolol; triazolam
Hepatic oxidation	Diazepam
(No change in hepatic conjugation)	(Lorazepam)
Serum albumin	Warfarin; sulfonylurea

Note: These changes and their effects on the selected drugs are not universal. A
wide scatter exists in the geriatric population.

Table 1–2. Pharmacodynamic Alterations in the Elderly

Alteration	Drug	Possible Outcome
Impaired barorecep-tor function; venous insufficiency	Diuretics; tricyclics; methyldopa; others	Orthostatic hypoten-sion
Decreased beta recep-tor sensitivity	Beta blockers	Inadequate control of hypertension or heart rate
Impaired coun-terregulatory mech-anisms	Hydralazine	No reflex tachycardia
Altered temperature regulation	Phenothiazines	Hypo- or hyperthermia
Increased ADH secre-tion	Chlorpropamide; others	Hyponatremia
Decreased androgenic hormones (males)	Digoxin; spironolactone	Gynecomastia

Underlying Disorder*	Drug	Possible Side Effect
Atrophic gastritis	Aspirin; NSAIDs	Gastric hemorrhage
Immobility; cathartic bowel	Many	Constipation
Alzheimer's disease	Many	Confusional state
Sinus or AV nodal dis-ease	Digoxin; verapamil	Bradycardia
Venous insufficiency	Nifedipine	Edema
Cataracts	Corticosteroids	Accelerated formation of cataract
Unstable bladder	Diuretic	Incontinence
Prostatic hyperplasia	Anticholinergics; tricy-clics; diisopyramide	Urinary retention
Parkinson's disease	Metoclopramide; neuro-leptics	Parkinsonian symp-toms

*May be subclinical.

PHARMACOKINETIC CHANGES

Gastrointestinal absorption of drugs does not decline, as a rule, with age. Reduction in parietal cell mass leads to an increased incidence of gastric hypochlorhydria with age. However, other factors may compensate and the net effect is generally slight. Increased gastric pH lowers the solubility of certain agents, impairing their absorp-tion in the intestine. Calcium carbonate is poorly absorbed in the presence of hypochlorhydria, but when taken with meals, absorption is adequate. Gastric absorption of salicylate is reduced in the less acid environment, but dissolution rate is increased so that no net change in absorption occurs. Finally, levodopa is decarboxylated in an acid environment to dopamine, which reduces its entry into the central nervous system, with the result that older patients have increased serum levels of levodopa and a tendency to greater peripheral toxicity. For this reason, levodopa is routinely given in combination with carbidopa, which postpones decarboxylation until the substance enters the brain.

Delayed gastric emptying, decreased gastrointestinal motility, and decreased splanchnic blood flow are other factors that contribute to altered drug handling in a proportion of the elderly. The various effects that could occur as a result are probably offset by the great capacity for passive absorption by the upper small intestine. With the exception of a few drugs, gastrointestinal absorption does not appear to be significantly altered as a consequence of normal aging.

Distribution of certain drugs is altered with age. The volume of distribution (V_d) is the hypothetical volume in which a drug exists at equilibrium; it is derived by computing the total amount of drug in the body relative to its concentration in plasma. The V_d tells us how widely the drug is distributed beyond what is represented by measuring its concentration in plasma. The distribution is dependent on the drug's extent of binding to plasma proteins (which will prevent it from being released from the plasma compartment, thereby reducing the V_d), its degree of lipid solubility (which enables it to traverse lipid membranes and enter tissues, thereby increasing the V_d), and its degree of binding to various body tissues. With age, total body fat increases and lean body mass tends to decrease as a percentage of total body weight. Therefore, the V_d for fat-soluble drugs tends to increase with age, whereas for water-soluble drugs it tends to decrease. Alterations in protein binding are common in old age (see below), affecting the V_d of highly bound drugs in certain situations.

The larger the V_d, the lower the peak plasma levels and the greater the elimination half-life, all other factors remaining equal. Lipid-soluble drugs tend to distribute widely in geriatric patients. Although peak plasma level might not be increased for a lipid-soluble drug such as diazepam, the drug can accumulate in tissues and the likelihood of toxicity could increase over time with daily dosing, and might present in a delayed manner. This is a troubling problem in geriatrics since delayed toxicity can be mistaken for other problems. However, with a water-soluble substance such as alcohol, peak plasma levels would be higher after a given initial dose, and the acute effect might be accentuated. For both lipid- and water-soluble drugs, the situation is actually far more complex, affected by factors such as hepatic metabolism, renal excretion, and increased sensitivity to the agent.

Protein Binding

Drugs are bound to plasma proteins, notably albumin, alpha$_1$ A glycoprotein (AAG), which circulates in the globulin fraction, and certain other globulins. The intensity of protein binding (represented by the dissociation constant, K_d) probably does not change with age. Protein synthesis declines in normal aging, resulting in plasma albumin levels that are lower but still within the normal range. Levels may decrease rapidly, however, when elderly patients become sick.

When protein binding decreases acutely, the amount of drug that circulates freely in plasma (free fraction) increases. Free drug is able to move out of the extracellular fluid and distribute to tissues, and could result in enhanced pharmacologic effect. However, free drug can also reach organs of elimination such as the liver and kidney, and be made more available for metabolism and excretion, eventually offsetting the acutely increased pharmacologic effect. Decreased protein binding that occurs in normal aging probably has little clinical significance, but in acute and chronic illness, or when drugs displace one another at protein binding sites, enhanced drug effects may occur.

AAG levels increase with age. Since this protein is an acute phase reactant, it may be higher than normal in elderly populations because of underlying disease. Basic drugs, such as propranolol, lidocaine, and quinidine, are bound to AAG rather than to albumin, which binds primarily acidic drugs. However, the importance of this has not yet been fully delineated.

Metabolism of drugs takes place primarily in the liver, with a small amount occurring in the kidney, small intestine, and lungs.

Drugs are classified as **high extraction** or **low extraction**, depending on the rate with which they are removed from the blood as they pass through the liver. Hepatic blood flow tends to decline with age. Thus, drugs that depend on extraction for metabolism should be cleared more slowly with age. Although this is true for one high extraction drug, propranolol, it is not true for all, e.g., lidocaine. The clearance of low extraction drugs is relatively more dependent on hepatic enzyme activity. Low extraction drugs that are highly protein-bound (warfarin and tolbutamide) may also depend on the degree of protein binding for their clearance, since an increase in the free fraction would allow more drug to be presented to the liver for metabolism.

In the liver, enzymatic transformation of drugs can occur by several mechanisms. The traditional schema separates these mechanisms into Phase I and Phase II metabolism. Some drugs undergo sequential metabolism by more than one process. Many, but not all drugs that undergo primarily Phase I metabolism (oxidation) tend to be cleared more slowly with age, whereas those dependent on Phase II metabolism (conjugation) tend to have unaltered, and in some cases enhanced, clearance.

In general, hepatic transformation can involve the microsomal enzyme (mixed function oxidase or cytochrome P-450) system, or nonmicrosomal enzymes. Microsomal enzymes can be induced or inhibited by a number of drugs and other exogenous agents. There is a large genetic variation in the activity of the system and its inducibility. This genetic variation probably accounts somewhat for the inconsistencies that have been observed in aging research of this system. At present, the consensus is that the activity of the microsomal system declines with age, either because the enzymes themselves change or because the hepatocellular milieu changes in some way. There is general disagreement over whether induction of this system grows sluggish.

There is also conflicting evidence with regard to Phase II processes, but the bulk of evidence suggests that this function does not decline with age, and in some cases (e.g., glucuronidation of some drugs) increases with age.

In short, there is controversy as to the nature of age changes in hepatic drug metabolism, which are difficult to measure in the clinical setting. The functions that seem to decline with age are associated with significant variability among individuals as well as among drugs.

Excretion

Renal excretion tends to decline significantly with age, glomerular filtration rate decreasing by nearly 50% on the average between the ages of 20 and 70. However, there is great interindividual variation in this decline, renal function remaining youthful in many older individuals.

Drugs that depend on renal function for their clearance (e.g., digoxin), or that have active metabolites that are renally excreted (e.g., chlorpropamide), must be given cautiously in the elderly. Serum creatinine is a poor predictor of renal function in late life because the level of creatinine in the serum depends on muscle mass and muscle mass declines with age. Thus, serum creatinine may be normal even in the face of significantly reduced creatinine clearance. Creatinine clearance can be accurately measured only when a 24-hour urine collection is analyzed, but this is a difficult specimen to obtain in many elderly patients. Thus, one should assume that a renally excreted drug is eliminated slowly by a given elderly patient until proven otherwise, and the dosage should be decreased accordingly. This is particularly important for agents with a narrow therapeutic index, such as digoxin and gentamicin. It may be less important for a medication such as penicillin, which has a wide therapeutic index, or for an agent such as insulin, for which there is a readily measurable end point, namely, blood sugar.

In many cases, it is helpful to have a clear estimate of renal function before prescribing a drug, as in a seriously ill patient who requires a potentially toxic antibiotic such as gentamicin. In such situations, the Cockcroft-Gault equation for estimation of creatinine function can be used. When estimating creatinine clearance in this way, it is important to know that dose adjustments for renal function are made only when maintenance dose is being calculated. It is most often an excessively high maintenance dose, rather than a loading dose, that leads to drug accumulation and dose-related toxicity. Loading doses tend to produce toxicity as a result of pharmacodynamic factors.

Rapid Assessment of Creatinine Clearance: Utility and Pitfalls of the Cockcroft-Gault Equation

Rapid assessment of creatinine clearance is done via the following equation (see Cockcroft & Gault):

$$\text{Creatinine Clearance} = \frac{\text{Weight(kg)} \times (140 - \text{Age})}{72 \times \text{Serum Creatinine (mg /dl)}}$$

For women, multiply result × 0.85

This widely used equation was derived from a group of hospitalized men studied in a retrospective manner. The correction factor for women is based on estimates of altered body composition. Though a crude method of estimating renal function, the data used for this equation correlate well with data derived elsewhere and reflect the fact that, on the average, creatinine clearance declines by 50% from the third to the eighth decade of life.

For the significant minority of older patients who do not have age-related decline in renal function, reliance on this equation poses a risk of underdosing. Conversely, the equation will overestimate creatinine clearance in some patients and is not reliable in severe renal failure, i.e., when GFR is less than 10 ml/min. The dilemma is confounded by the fact that creatinine clearance as well as serum creatinine may change daily in sick patients.

Unknowns
Certain drugs and their metabolites are excreted through the hepatobiliary system and may undergo enterohepatic circulation. The degree to which function of this system changes with age requires further study.

Summary
The consequences of the many age-related pharmacokinetic changes are that many drugs reach higher concentrations and remain in the body for longer periods in older individuals than in younger adults. In addition, because the steady-state concentration of a drug is achieved only after 5 half-lives have passed, steady state at a given dosage may be achieved much later than expected. A physician may mistakenly prescribe dose increases sooner than indicated and, with some drugs, adverse effects may appear long after the drug was first initiated. When this happens the side effect can be mistaken for a non-drug-related problem.

Drug-Drug and Nutrient-Drug Interactions
Interactions can occur and interfere with drug disposition. Elderly outpatients take an average of two to three drugs daily, and institutionalized patients an average of seven. Drugs may compete for gastrointestinal absorption or renal excretion, may induce or inhibit the activity of hepatic enzymes, and may displace one another from protein binding sites. Vitamins, minerals, and over-the-counter preparations participate in these interactions as well. Geriatric patients are more likely to be exposed to these interactions because of the large number of agents that they are ingesting. Unfortunately, although many interactions can be predicted, others cannot.

PITFALLS IN DOSAGE CALCULATION
In view of the fact that drug metabolism and excretion is often decreased with age, it is wise to start with a low dose and increase slowly until therapeutic effect is achieved, unless the clinical situation demands that therapeutic levels are achieved promptly. Because a drug's loading dose is dependent on its V_d, it is difficult to calculate an age-adjusted loading dose, and one generally has to make an educated guess, starting with the usual adult loading dose. In most cases, inappropriately high maintenance doses are more likely to produce dose-related toxicity than the loading dose. However, elderly patients are often exquisitely sensitive to the high plasma levels attained acutely when a loading dose is given, so that potentially toxic drugs like theophylline, digoxin, and lidocaine should be given slowly, the patient should be clinically monitored, therapeutic drug levels should be performed, and appropriate dosage intervals of the drug observed.

Drug dosages are often calculated on the basis of lean body weight or ideal body weight, or body-mass index (weight in kilograms divided by height in meters squared). Body weight that is ideal for height cannot be predicted accurately in late life, since height decreases with age, particularly in women. Standards of ideal body weight and body-mass index that have been adopted for adults in general can lead to erroneous assumptions about the geriatric patient. If a certain drug dose is supposed to be calculated on the basis of lean body weight but the patient is obese, simply weighing the patient may dangerously overestimate the drug dose. Caution dictates that lean body weight be estimated, but this is done by measuring height and checking ideal body weight tables. These tables do not take into consideration the aged patient with loss of height due to skeletal changes such as vertebral osteoporosis or increased flexion at the knee and hip. Using these tables will then define the patient as being overweight and the dose will be determined on a lean body weight for a much shorter person, resulting in underdosing.

In the absence of guidelines in this situation, caution must be observed. At the very least, one should make an effort to determine what the patient's height was at the age of 40.

THE PROBLEM OF POLYPHARMACY

The elderly take far more prescription and over-the-counter drugs than do younger patients. This problem of **polypharmacy** results in a greater number of adverse drug reactions because of the numeric exposure itself, and because of drug-drug interactions. In addition, a patient who is overwhelmed by a complicated medical regimen is more likely to make medication errors, which can lead not only to toxicity but to lower therapeutic effect. A medication regimen can almost always be simplified if the following measures are observed.

1. Obtain a geriatric drug history. Geriatric patients often take over-the-counter preparations, eye drops, injectables, suppositories, and transdermal medications, but will not report these when asked about "medicines" or "pills." All active agents can produce side effects and participate in drug interactions, regardless of the route of delivery. A complete and accurate history can often be achieved only if the patient or family member brings in all medications for inspection. A home visit is often revealing.

Asking the right questions prevents pills from being taken for the wrong reason. Patients who are told to discontinue a diuretic may resume the medication because without it they were "not urinating enough." Sleeping pills are often mistakenly prescribed to patients kept awake by dyspnea, pain, or nocturia. One patient begged for sleeping pills because she couldn't sleep past 2 A.M., but when finally asked, reported that she went to bed (and slept) by 8 P.M., but she was socially isolated and suffered from low vision so she had nothing to do after dark but sleep.

Elderly patients often visit a number of physicians and may obtain prescriptions from all of them. One patient who received warfarin from her cardiologist developed gastrointestinal hemorrhage when she was given trimethoprim-sulfamethoxasole by her urologist. A glaucoma patient with hypertension who was given hydrochlorothiazide by her internist developed severe hypokalemia when acetazolamide was added by the ophthalmologist. All physicians involved in the care of the patient should be fully informed about the drug regimen so that harmful interactions can be avoided. This task often falls to the primary care physician, who is in a position to act as gate keeper.

2. If an adverse effect occurs, don't add a drug. Take one away. Identify all problems that could be drug side effects. These of course are best managed by stopping the offending agent rather than writing yet another prescription. Unfortunately, the latter approach is often used, probably because drug effects mimic geriatric problems. Table 1–3 summarizes some drug effects that tend to be erroneously managed.

3. Discontinue all drugs deemed unnecessary or of questionable therapeutic efficacy. The patient may resist at first, often tenaciously, so it is sensible to attempt this in steps. One patient was successfully withdrawn from five medications but insisted on the sixth because she felt that she needed to be taking "at least *some* medicine." Although innocuous agents can be discontinued abruptly, others, such as cardiovascular, psychotropic, and neurotropic agents, should be withdrawn slowly.

Drugs and their faulty indications are summarized in Table 1–4.

4. Identify the overtreated patient. Blood pressure need not be lowered to 120/80 in the geriatric patient. Digoxin need not be "pushed to toxicity" for inotropic effect. Simple ventricular arrhythmias do not need to be completely suppressed and may require no treatment. Mild peripheral edema usually does not have to be treated out of hand and often requires only reassurance.

5. Employ nonpharmacologic treatments whenever feasible. Nonpharmacologic approaches can reduce or even eliminate the need for drugs in many disorders and are given throughout this book. Although physical exercise generally has to be modified in the elderly, many patients express delight in playing an active part in their treatment and knowing that something still can be done "at that age." Dietary modifications may be extremely difficult, should be imposed cautiously if there is evidence that the patient's nutritional status is marginal, and should be avoided if they reduce the patient's quality of life.

Patient education is itself an important nonpharmacologic ap-

Table 1–3. Some Erroneously Managed Drug Effects

Side Effect	Offering Agent	Common Error
Gout	Nonessential diuretic	Hypouricemic agent
Bladder dysfunction	Diuretic	Antispasmodic
Urinary retention	Diisopyramide; tricyclics; anticholinergics	Urecholine
Hyperglycemia	Thiazides; corticosteroids	Hypoglycemic agents
Constipation	Antihypertensives; tricyclics; others	Laxative
Loose bowels	Antacids; fecal impaction	Antidiarrheal agent
Confusion	Many	Extensive workup
Arrhythmia	Timolol eye drops; adrenergic agents; bronchodilators	Pacemaker; antiarrhythmic
Restlessness (akathesia)	Neuroleptic	Increased dose

Table 1-4. Drugs and Their Faulty Indications

Agent	Faulty Indication
Megavitamins	Probably all
Multivitamins	Energy; appetite; "health"
Choline and lecithin	Memory
Zinc	Idiopathic or structural hyposmia
Vasodilator	Memory loss
Diuretic	Minimal dependent edema; "to urinate"
Laxatives	Regularity
Digoxin	Edema; sinus tachycardia
Hypnotics	Sleeplessness due to nocturia, PND, or pain
Androgens	Involutional or vascular impotence
Hypoglycemic agents	Nondiabetic glucose intolerance; secondary hyperglycemia with cause removed
Antacids	Constipation
Anti-arrhythmics	Benign atrial or ventricular ectopics
Thyroid hormone	Fatigue; obesity; abnormal basal metabolic rate, protein bound iodine, or low T_3

proach. Patients often assume that pills increase appetite, make them energetic, and improve memory or sexual potency. Others may not know that it is harmless to move the bowels less than once a day, that essential tremor is not harmful, that their heart is fine, or that they do not need to sleep 8 hours every night. Patients may share pills with one another, believing that what works for one person will work for others. Although major changes in diet may be hard to achieve, small dietary tips can be very helpful: Unaware diabetic patients are known to quench their thirst with large amounts of fruit juice; one diabetic patient was unaware that 4 pounds of grapes a day was inadvisable.

THE PROBLEM OF COMPLIANCE

The actual medical regimen and the prescribed medical regimen are often at odds in geriatric practice. This is due to unrealistically complicated prescribing; the presence of disease adversely affecting memory, vision, or manual dexterity; and physical or financial factors limiting access to the prescribed items. The following guidelines will help to maximize compliance and minimize medication errors.

1. **Don't assume that every patient can remember a complicated medication regimen.** If appropriate, enlist family members, the visiting nurse, or other involved parties to assist the patient by dispensing medications, preparing them and setting them out, putting up notes in strategic locations, and calling on the phone to remind. Periodic pill counts can help determine if the regimen is being adhered to. Mnemonic devices and specialized drug dispensers can be

devised or purchased at most pharmacies to assist the patient in this. It is often helpful when the medicine bottle is relabeled in large lettering giving instructions and the reason the pill is being taken.

2. Quiz the patient periodically to see if medication is being taken correctly. Some patients can be asked to recite the regimen from memory, but others should be asked to identify medications brought to the office.

3. Be aware that neither generic nor brand-name prescribing is a superior method. A generic drug is usually much cheaper than a brand name. However, a cheaper price is not guaranteed by the dispensing pharmacist. Two tablets of 200-mg over-the-counter brand-name ibuprofen may be less expensive than the generic 400-mg prescription variety. In some circumstances, generic prescribing may create inconsistency, since different manufacturers produce the same drug in their own version of color or shape. If the pharmacist stocks a new brand, or if a patient shops in more than one pharmacy, each new prescription may be unfamiliar, or may closely resemble another drug in the regimen. In the patient with poor vision, a little dementia, or an overwhelming regimen, prescribing by brand name occasionally confers just enough consistency to the regimen to make it manageable.

4. Observe the patient opening bottles and other pill containers, identifying medications, using inhalers, and administering insulin and eye drops. These demonstrations are always highly revealing.

5. Inspect the contents of the patient's medication bottles. Bottles sometimes contain unpleasant surprises, such as the wrong pill, the wrong dose, or a mixture of several look-alikes, which generally have been placed there by the patient or a well-meaning caregiver. I have found mixtures of agents such as furosemide, digoxin, aminophylline, and thyroxine in the same bottle, labeled and ingested as a single drug. All containers should be brought in at each office visit.

6. Utilize nonchildproof containers if necessary, instructing the patient and family to take other precautions if children are in the household. In most states, pharmacists are legally required to dispense childproof containers unless otherwise specified. These containers and other elaborate packaging methods can be a curse to the geriatric patient.

7. Consider combination agents when medically (and financially) appropriate. Although commercial combinations are more expensive than two pills taken separately, a complicated medical regimen can be made simpler by these formulations.

8. Attempt to treat specific conditions with monotherapy or groups of diseases with the same medication. Hypertension can often be treated with one medication, not necessarily a diuretic. In contrast, a diuretic should be considered in the hypertensive patient with significant fluid-retaining states. One calcium channel blocking agent may improve angina, hypertension, and tachyarrhythmias simultaneously.

9. Avoid qid and tid regimens if possible. Agents that are excreted slowly in the elderly can and should be given less frequently than prescribed for younger patients, harnessing this physiologic factor to uncomplicate a medical regimen. Antibiotics can be taken tid or less, captopril bid, clonidine and naproxen once a day. Extremely long acting ("one a day") agents such as piroxicam or chlorthalidone, if used at all, can sometimes be given on a less-than-daily basis (e.g., Monday, Wednesday, and Friday; Mondays only; etc.).

When medically feasible, separate drugs should be scheduled to the same dosage interval unless doing so would cause a counterproductive drug-drug interaction.

10. Reevaluate the regimen periodically. Opportunities often arise that allow the regimen to be simplified. New commercial preparations are constantly arriving on the market.

11. Be aware that the prescriber's job does not end with the prescription. The realities of a busy practice cannot excuse the practitioner from the responsibility of ensuring that the patient understands the instructions and from finding out whether the patient will be able to take the medication properly. If necessary, the nurse or other well-trained personnel should be given some of these responsibilities.

BIBLIOGRAPHY

Cockcroft, D.W., and Gault, M.H. Prediction of creatinine clearance from serum creatinine. *Nephron* 16:31–41, 1976.

Greenblatt, D.J., Sellers, E.M., and Shader, R.I. Drug disposition in old age. *N. Engl. J. Med.* 306:18, 1982.

Montamat, S.C., Cusack, B.J., and Vestal, R.E. Current concepts—geriatrics: Management of drug therapy in the elderly. *N. Engl. J. Med.* 321:303–308, 1989.

Yuen, G.J. Altered pharmacokinetics in the elderly. *Clin. Geriatr. Med.* 6:257–262, 1990.

Nonsteroidal Anti-Inflammatory Agents and Acetaminophen

Nonsteroidal anti-inflammatory agents (NSAIDs) exert their pharmacologic and toxic effects by inhibiting the synthesis of prostaglandins (PGs). Although individual agents may have additional actions, the mechanism that all these agents seem to have in common is the antiprostaglandin effect. All could be classified as NSAIDs, but popular terminology differentiates among three major categories: aspirin, nonacetylated salicylates, and NSAIDs. This terminology is in part historical, the groups of agents popularly referred to as NSAIDs being the most recently developed. Their pharmacologic actions tend to differ quantitatively rather than qualitatively, as summarized in Table 2-1.

Acetaminophen, a related drug, may inhibit prostaglandin to a certain extent. However, it differs vastly from NSAIDs in its therapeutic and toxic spectrum, and is dealt with separately (see below).

PHARMACOLOGIC CONSIDERATIONS

Mechanism of Action

Prostaglandins are a group of substances synthesized in a complex process stemming from the metabolism of arachidonic acid, an essential fatty acid component of cell membranes (Figure 2-1). Most prostaglandin inhibitors deactivate cyclooxygenase, the enzyme responsible for the conversion of arachidonic acid to prostaglandins. Cellular damage produces release of many local chemical mediators, including PG. Chemical mediators have vasoactive and chemoattractant properties that result in leakage of vascular endothelium, influx of phagocytic cells, and release of cytotoxic enzymes. This inflammatory response is altered by PG inhibition. The analgesic effect of these agents is related to the fact that PGs sensitize peripheral nerve endings to many of the local mediators that are released, as well to mechanical factors. However, analgesics that work through prostaglandin inhibition tend to be more effective against dull pain associated with inflammation than against sharp pain due to direct stimulation of sensory nerves. It has been suggested that these agents operate via central mechanisms as well, perhaps by inhibiting central prostaglandin synthesis, but the importance of this mechanism is not known.

As analgesics, NSAIDs are characterized by a **ceiling effect**, a dose above which further analgesic efficacy cannot be achieved. Unlike narcotic analgesics, tolerance does not develop to the therapeutic or toxic effects of NSAIDs. Although the analgesic mechanism of action is complex, NSAIDs may have a specific effect on bone pain produced by metastatic cancer, modifying important PG-mediated processes of osteoclastic lesions. The analgesic and anti-inflammatory potency of these agents varies, often unpredictably, a feature that may have more to do with the host than with the specific drug. They are used in the treatment of inflammatory and noninflammatory arthritis, soft tissue rheumatism, trauma, and other pain syndromes.

With the exception of most nonacetylated salicylates, NSAIDs re-

Table 2–1. Actions of Anti-Inflammatory Agents and Acetaminophen

Action	Aspirin	Nonacetylated Salicylates	Other NSAIDs	Acetaminophen
Anti-inflammatory	Potent	Potent	Potent	No
Analgesic	Moderate	Moderate	Moderate	Moderate
Antipyretic	Yes	Yes	Yes	Yes
Antiplatelet	Potent; prolonged	Negligible	Potency & duration vary (see text)	No
Gastrotoxicity	Potent	Mild to moderate	Potent	No
Acute renal syndromes	Unlikely	Weak	Moderate	Not reported
Chronic analgesic nephropathy	?	?	?	Doubtful
Confusion	In overdose	Not reported	Occasional	No
Hepatotoxicity	Questionable in adults	Not reported	Occasional	In overdose
Aspirin allergy	Yes	Rare	Occasional	Rare
Other	Salicylism	Salicylism	See text	—

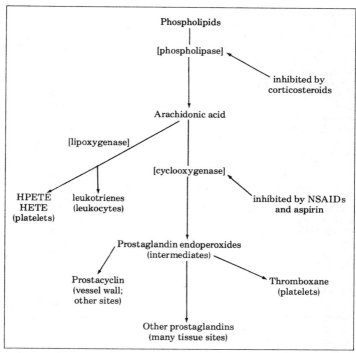

Figure 2-1. Prostaglandin Synthesis

duce platelet adhesiveness. Aspirin irreversibly acetylates cyclooxygenase, effectively altering the platelet for its entire life span. Phenylbutazone, indomethacin, and naproxen are relatively potent platelet
inhibitors; other NSAIDs have intermediate effects; and the nonacetylated salicylates have little effect on platelets. Platelet inhibitors are discussed in Chapter 14.

Although most if not all NSAIDs have an antipyretic effect, selective treatment of fever is generally given with aspirin or acetaminophen, the former because of its low cost, the latter because of its
safety.

Other Actions

Different prostaglandins are produced in different tissues and act as
mediators of local physiologic processes, such as dilation or constriction of smooth muscle in the gastrointestinal tract, cardiovascular
system, and genitourinary system. In the gastrointestinal tract,
PGs inhibit gastric acid secretion and protect against mucosal damaging agents, an effect that has been termed **cytoprotection**. In
blood vessels, the PG prostacyclin acts as a vasodilator and platelet
antiaggregant, balancing the effect of thromboxane A-2, which is a
local vasoconstrictor and powerful platelet aggregant. In the kidney, prostaglandins mediate salt and water balance and potassium

disposition, and produce selective vasodilatation in response to decreased effective arterial pressure, diverting renal blood flow to areas of hypoperfusion. In the uterus, prostaglandin produces myometrial contraction, an effect that has been harnessed in the treatment of dysmenorrhea, but thus far has no application in the postmenopausal patient.

Since inhibitors of prostaglandin synthesis are generally nonselective in their effect, a variety of organ functions can be affected by treatment with this group of agents. Likewise, when cyclooxygenase is inhibited, arachidonic acid may be preferentially converted to leukotrienes and other agents that are synthesized under the direction of the enzyme lipooxygenase. Products of the lipooxygenase pathway are potent mediators of inflammation and may exert various forms of mucosal and tissue damage. NSAIDs differ fundamentally from corticosteroids, which inhibit both cyclooxygenase and lipoxygenase and produce a vastly different array of effects (see Chapter 3).

Although the synthesis of PG may decline in some organ systems in some species, it is not known if there is a generalized decline in PG synthesis with age. Whether or not PG synthesis is altered, age-related changes in a variety of organ systems increase the likelihood that inhibition of protective prostaglandins will produce unwanted effects.

ADVERSE EFFECTS

Because of the ubiquitous nature of prostaglandins, adverse effects can occur in virtually every organ system. The frequency with which specific organs are affected varies somewhat, depending on the class or subclass of anti-inflammatory agent, and is in part related to the intensity with which specific agents inhibit a particular subclass of prostaglandin. Host response, end organ dysfunction, concomitant use of other medications, and probably unknown factors operate as well. In general, it is prudent to assume that all nonsteroidal inflammatory agents are capable of producing the adverse effects to be discussed in this section, so that the proper vigilance can be observed. Toxicity unique to specific agents will be discussed in the separate sections below.

Gastrointestinal Toxicity

By inhibiting cytoprotective prostaglandin produced by gastric mucosal cells, NSAIDs are capable of causing gastric mucosal erythema, erosive or diffuse gastritis, and gastric ulcer, a group of conditions collectively referred to as NSAID gastropathy. Duodenal lesions may also occur but are less common than gastric disease, probably because the development of duodenal ulcer depends on a different mechanism, namely, delivery of acid to the duodenum. Symptoms of NSAID gastropathy range from mild dyspepsia to painful or painless bleeding ulcer. It has been claimed that the elderly are up to seven times more likely to develop NSAID gastropathy than are younger adults. This observation should not be ascribed to the fact that older adults are the chief consumers of NSAIDs, but to a true biologic propensity, namely, the frequent coexistence of underlying gastric mucosal atrophy. Short-term or "prn" ingestion of NSAIDs is less likely to produce serious symptoms than continuous full-dose use.

By producing gastritis, which can result in delayed gastric emptying, NSAIDs also predispose to the development of **reflux esophagitis**. **Enterocolitis** and **nonspecific diarrhea** may also occur in susceptible individuals; this has been attributed to decreased production of intestinal cytoprotective PG. **Inflammatory bowel disease** may be reactivated by NSAIDs. Nonacetylated salicylates are less likely to be toxic to the gastrointestinal tract.

Renal Syndromes

NSAIDs are capable of producing a variety of renal syndromes. Several prostaglandins are produced in the kidney and function in complex physiologic processes that maintain internal renal homeostasis, which may be upset by NSAIDs. Except in the case of hypersensitivity reactions, NSAIDs probably do not produce renal syndromes de novo, but rather in the host whose homeostatic safeguards are already maximally expended. Any factor that can produce decreased effective arterial volume in the renal arteriole triggers a physiologic response that consists of increased secretion of catecholamines and stimulation of the renin-angiotensin system, effects that serve to preserve renal hemodynamics. Insults such as hypotension, dehydration, or volume contraction in cirrhosis or nephrosis can have this effect. Although NSAID-induced inhibition of renal PG produces no adverse effects on the truly normal kidney, renal insufficiency may be produced when extrinsic insults or underlying renal disease exist. Among the syndromes that have been described are **azotemia, proteinuria, acute renal failure, papillary necrosis, interstitial nephritis,** and **nephrotic syndrome.** The precise mechanisms of these conditions probably vary, and PG inhibition is not necessarily implicated in all.

Prostaglandin takes part in the regulation of the renin-angiotensin-aldosterone system and promotes normal disposition of potassium. NSAIDs have been implicated in the production of hyperkalemia in susceptible individuals. The risk is increased by concurrent use of the potassium-sparing diuretic triamterene. In addition, **hyperkalemia** can result when these agents produce acute renal failure.

By inhibiting the action of antidiuretic hormone and by regulating medullary function, renal PG also influences water metabolism. Ingestion of NSAIDs may impair clearance of free water, resulting in **hyponatremia.** More commonly, NSAIDs inhibit the natiuretic properties of renal prostaglandins, and produce edema. It is not known if NSAIDs **elevate blood pressure** de novo, but they are capable of reducing the efficacy of antihypertensive agents.

Fortunately, serious renal syndromes are unusual. However, elderly patients seem to be at an increased risk of developing renal insufficiency from NSAIDs. This is probably because of the coexistence of factors such as the tendency to develop volume contraction and sodium depletion, and to concurrent use of diuretics.

Analgesic nephropathy is a well-known, but poorly understood form of chronic renal failure that has been attributed to "analgesic abuse," and in years past was blamed on chronic ingestion of phenacetin. Newer information has tended to place the blame on aspirin and other NSAIDs. Whether or not specific agents can be implicated remains controversial, since confounding factors are almost always present in patients who develop this syndrome.

Sulindac, which is thought to be relatively sparing of renal PG, has been implicated in fewer renal problems. However, all non-salicylate NSAIDs should be assumed to be capable of producing renal dysfunction and appropriate monitoring observed. Less is known about the renal effects of nonacetylated salicylates and it is too soon to say with certainty, as is sometimes claimed, that these agents are completely safe in this regard. Acute renal toxicity of aspirin may be limited by the fact that it is difficult to comply with a full dose regimen for prolonged periods, but this is not certain.

Central Nervous System Effects

A variety of central nervous system effects have been ascribed to NSAIDs. Although dizziness and headaches have been reported in adult patients of all ages, the elderly are more prone to develop reversible confusional states, impaired concentration and memory, depression, and psychotic reactions. The precise way by which NSAIDs produce such symptoms is not known. The greater susceptibility of the elderly undoubtedly has to do with underlying compromise of brain function, including early or subclinical dementia. Rare central effects include aseptic meningitis and visual disturbances.

Salicylates have a different spectrum of CNS effects. They produce tinnitus at high doses and may produce delirium at toxic doses.

Aspirin-Like Hypersensitivity

The classic triad of nasal polyps, asthma, and aspirin hypersensitivity is now recognized as a phenomenon, with or without the presence of nasal polyps, that occurs in a small proportion of asthmatics, and that may be brought about by virtually all NSAIDs. Symptoms range from rhinitis or urticaria to severe bronchospasm, angioneurotic edema, or anaphylaxis. These occur in susceptible individuals because inhibition of cyclooxygenase sometimes pushes the lipoxygenase pathway to produce leukotriene C, D, and E (slow reacting substance A), mediators of bronchospasm and asthma. Because the tendency to inhibit cyclooxygenase varies, those NSAIDs with weak inhibiting activity would be less likely to trigger a reaction.

Acetaminophen in high doses and nonacetylated salicylates have rarely been reported to cross-react and are usually offered as alternatives to aspirin-sensitive individuals. In general, all prostaglandin inhibitors should be avoided in patients known to have this condition. In some circumstances, desensitization may be attempted by an experienced allergist.

Hepatotoxicity

Hepatic problems are unusual side effects of NSAIDs at ordinary doses in adults. There is a suggestion that the elderly may be at increased risk of dose-related hepatotoxicity. Benoxaprofen, a propionic acid derivative, was removed from the market because of a high incidence of liver and renal damage in elderly patients. This was an ultra-long-acting agent and a direct toxic effect from accumulation of drug metabolites was implicated. Hepatotoxicity from classic NSAIDs is rare. Most cases are hypersensitivity reactions that develop shortly after the drug is instituted. Hepatotoxicity has been reported to occur somewhat disproportionately, though rarely, with sulindac and diclofenac as compared to other NSAIDs. Case reports suggest a hypersensitivity reaction, female predilection, and possible coexistence of other predisposing factors. Phenylbutazone also produces hepatic dysfunction, which may be related to hypersensitivity or to direct, dose-related toxicity, with liver damage being a typical outcome of acute overdose.

A number of additional hepatic syndromes have been described with the use of aspirin and possibly the other salicylates, including a warfarin-like coagulopathy, but these syndromes are very unusual.

Miscellaneous Adverse Effects

NSAIDs have been noted to produce a wide variety of side effects, most fortunately rare. These include bone marrow aplasia, proctocolitis, pancreatitis, urinary dysfunction, aseptic meningitis, visual disturbances, and dermatologic reactions ranging from minor rash to fulminant exfoliative dermatitis. Unusual effects are discussed in the Bibliography references (see O'Brien & Bagby).

In summary, it can be said that the range of effects is as wide as the distribution of prostaglandins in the body, and the possibilities are as unpredictable and exotic as the patient's underlying susceptibilities. The vast majority of patients tolerate short-term use of these agents quite well. Prolonged use demands careful monitoring. The elderly have an increased likelihood of developing gastropathy, azotemia, and CNS symptoms.

IMPORTANT DRUG INTERACTIONS

All NSAIDs are highly protein-bound and capable of displacing other protein-bound drugs from shared binding sites. However, displacement interactions are probably clinically important in only a few circumstances. Aspirin displaces other nonsalicylate NSAIDs from protein-binding sites, increasing the free, active fraction of the latter. Since the free fraction is more rapidly excreted, plasma levels of the displaced agent are ultimately reduced and the clinical significance of this interaction is probably less than the adverse pharmacodynamic consequences of combining two PG inhibitors. A more important displacement interaction occurs when aspirin or phenylbutazone is given with warfarin, resulting in temporarily increased anticoagulant effect. Although most other anti-inflammatory agents do not participate in displacement reactions with warfarin, they should not be coadministered because of their antiplatelet effect, which disrupts an essential hemostatic mechanism, and because their gastrotoxicity increases the risk of gastrointestinal bleeding.

Aspirin and phenylbutazone may also displace phenytoin and the first-generation oral hypoglycemic agents, increasing their effect, though transiently.

Many NSAIDs decrease renal lithium clearance, which may lead to lithium toxicity.

Some NSAIDs reduce renal tubular secretion and clearance of methotrexate, increasing its concentration. This is probably only an important interaction in cancer patients who take high doses of methotrexate and may not occur in patients with rheumatoid arthritis who receive much smaller amounts of the drug. Competition for renal clearance of drugs seems to be more likely with phenylbutazone, fenoprofen, naproxen, and tolmetin than other NSAIDs.

Phenylbutazone may alter the metabolism of drugs that are degraded by microsomal enzymes and has been reported to increase the metabolism of digitoxin, but to decrease the metabolism of others, including warfarin. Such activity has not been described for the other NSAIDs.

NSAIDs block the natiuretic and renal vasodilating effects of furosemide, both PG-mediated processes, resulting in decreased diuretic effect. The diuretic and hypotensive action of the thiazides, which produce natiuresis by a different mechanism, are less consistently affected. The combination of NSAIDs and triamterene has been reported to result in renal failure; older individuals with underlying renal insufficiency seem to be particularly at risk for this interaction.

NSAIDs are capable of counteracting the hypotensive effect of antihypertensive agents. This effect is generally modest (on the order of 10 mm Hg or less). It has been described with thiazide diuretics, beta blockers, captopril, and others, and may be due simply to antinatiuresis. In the case of captopril, and presumably the other angiotensin-converting enzyme inhibitors, NSAIDs counter their ability to release vasodilating PGs. In general, it is prudent to monitor the blood pressure of any patient receiving NSAIDs.

For further discussion of drug interactions, the reader is referred to the Bibliography (see Furst).

PRECAUTIONS

Elderly patients who are expected to ingest NSAIDs on a long-term basis should have baseline and periodic monitoring of renal function, blood pressure, and occult blood in stool, as well as other physical and laboratory parameters when indicated.

The physician should maintain a high index of suspicion of occult bleeding in geriatric patients if they present with subtle signs or symptoms.

NSAIDs should be avoided or used with extreme caution in patients with a history of aspirin hypersensitivity.

USE OF NSAIDS IN ULCER DISEASE

Patients with a history of peptic ulcer should avoid NSAIDs if possible. If NSAIDs are required, they should not be given without concomitant use of full anti-ulcer treatment. A variety of anti-ulcer agents have been recommended, but to date misoprostol (Cytotec) appears to offer the best protection against NSAID-induced gastropathy (see Chapter 26). Patients who cannot tolerate misoprostol should receive sucralfate or a histamine-2 blocker. It is uncertain if misoprostol is as useful in protecting the duodenal ulcer patient.

NSAIDs should not be given to patients with active or recent gastroduodenal disease. Those with a remote or vague history of peptic ulcer should be monitored carefully; although anti-ulcer prophylaxis is not mandatory in such cases, it should be strongly considered because of the often painless or subtle presentation of NSAID gastropathy in the elderly.

GENERAL DOSING GUIDELINES

For analgesia, the smallest effective dose should be given. If a dosage increase does not result in additional analgesia, another agent should be considered. Maximum doses of all of these agents are generally lower for elderly people than younger adults.

Initial and maintenance anti-inflammatory doses are higher than analgesic doses. Anti-inflammatory effect may not be achieved for as long as 1 to 2 weeks of regular dosing, so dose increments should not generally be made until 2 weeks have elapsed. If additional analgesia is required during that time, adjunctive treatment may be given with drugs outside of the NSAID family, or by nonpharmacologic means.

Doses are summarized in Tables 2-2 and 2-3. Dosing for ketorolac and acetaminophen is found under the appropriate text headings.

INDIVIDUAL AGENTS

Aspirin

Aspirin (acetylsalicylic acid) exerts its anti-inflammatory effect by inhibiting the synthesis of PG. The acetyl moiety of aspirin is responsible for deactivation of cyclooxygenase. This moiety is not shared by other salicylates or NSAIDs and is responsible for aspirin's potent and prolonged antiplatelet activity (see Chapter 15). In antiprostaglandin, anti-inflammatory, and analgesic potency, however, aspirin is relatively comparable to the other agents.

Aspirin is rapidly absorbed from the stomach and upper small intestine, and reaches a peak plasma concentration in 15 to 20 minutes. It requires an acid environment for absorption. Although gastric pH is often higher than normal in the elderly because of gastric mucosal atrophy, the rate and extent of absorption of aspirin is not affected by age. Food and antacids delay but do not decrease the rate of absorption. The rate of absorption does depend on tablet formulation, effervescent preparations being the most rapidly (peak levels 15–40 minutes) and enteric-coated tablets the most slowly absorbed (up to 6 hours). Time to peak salicylate levels ranges from 30–60 minutes to 8–14 hours.

Aspirin is rapidly hydrolyzed to salicylate. Part of this process takes place in the gut wall, part in the liver, and the proportion that reaches the systemic circulation is hydrolyzed by enzymes in plasma and red cells. Thus, aspirin circulates in plasma primarily as salicylate. The elimination of salicylate is complex, part being excreted unchanged by the kidney, and part being converted in the liver to renally excreted metabolites. The proportion of each metabolite produced and excreted depends on a number of factors, including

Table 2-2. Some Commonly Used Salicylates

Agent (Brand)	Dose	
	Analgesia	Anti-Inflammatory*
Aspirin (Many)	325–650 qid prn	650 qid or 950 tid
Choline magnesium trisalicylate (Trilisate)	500–1000 bid	750 tid
Salsalate (Disalcid)	500–1000 bid	750 tid

*Dose is best estimated according to serum salicylate levels. Anti-inflammatory concentration ranges from 100 to 300 μg/ml. Some patients may tolerate higher doses than given in the table.

Table 2-3. Classic Nonsteroidal Anti-Inflammatory Agents

| Propionic Acid Derivatives | Dose (mg) | |
	Initial	Anti-Inflammatory (total daily)*
Ibuprofen (Motrin, others)	200-400 bid-qid	1200-2400 in 2 to 4 divided doses
Fenoprofen (Nalfon)	200 qid	900-2400 in 3 to 4 divided doses
Ketoprofen (Orudis)	25 bid	100-150 in 3 to 4 divided doses
Flurbiprofen (Ansaid)	50 bid	200 in 3 to 4 divided doses
Naproxen (Naprosyn)	250 once or twice daily	500-1000 in 2 to 3 divided doses
Naproxen sodium (Anaprox)	275 once or twice daily	550-1100 in 2 to 3 divided doses
Oxicam		
Piroxicam (Feldene)	10 once daily	10-20 daily or alternate days
Indoles/Indenes		
Indomethacin (Indocin, others)	10 bid-qid	100-150 in 2 to 4 divided doses
Sulindac (Clinoril)	150 daily	150-300 in 2 divided doses
Others		
Tolmetin (Tolectin)	200 tid	600-1800 in 2 to 4 divided doses
Meclofenamate sodium (Meclomen)	50 bid	200-400 in 3 to 4 divided doses
Diclofenac (Voltaren)	25 bid	150-200 in 3 to 4 divided doses
Phenylbutazone (Butazolidin)		see text

*Higher doses may be required for full effect in patients with inflammatory arthritis. Dose should be strictly individualized. Full anti-inflammatory dose is less often required in osteoarthritis than in rheumatoid and rheumatoidlike arthritis.

urine pH and dose. At low doses (roughly 325 mg or less) aspirin is rapidly metabolized, little salicylate is excreted unchanged in the urine, and the plasma half-life is 2-3 hours. At high doses, the capacity of the liver to produce certain metabolites may be exceeded and more unchanged salicylate remains for renal excretion. Elimination half-life of salicylate thus increases with increasing dosage. In practice, doses greater than 650 mg are not given at once because of immediate toxicity, but regardless of dose, salicylate levels are higher in elderly as compared to younger adults.

Aspirin itself binds poorly to plasma proteins, but salicylate is 80%-90% bound. The extent bound to serum proteins increases in a dose-dependent fashion. Despite high protein binding, salicylate distributes into most tissues, including synovial fluid.

Adverse Effects

Gastrointestinal irritation is the most common adverse effect of aspirin and is dose-dependent. The most common symptoms are nausea, stomach pain, and heartburn. Bleeding may manifest as chronic occult blood loss, hematemesis, or melena due to hemorrhagic gastritis or peptic ulcer.

Gastrointestinal symptoms are most likely to occur in patients taking 900 mg/day or more, and may be extremely uncommon (i.e., barely higher than placebo) at doses of 325 mg/day or less. However, pre-existing lesions, whether overt or occult, may become clinically apparent even at small doses. This is partly related to the antiplatelet effect of aspirin, which interferes with hemostasis of bleedable lesions.

Gastrointestinal toxicity occurs indirectly, as the result of inhibition of cytoprotective PG, but may also occur directly when aspirin comes in contact with the mucosal lining. Intact gastric mucosa requires an acid environment for aspirin to initiate damage. Although gastric achlorhydria is a common finding in late life, this is found in association with atrophic gastritis and a disrupted mucosal barrier, which facilitates and perpetuates aspirin-induced injury.

The direct irritative effect of aspirin is minimized by the use of enteric-coated preparations. Buffered aspirin does not contain enough buffering capacity to make it more effective in most cases than ordinary aspirin, although individual patients may report reduction of symptoms with these preparations.

As a powerful platelet inhibitor, aspirin increases the risk of **bleeding.** In addition to gastrointestinal bleeding, geriatric patients may be at increased risk of epistaxis and subdural hematoma. The tendency to epistaxis may be related to thinning and friability of the nasal mucosa. Subdural hematoma is only partly related to the tendency to fall and may occur spontaneously. Aspirin probably also increases the risk of senile purpura, a benign ecchymosis that is common in older patients whether or not they are taking antithrombotic agents. Platelet inhibition occurs readily at doses of 325 mg/day and probably at doses as low as 80 mg.

Dose-related symptoms of **salicylism,** such as tinnitus, dizziness, and confusion, may occur. Because of age-related alterations in the pharmacokinetics of salicylates, the elderly may develop these side effects on lower doses than expected. The development of tinnitus, which is often a warning sign of other symptoms of salicylism, may be less reliable in the elderly if there is pre-existing neurosensory hearing loss.

Salicylates increase renal excretion of urate at very high doses, but decrease excretion at low doses. Thus, ordinary doses of aspirin may **increase serum uric acid levels** and occasionally promote acute gouty attacks. The incidence of this complication is low; antigout prophylaxis is not warranted in patients with asymptomatic hyperuricemia.

Other side effects of aspirin are shared by other NSAIDs and are discussed earlier in this chapter.

Important Drug Interactions

Aspirin should not be given with anticoagulants. It may prolong the prothrombin time (PT) when given with warfarin. This interaction

has been attributed to displacement of warfarin from protein binding sites. Although the PT is usually not elevated with doses of
less than 1 g/day of aspirin, the two agents should not be given concurrently because of aspirin's antiplatelet effect as well as its corro-
sive effect on the gastric mucosa. Aspirin does not participate in
pharmacokinetic interactions with heparin, but heparin itself is
known to prolong the bleeding time and this effect is magnified by
aspirin.

Aspirin may enhance the hypoglycemic effect of sulfonylurea
agents, possibly by displacing them from plasma proteins. Displacement interactions have not been described with the newer sulfonylurea agents, glipizide and glyburide.

Antacids are commonly given with aspirin, but there is no rationale for giving them with the enteric-coated variety. In fact, by increasing gastric pH, antacids may cause premature release of aspirin from its enteric coating, enhancing its gastrointestinal toxicity
as well as its excretion. Antacids probably do not impair overall absorption of aspirin, but do increase excretion.

Drug interactions of NSAIDs in general are discussed earlier in
this chapter.

Indications

Aspirin is indicated for the treatment of mild to moderate pain syndromes, including osteoarthritis. It is also highly suitable for the
management of fever. However, for both of these indications acetaminophen is generally preferred, because it does not produce bleeding.

The place of aspirin in the management of stubborn osteoarthritis,
rheumatoid arthritis, and soft tissue rheumatism is being taken over
increasingly by more convenient NSAIDs and apparently less toxic
nonacetylated salicylates.

Use of aspirin for the prevention of thromboembolic disease is discussed in Chapter 15.

Doses are found in Table 2-2.

Nonacetylated Salicylates

The nonacetylated salicylates differ from other inhibitors of PG in
that they do not inhibit cyclooxygenase. For this or other reasons,
they have a sparing effect on certain prostaglandins, and do not
seem to produce as much gastropathy or renal toxicity at ordinary
doses. These agents do not contain the acetyl moiety of aspirin and
do not impair platelet function by this or other mechanisms at ordinary doses. In addition, they are less likely than other NSAIDs to
cross-react with aspirin in producing asthma and other hypersensitivity phenomena. As salicylates, however, they share specific properties with aspirin.

It has been recognized recently that nonacetylated salicylates are
as effective as aspirin in relieving pain. Because at equipotent doses
they are less toxic than aspirin, and because they can be given less
frequently than aspirin, they may be more useful for the treatment
of chronic and recurrent pain syndromes, such as arthritis. For occasional prn use in fever, headache, and other mild pain syndromes,
aspirin and over-the-counter ibuprofen may be preferred on the basis
of cost, availability, and dosage flexibility.

Nonacetylated salicylates participate in the same drug-drug interactions as aspirin. These interactions could be due to displacement

of drugs from protein-binding sites, which temporarily enhances the activity of the displaced drug. Interactions occur with warfarin and first-generation oral hypoglycemic agents. Salicylate also antagonizes the uricosuric effect of probenecid and sulfinpyrazone, perhaps by competing for renal elimination.

Doses are summarized in Table 2–2.

Choline Magnesium Trisalicylate (Trilisate)

Choline magnesium trisalicylate is a mixture of choline salicylate and magnesium salicylate. The salicylate moiety is rapidly absorbed and undergoes typical salicylate pharmacokinetics. Thus, as dosage is increased, salicylate levels in plasma increase in a nonlinear fashion, and at higher doses elimination half-life of the active portion is up to 17 hours. This half-life is probably longer in older people.

ADVERSE REACTIONS. Dose-related symptoms of **salicylism** may occur, as with aspirin, and may go unrecognized. Ironically, because this agent is well tolerated at relatively high doses, toxic salicylate levels are more likely to be attained than with an agent such as aspirin.

Because of the magnesium content of this agent, there is a risk of **hypermagnesemia** in patients with renal insufficiency. This property is not shared by other salicylates.

Although renal and gastrointestinal syndromes are less likely to occur with nonacetylated salicylates than with other NSAIDs, vigilance should be observed.

Platelet function is not altered by this agent or other nonacetylated salicylates. Aspirinlike hypersensitivity symptoms have only rarely been reported.

CONTRAINDICATIONS AND PRECAUTIONS. Because of its magnesium content, this agent is best avoided by patients with renal failure.

Other properties of this agent are discussed in connection with all NSAIDs earlier in this chapter.

Salsalate (Salicylsalicylic Acid; Disalcid)

Salsalate consists of two linked molecules of salicylic acid. It is insoluble at acid pH and is largely absorbed in the upper small intestine. The parent dimer rapidly undergoes hydrolysis in the small intestine or in the plasma, forming two molecules of salicylic acid, which undergo typical salicylate disposition. A portion of the parent compound is not hydrolyzed before undergoing hepatic conjugation, and is not subject to saturable pharmacokinetics seen with other salicylates. Nonetheless, substantial salicylate is formed, and at anti-inflammatory doses the half-life of active salicylate is as long as 17 hours. As a salicylate, the elimination half-life may be somewhat prolonged in the elderly.

ADVERSE REACTIONS. Salsalate shares the same spectrum of potential adverse reactions and precautions as does choline magnesium trisalicylate, except that hypermagnesemia does not occur.

Other Nonacetylated Salicylates

Diflusinal (Dolobid) is a nonacetylated salicylate with a somewhat different range of actions. It has only slight antipyretic effect but has potent antiplatelet activity and may produce greater gastric irritation and other forms of toxicity than other nonacetylated salicylates. It will not be considered here.

Several compounds are available without prescription. These include choline salicylate (Arthropan), magnesium salicylate (Doan's pills), and others. The same precautions should be observed with these over-the-counter agents as with salsalate and choline magnesium trisalicylate.

Classic Nonsteroidal Anti-Inflammatory Agents

Members of this ever-expanding group of agents differ from the salicylates in a variety of ways, as summarized in Table 2-1. For purposes of clarity, they are discussed separately and will hereafter be referred to as the NSAIDs.

Are All NSAIDs Alike?

The spectrum of activity and potential toxicity of all NSAIDs are relatively the same, with exceptions to be pointed out in the discussions of individual agents. Assertions that individual agents differ in analgesic efficacy are based on observations made under experimental conditions, often in animals. These results are not directly applicable to arthritic and uncomfortable humans, who vary immensely on a clinical level. Clinical studies are, furthermore, able to compare two or at the most three agents at once.

There does seem to be interindividual variation in response to different agents. Thus, one patient may respond poorly to sulindac but well to ibuprofen, whereas another patient may report the opposite outcome. These reports are not well understood but have led rheumatologists and pain experts to recommend that failure to respond to one NSAID should prompt a switch to one or more NSAIDs of another class or subclass before abandoning this group of drugs.

NSAIDs are listed by class in Table 2-3.

Potential toxicity is generally shared by all NSAIDs, as discussed earlier in this chapter. Although various claims have been made that one agent is less likely than another to produce problems such as gastric, renal, or hepatic toxicity, this cannot be guaranteed in advance. Thus, patients who have experienced serious side effects from one NSAID may be at risk of experiencing the same problem with another. Only when side effects are mild is it wise to consider trying an alternative NSAID rather than abandoning this group of drugs.

Pharmacokinetics

Most NSAIDs are well absorbed orally. In general, food or concurrent administration of antacids delays but does not diminish total absorption. All are highly protein-bound. The nature and location of binding varies, but differs from that of aspirin.

NSAIDs enter synovium slowly but, once there, concentrations tend to be maintained for a considerable period after the drug has left the plasma compartment, and prostaglandin inhibition in the synovium may last even longer. For this reason, circulation time in plasma does not necessarily correlate with the drug's therapeutic action. However, antiplatelet activity, which is dependent on reversible inhibition of cyclooxygenase in platelets, correlates well with the presence of the drug in plasma.

The NSAIDs currently in use tend to be highly metabolized with little unchanged drug being excreted by the kidney, and serum half-lives tend to be only slightly prolonged with age. However, there are exceptions to this, which are noted in the discussions of specific agents.

Specific Agents

IBUPROFEN (MOTRIN, OTHERS). Ibuprofen is the first of the new generation of NSAIDs to come into general use and, in low doses, is the only NSAID that is available over the counter. Its early and sustaining popularity derives from the fact that it is better tolerated than its predecessors, phenylbutazone and indomethacin. However, in equipotent doses, there is no evidence that ibuprofen is safer than newer NSAIDs.

Ibuprofen is structurally related to fenoprofen, ketoprofen, flurbiprofen, and naproxen.

Peak plasma levels occur within 1 to 2 hours of administration and serum half-life is short at roughly 2–3 hours. The agent is 99% bound to plasma proteins and enters synovium slowly, but, once within the synovium, concentrations are maintained well after ibuprofen has left the plasma compartment. Despite its significant protein binding, ibuprofen occupies only a few binding sites. This property is probably shared by most other NSAIDs and is the probable explanation for the lack of displacement interactions observed with most of these agents. A probable exception to this is phenylbutazone (see below).

Plasma half-life is slightly prolonged in elderly subjects. As with many of the NSAIDs, dose recommendations for elderly patients should depend less on pharmacokinetic changes than on clinical response and potential toxicity. When ibuprofen is given on the short term, the slight prolongation of half-life that may occur is not clinically significant; since the presence of the drug in the synovium outlasts its presence in plasma, dose intervals do not necessarily depend on plasma half-life.

FENOPROFEN (NALFON). Fenoprofen is well absorbed orally, with peak plasma levels being reached within 2 hours. When taken with food, peak plasma levels may be slightly lower than when taken on an empty stomach, whereas antacid may retard but not reduce peak plasma levels. Fenoprofen is highly bound to serum proteins and has a half-life in serum of 2–3 hours. Very little unchanged drug is recovered in the urine.

Drug Interactions. Coadministration of barbiturate, an inducer of hepatic microsomal enzymes, has been observed to increase hepatic metabolism of fenoprofen; this may require dose adjustment. Other enzyme inducers could theoretically have the same effect.

KETOPROFEN (ORUDIS). Ketoprofen has many similarities to ibuprofen and fenoprofen. It is well absorbed, with peak plasma levels being attained in 1 hour, and is highly protein-bound. Plasma half-life ranges from 1.2 to 4.0 hours. It is conjugated to a renally excreted metabolite with only a small amount of unchanged drug being excreted in the urine. At high doses, metabolism is saturated. Unlike ibuprofen and fenoprofen, plasma half-life of ketoprofen has been observed in some studies to increase significantly with age. The peculiar pharmacokinetic profile of this drug has been attributed to a **futile cycle,** an in vitro phenomenon that is believed to occur in renal failure: the glucuronide metabolite recirculates and is ultimately deconjugated to the parent compound, a process that could theoretically occur to a certain extent in age-related renal decline. It is possible that this process occurs with other NSAIDs as well, but more study is needed.

FLURBIPROFEN (ANSAID). This fluorinated compound is a recently introduced member of the propionic acid family. Peak plasma levels are achieved in roughly 1.5 hours. It is metabolized primarily by hepatic conjugation, with only a small amount of parent compound being excreted in the urine. Elimination is biphasic, with the terminal half-life in plasma being approximately 5–6 hours. As with most NSAIDs, the duration of action outlasts its plasma half-life. This agent has not been well studied in the elderly. Dosing precautions should be observed.

NAPROXEN (NAPROSYN). Peak plasma levels of naproxen are achieved within 2 to 4 hours. The half-life is much longer than that of the other propionic acid derivates, averaging 14 hours. It is converted to inactive metabolites that are excreted in the urine. Conjugated metabolites are thought to undergo a futile cycle (see **ketoprofen** above), which could prolong its half-life further in geriatric patients.

Naproxen is a potent inhibitor of cyclooxygenase, giving it significant antiplatelet activity. As with other nonacetylated NSAIDs, the effect on cyclooxygenase is reversible, but the relatively long serum half-life of naproxen confers a somewhat longer antiplatelet effect than other NSAIDs.

Naproxen is also available as the sodium salt (Anaprox), which differs from naproxen in its rapidity of absorption, peak plasma levels being achieved in only 1 to 2 hours. Otherwise, the pharmacokinetics are the same. Because of quicker onset of action, the salt is promoted as an analgesic, with a marketing emphasis on the treatment of dysmenorrhea. It is mentioned here because the prescribing dose for each compound differs. The salt contains 25 mg of sodium (approximately 1 mEq) per 200 mg of naproxen (275 mg salt = 250 mg naproxen). Product selection should probably be made on the basis of cost and formulation. Naproxen is available in liquid form whereas the salt is not.

PIROXICAM (FELDENE). Piroxicam is well absorbed orally and reaches peak plasma levels within 2 to 4 hours. It is highly protein-bound. It is hydroxylated in the liver and then conjugated, both metabolites being excreted in the urine. The drug undergoes enterohepatic circulation with a mean plasma half-life of nearly 50 hours. Although the half-life of piroxicam is apparently not further prolonged with age, there is interindividual variation in half-life at all ages to a maximum of 86 hours in some subjects. With daily administration, piroxicam levels in blood could continue to rise for more than a week, so that the therapeutic effect and toxicity could present in a delayed fashion. Despite its prolonged half-life, there is surprisingly no evidence that piroxicam is less well tolerated in older individuals than other NSAIDs, perhaps because published studies of this drug have been short-term.

Once steady state and clinical response have been achieved, this agent can theoretically be given less than once daily. Such dosage scheduling should be considered when long-term use is intended.

INDOMETHACIN (INDOCIN, OTHERS). Indomethacin is an extremely potent inhibitor of cyclooxygenase. As such, it is a very potent inhibitor of platelet aggregation, but the duration of this effect is brief when compared to aspirin, paralleling its presence in serum. In addition, indomethacin inhibits leukocyte motility, resembling colchicine in this regard (see Chap. 5).

Indomethacin is well absorbed with peak plasma levels being attained in 2 hours. Several hepatic metabolites are produced by microsomal and nonmicrosomal processes, and the drug undergoes enterohepatic circulation. A second phase of metabolism occurs when unchanged indomethacin is released from tissue sites such as the synovium. Serum half-life is variable, ranging from 2 to 11 hours, but does not seem to change significantly with age. The amount of unchanged indomethacin recovered in the urine may increase with age, but the short half-life of the drug lessens the clinical importance of this.

Adverse Effects. Indomethacin has been associated with CNS side effects more often than other NSAIDs. In addition to causing the characteristic effects such as **dizziness, headaches,** and **memory deficits,** indomethacin has been reported to cause **psychosis, hallucinations,** and **depression.** This propensity has been attributed to its structural similarity to serotonin, but this mechanism is speculative.

Otherwise, the spectrum of side effects attributed to indomethacin is similar to that seen with other NSAIDs, but the incidence is quite a bit higher.

SULINDAC (CLINORIL). Though structurally related to indomethacin, sulindac is less potent and tends to be better tolerated. A prodrug, sulindac is a sulfoxide. It is oxidized in the liver to a sulfone, which is conjugated and excreted in the urine. Unconjugated sulfone undergoes reversible reduction to a sulfide, the active form, which peaks in plasma 2–3 hours after ingestion of the pro-drug. Sulindac has a serum half-life of 7 hours, but the half-life of the active sulfide is as long as 18 hours, with steady state levels being reached in about 5 days. Active and inactive drug are highly protein-bound and undergo enterohepatic circulation, and sulfide does not undergo significant renal excretion. Sulindac and its metabolites may accumulate more rapidly over time in the elderly than in the young, although the precise way in which this occurs is not known.

Adverse Effects. Central nervous system side effects may resemble those of indomethacin to a limited extent, but are not as common perhaps because its structural similarity to serotonin is less. In general, the spectrum of side effects is the same as with the other NSAIDs. Claims that sulindac is less likely to cause gastrointestinal or renal toxicity are controversial.

TOLMETIN (TOLECTIN). Tolmetin is structurally related to indomethacin and sulindac. It is well absorbed with peak plasma concentrations being achieved in less than 1 hour. The half-life in nonelderly adults is short, averaging 1–2 hours, but it suppresses synovial fluid prostaglandin for a much longer period of time. It is extensively protein-bound and is eliminated in a biphasic manner. It is oxidized in the liver to inactive metabolites.

MECLOFENAMATE SODIUM (MECLOMEN). Meclofenamate sodium is not considered a first-line drug for arthritis in that it has a reputation for enhanced toxicity. However, part of its reputation may derive from its association with a related but more toxic agent, mefenamic acid (Ponstel), which is an analgesic marketed for use in dysmenorrhea.

Adverse Effects. As with other NSAIDs, gastrointestinal symptoms occur commonly with meclofenamate. **Diarrhea** may be particularly common with this agent, and is at least as common in older as in younger adults.

DICLOFENAC (VOLTAREN). Diclofenac is structurally similar to meclofenamate and to acetic acid derivatives such as indomethacin. It is well absorbed from the gastrointestinal tract, with peak plasma levels being achieved within 2 to 3 hours. Extensive first-pass metabolism occurs, reducing bioavailability of a given dose. Despite this, no decrease in clearance rate has yet been demonstrated in elderly subjects, and the drug does not accumulate. Diclofenac is metabolized in the liver to active and inactive metabolites, which are excreted in urine and bile. Only small amounts of unchanged diclofenac is excreted in the urine. Plasma half-life averages 1 to 2 hours, but the drug remains in synovium longer than in serum.

Adverse Effects. Autoimmune hemolytic anemia has been reported and agranulocytosis may be a significant risk. In general, the toxicity spectrum seems to be similar to other NSAIDs, but further experience with this agent is required before any definite conclusions can be reached.

PHENYLBUTAZONE (BUTAZOLIDIN). The use of phenylbutazone, one of the oldest NSAIDs, has declined in recent years because of its potential toxicity. It is no longer approved as a first-line agent, and it is not approved for long-term use in patients over 60. Phenylbutazone is not similar in structure to other classes of NSAIDs, but shares structure and some pharmacologic properties with the antiplatelet and uricosuric agent sulfinpyrazone. It has potent antiinflammatory and antiplatelet effects.

Phenylbutazone is well absorbed, with peak plasma levels being attained in 2 hours. Average serum half-life is greater than 50 hours, and the drug remains in the synovium for up to 3 weeks after it is discontinued. It is oxidized and conjugated in the liver to active and inactive metabolites. One active metabolite, oxyphenbutazone, has a serum half-life of several days, and was previously marketed as a separate agent (Tandearil). Because of its prolonged half-life, tendency to accumulate, and consequent toxicity, oxyphenbutazone is no longer used. Both phenylbutazone and oxyphenbutazone are extensively bound to plasma proteins.

Pharmacokinetic studies of phenylbutazone in the elderly demonstrate a somewhat increased average serum half-life as compared to younger subjects. This may be a partial explanation for the fact that toxicity is more common in the elderly. Drug-drug interactions and pharmacodynamic effects most likely also play an important role.

Adverse Reactions. Phenylbutazone shares the spectrum of toxicity of the other NSAIDs, although the incidence of side effects is probably higher. In addition, it has been associated with irreversible bone marrow aplasia with agranulocytosis, thrombocytopenia, or aplastic anemia, side effects that have been reported most often in elderly patients. These side effects have, however, rarely been reported with short-term use.

Phenylbutazone also inhibits renal reabsorption of uric acid and can produce uricosuria. Obstructive uropathy due to uric acid stone formation has been reported.

Drug Interactions. In addition to the typical pharmacodynamic interactions that can occur with other NSAIDs, phenylbutazone and its metabolite oxyphenbutazone displace a number of substances from plasma proteins and displacement interactions with agents such as warfarin and the sulfonylurea agents occur. Phenylbutazone may also interfere with the hepatic metabolism of warfarin, phenytoin, and oral hypoglycemic agents.

The Place of Phenylbutazone in Therapy. Phenylbutazone is a potent anti-inflammatory agent that produces little toxicity when used in the short term, even in geriatric patients. As such, it has been found to be particularly suitable for the treatment of acute gouty arthritis in patients unable to take colchicine. However, many NSAIDs may be useful in gout. In the absence of controlled studies, it is not known how phenylbutazone compares to these or other alternatives.

Because serious toxicity with long-term phenylbutazone use is most likely to occur in the elderly, this drug should not be used for longer than 1 week at a time in such patients. In practice, the present medical legal climate has curtailed the use of phenylbutazone even in the short term.

KETOROLAC: A PARENTERAL NSAID. Ketorolac (Toradol) is the first NSAID available for parenteral use. It has the same spectrum of activity and potential for toxicity as other classic NSAIDs, but it is intended for the management of acute pain syndromes, such as postoperative pain and perhaps for renal or biliary colic. A substantial portion of this drug is eliminated by the kidney and the serum half-life of 4 to 6 hours is prolonged with advanced age.

Short-term use has not been reported to cause gastrointestinal bleeding, but the drug has not been adequately studied in geriatric patients. Presently it should be reserved for patients who cannot tolerate appropriate doses of parenteral opioid analgesics.

Dosing. Usual dose: 30 mg IM, followed by 15 mg every 6–8 hours if needed. Some patients may require higher doses but the safety of higher doses in the elderly is not known.

ACETAMINOPHEN

In ordinary doses, acetaminophen has virtually no acute toxicity. Unlike the NSAIDs, it does not impair platelet function and does not produce gastropathy, renal syndromes, or confusional states. Unlike the salicylates, acetaminophen has no effect on the excretion of uric acid. Nor is there significant cross-reactivity with aspirin in aspirin-induced asthma and related syndromes. Long-term toxicity in healthy individuals has not been described.

Pharmacologic Considerations

Acetaminophen is a metabolic by-product of phenacetin, and is thought to be the active principle of its parent drug. Phenacetin, which may itself have inherent analgesic properties, will not be discussed here. Although it may be less toxic than previously suggested, its use has been eclipsed by other analgesics in recent years.

Mechanism of Action

The mechanism of analgesic action of acetaminophen is not completely understood, but it is believed to inhibit prostaglandin synthesis in the CNS without doing so to a significant degree in the periphery. It is not known why such a disparate effect on prostaglandin synthesis might occur, but this characteristic is offered to explain why it has antipyretic and analgesic activity without exerting important anti-inflammatory activity. Lacking anti-inflammatory activity, acetaminophen tends to produce somewhat less analgesia than other NSAIDs in conditions where pain is in part mediated by inflammation. Otherwise, acetaminophen has analgesic potency approximately equal to aspirin.

Pharmacokinetics

Acetaminophen is rapidly absorbed from the upper small intestine and peak plasma levels are reached within 1 to 2 hours. The drug is extensively metabolized by the liver, primarily by conjugation to inactive metabolites. However, some metabolites are produced by the microsomal enzyme system. One of these, n-acetyl-p-benzoquineoneamine, is a highly reactive intermediate, which is capable of binding to hepatocytes. Under ordinary circumstances, this intermediate is further metabolized and excreted uneventfully; but in overdose, metabolic capacity is overwhelmed, the toxic intermediate lingers, and hepatic necrosis may occur (see Adverse Effects below).

On the average, the plasma half-life of acetaminophen is 2–3 hours. Clearance is slightly prolonged in older subjects, but the therapeutic index of acetaminophen is probably wide enough that dose adjustments do not have to be made when use is casual. Although it is not known whether this is the case when the drug is to be taken for prolonged periods, there is no evidence that the elderly are at increased risk of toxicity under these circumstances.

Adverse Effects

Few if any adverse effects have been attributed to short-term acetaminophen. Skin rashes and urticaria have been reported occasionally and various blood dyscrasias rarely. Individuals with aspirin-induced asthma and related immunological reactions have only rarely been reported to exhibit clinical cross-reactivity with acetaminophen.

Although it has been suggested that acetaminophen might be the substance responsible for so-called analgesic nephropathy, long ascribed to its parent compound phenacetin, neither the role of acetaminophen nor a central role of phenacetin has been substantiated. Analgesic nephropathy is a form of chronic renal failure associated with chronic abuse of certain analgesics. Current thinking on this long-debated issue supports the conclusion that salicylate analgesics are more likely than phenacetinlike drugs to produce pathology such as papillary necrosis, and acetaminophen may be one of the safest available agents in this regard. Nor does acetaminophen produce the renal syndromes associated with NSAID use, such as edema, elevation of blood pressure, hyperkalemia, or acute renal insufficiency.

Acetaminophen overdose (a single dose of 7.5 g or more in non-elderly adults) may produce hepatic necrosis and, less frequently, renal failure. This reaction may be fatal, but surviving patients usually recover normal hepatic function. The risk of this toxicity is increased in patients with underlying hepatic disease and alcohol abuse, and, theoretically, by concurrent use of drugs other than alcohol that induce hepatic microsomal enzymes, such as barbiturates and phenytoin. The risk of hepatic necrosis is not increased by old age per se. Acetaminophen overdose is treated supportively and with administration of acetylcysteine (Mucomyst).

Drug Interactions

Few if any important drug interactions with acetaminophen have been described. Absorption may be delayed but not reduced by concurrent administration of agents that reduce gastric emptying. Metoclopramide increases the rate of gastric emptying and may increase the rate of absorption, a desirable but minimally important effect. Enzyme-inducing drugs, including alcohol, are known or feared to increase acetaminophen hepatotoxicity in overdose. It is possible that such agents might act in concert with chronic high-dose (more than 4 g per day) ingestion of acetaminophen to produce hepatotoxicity, but such cases are likely to be unusual.

Contraindications

Acetaminophen is contraindicated in individuals with a history of severe aspirinlike hypersensitivity reactions who have demonstrated a clear-cut reaction **to acetaminophen itself.** It is not otherwise contraindicated in aspirin-sensitive patients, although caution should be observed when the drug is first instituted.

Indications

Acetaminophen is indicated as first-line treatment of conditions where mild to moderate analgesia is required, and is the antipyretic of choice. It is considered first-line treatment for the pain of osteoarthritis and soft tissue rheumatism unless there is a significant inflammatory component.

Dosing

Casual use: 325 to 650 mg prn every 4–6 hours, up to a total dose of 2600 mg in 24 hours. In exceptional circumstances, a total daily dose of 4 g in 4 to 6 divided doses may be given.
Chronic use: A total dose of 2600 g over 24 hours should not be exceeded in most circumstances.

NONPHARMACOLOGIC MANAGEMENT

Anti-inflammatory agents should not be the first management technique in the patient with osteoarthritis. The patient should be asked whether the pain is severe enough to require medication, since many patients will passively accept the prescription on the notion that it will be good for or even cure the arthritis. If medication is desired, acetaminophen may be as effective as nonanti-inflammatory doses of NSAIDs in this generally mild, noninflammatory disease. Use of a cane or other assistive device may reduce the need for or dose of analgesics. Patients with chronic or recurrent pain due to arthritis of the joints or of the spine may also obtain partial relief with strengthening exercises, and some report relief with local heat, counterirritant rubs (Ben-Gay, others), and coolant sprays (ethyl chloride). Specific guidelines on the use of biofeedback, acupuncture, and transcutaneous electrical nerve stimulation (TENS) require further controlled study. A multispecialty pain clinic is a good resource for the various modalities of pain management. When these methods have failed or are not appropriate, orthopedic surgery should be considered. Many elderly patients are excellent candidates for total joint replacement, although they may not be aware of this fact, thinking that they are "too old" for the procedure.

BIBLIOGRAPHY

Bailey, R.B., and Jones, S.R. Chronic salicylate intoxication. A common cause of morbidity in the elderly. *J. Amer. Geriatr. Soc.* 37:556-561, 1989.

Clive, D.M., and Stoff, J.S. Renal syndromes associated with nonsteroidal antiinflammatory drugs. *N. Engl. J. Med.* 310:563-572, 1984.

Day, R.O., et al. Variability in response to NSAIDs, Fact or Fiction? *Drugs* 36:643-651, 1988.

Furst, D.E. Clinically important interactions of nonsteroidal anti-inflammatory drugs with other medications. *J. Rheumatol.* 15(Supp 17):58- 62, 1988.

Jackson, C.H., MacDonald, N.C., and Cornett, J.W. Acetaminophen: a practical pharmacologic overview. *Can. Med. Assoc. J.* 131:25-37, 1984.

Lamy, P.P. Renal effects of nonsteroidal antiinflammatory drugs. Heightened risk to the elderly? *J. Amer. Geriatr. Soc.* 34:361-367, 1986.

Lanza, F.L., et al. Double-blind placebo-controlled endoscopic comparison of the mucosal protective effects of misoprostol versus cimetidine on tolmetin-induced mucosal injury to the stomach and duodenum. *Gastroenterol* 95:289-294, 1988.

Levy, G. Clinical pharmacokinetics of salicylates. *Brit J. Clin. Pharm.* 10:285S-290S, 1981.

O'Brien, W.M., and Bagby, G.F. Rare adverse reactions to nonsteroidal antiinflammatory drugs. *J Rheumatol* 12:13-20,347-353,562-567,785-790, 1985.

Paulus, H.E. Aspirin versus nonacetylated salicylates. *J. Rheumatol.* 16:264-265, 1989.

Portenoy, R.K., and Farkash, A. Practical management of non-malignant pain in the elderly. *Geriatrics* 43:29-47, 1988.

Ravi, S., Keat, A.C., and Keat, E.C.B. Colitis caused by nonsteroidal anti-inflammatory drugs. *Postgrad. Med. J.* 62:773-776, 1986.

Roth, S.H., and Bennett, R.E. Nonsteroidal anti-inflammatory drug gastropathy: recognition and response. *Arch. Intern. Med.* 147:2093-2100, 1987.

Samter, M., and Stevenson, D.D. Reactions to aspirin and aspirin-like drugs. In M. Samter, D.W. Talmage, M.M. Frank, et al. *Immunological diseases* (4th ed.). Boston: Little, Brown, 1988. Pp. 1135-1147.

Corticosteroids

Systemic corticosteroids have a definite place in the management of the geriatric patient. However, toxicity of these drugs is accentuated in late life and they must be used with extreme caution, at the lowest possible dose, and for the shortest possible time.

The following discussion of corticosteroids focuses on prednisone, which differs only slightly from prednisolone but by convention is the most common agent used in the United States. The duration of action of prednisone lends itself well to alternate-day therapy and a simple tapering schedule.

PHARMACOLOGIC CONSIDERATIONS

Mechanism of Action

Corticosteroids are powerful anti-inflammatory agents, which act by inhibiting both the cyclooxygenase and the lipooxygenase pathways of prostaglandin synthesis (see Figure 2-1). Although these actions do not cure inflammatory disease, significant abatement is often possible. Thus, corticosteroids are most useful in diseases that are self-limiting, such as temporal arteritis, or are characterized by remissions and exacerbations, such as asthma.

Corticosteroids affect a wide range of tissues, and these effects have important ramifications for the geriatric patient. Corticosteroids stimulate hepatic gluconeogenesis and increase the secretion of glucagon, and may produce frank diabetes in susceptible individuals. It is this effect that has led to the use of the term *glucocorticoid*. They also have mineralocorticoid effects, however, leading to sodium retention and kaliuresis. Corticosteroids vary in the degree of mineralocorticoid action, with prednisone having an intermediate effect compared to other corticosteroids (Table 3-1). Corticosteroids increase protein breakdown and decrease protein synthesis, producing their most apparent clinical effects in skeletal muscle and bone. Their effects on leukocytes and other arms of the immune response increase the susceptibility to infection. They increase gastric acid secretion and through this or other mechanisms increase the susceptibility to peptic ulcer in certain patients. These well-known actions of corticosteroids produce toxicity that is more common or accentu-

Table 3-1. Comparison of Corticosteroids

Compound	Equivalent Dose (mg)	Mineralocorticoid Effect	Plasma half-life (min)
Cortisone	25.0	Significant	30
Cortisol	20.0	Significant	90
Prednisone	5.0	Moderate	60
Prednisolone	5.0	Moderate	200
Methylprednisolone	4.0	Little	180
Dexamethasone	0.75	Little	200

ated in elderly patients, who come to corticosteroid therapy predisposed to these effects.

Corticosteroids require tissue-specific receptors in order for hormone action to occur. Although aging is associated with reductions in the numbers of these receptor sites, it is not known whether this alters the therapeutic action of exogenous corticosteroids.

Pharmacokinetics

Absorption of prednisone is not reduced by food, and is apparently unaffected by small doses of antacid with which it is frequently administered. In the liver, prednisone is converted to its active 11-betahydroxy form (prednisolone), which is carried in plasma on steroid-hormone-binding globulin (transcortin) and albumin. Binding to albumin becomes more important at higher doses when transcortin sites are saturated. Although prednisolone is the active form of the drug, there is no convincing evidence that prednisone is ineffective in patients with liver disease.

Metabolism of active drug takes place in the hepatic microsomal enzyme system. Both activation and metabolic degradation are reduced in liver disease, which is perhaps the reason that it is not necessary to substitute prednisone with prednisolone in patients with liver dysfunction. The half-life of prednisolone and therefore prednisone is prolonged in liver disease. However, their half-lives are short, at 60 minutes for prednisone and 115–252 for prednisolone, and are far outdistanced by their long-lasting tissue effects, which can last for 24 to 36 hours depending on the dose administered. Pharmacokinetics and duration of action have not been defined for the elderly. It is generally accepted that toxicity is enhanced, but this may well be on the basis of age-related tissue susceptibility. As with younger adults, it is not possible to predict a patient's response to exogenous corticosteroids.

ADVERSE EFFECTS

Adverse effects of corticosteroids are generally dose-related and many are cumulative.

Long-term use of systemic corticosteroids may accelerate postmenopausal and involutional **osteoporosis**. Corticosteroid osteoporosis itself is characterized by both increased bone resorption and decreased bone formation, with particularly severe bone loss occurring at sites of trabecular bone, such as the spine. The mechanism is complex: corticosteroids impair bone collagen synthesis by inhibiting osteoblast function, decrease intestinal absorption and increase renal excretion of calcium, and, by suppressing ACTH, appear to reduce the nonovarian production of estrogen that accounts for most of that hormone in postmenopausal women. Although the risk of postmenopausal and involutional osteoporosis varies widely in the geriatric population, virtually all elderly patients should be assumed to be at risk for the development of corticosteroid osteoporosis, and preventive measures should be taken (see Contraindications and Precautions below and Chap. 21).

Corticosteroids **impair wound healing** by impairing collagen formation and by hindering the action of immune cells involved in healing mechanisms.

Corticosteroids **increase intraocular pressure** in susceptible individuals, patients with chronic open angle glaucoma or intraocular hypertension being at highest risk of this effect. Topical (ophthalmic) corticosteroids are somewhat more likely than oral agents to increase intraocular pressure. The precise mechanism of this corticosteroid sensitivity is not known. Corticosteroids have no known effect on the anterior chamber angle and therefore do not increase the risk of acute angle closure glaucoma per se.

Long-term use of systemic or ophthalmic corticosteroids accelerates the development of posterior subcapsular **cataracts.** This phenomenon seems to occur only in some patients. Although typical age-associated nuclear cataracts are not affected by steroids and age does not appear to be a separate risk factor, a posterior subcapsular cataract superimposed on an underlying nuclear cataract or other visual disability is likely to produce visual loss more rapidly, putting the elderly patient at increased risk of visual loss.

Psychosis is a recognized adverse effect of high-dose corticosteroid use and may occur after only two or three days of use. Geriatric patients are particularly susceptible to a variety of corticosteroid-induced **confusional states,** which may occur early on or after days to weeks of therapy. Mental status should be monitored throughout the course of treatment, particularly when high doses are being used.

Exacerbation of diabetes is a very common side effect of corticosteroid use in elderly patients.

Corticosteroids may **exacerbate peptic ulcer,** although the exact risk of this is subject to debate and they are probably safer in this regard than NSAIDs. Experimental evidence indicates that corticosteroids do not disrupt the gastric mucosal barrier to hydrogen ion diffusion as do NSAIDs and thus may not produce ulcers de novo. Nonetheless, corticosteroids do produce a modest increase in gastric secretion and may inhibit the protective alkaline response to mucosal injury. The risk of ulcer increases with increasing corticosteroid doses. Geriatric patients have not been identified as a group at higher ulcer risk from corticosteroid use per se, but they are theoretically more vulnerable since the risk of nonsteroid-related ulcer increases with age.

Systemic corticosteroids may produce **edema,** and patients with congestive heart failure or other fluid-retaining states may worsen clinically. Potassium loss may also occur but hypokalemia is unusual except in patients who are taking potassium-wasting diuretics. Corticosteroids may also **increase blood pressure,** although hypertension is probably more often associated with endogenous Cushing's syndrome than with exogenous drug.

Impairment of T-cell function by corticosteroids may result in **reactivation of tuberculosis.** This is a particularly important consideration in geriatric patients because as many as 30% of American elderly harbor subclinical *M. tuberculosis* as manifested by cutaneous reactivity. Latent herpes zoster is also prevalent in the geriatric age group and systemic corticosteroids may trigger the development of **cutaneous zoster** infection (shingles). **Other infectious complications** of corticosteroid use are most likely to occur in patients being treated with high doses for prolonged periods, often in connection with diseases that themselves increase the susceptibility to infection.

Other side effects of long-term corticosteroid use include **weight gain, moon facies, proximal myopathy,** and **avascular necrosis** of the hips, knees, or shoulders.

CORTICOSTEROID WITHDRAWAL

Long-term use of systemic corticosteroids suppresses the hypothalamic-pituitary-adrenal axis. Important suppression may occur as early as 5 days of therapy when daily doses exceed approximately 40 mg/day. Geriatric patients are fully capable of undergoing hypothalamic-pituitary-adrenal suppression.

Addisonian crisis is a well-known risk of abrupt withdrawal of corticosteroid therapy. Milder symptoms of corticosteroid withdrawal may occur, however, and may go unrecognized. Symptoms likely to be overlooked in elderly patients include aches and pains, lethargy, anorexia, weight loss, and others of a nonspecific nature.

IMPORTANT DRUG INTERACTIONS

The combination of NSAIDs and corticosteroids significantly increases the risk of peptic ulcer above the risk posed by either group of agents alone. This risk appears to increase with increasing corticosteroid dose.

Agents that stimulate hepatic microsomal enzymes, such as rifampin and anticonvulsants, increase the catabolism of prednisone and prednisolone. In one clinically apparent interaction, rifampin has been reported to produce exacerbations of corticosteroid-dependent asthma. Enzyme inducers could reduce the efficacy of corticosteroids more covertly in temporal arteritis, where corticosteroids are given in part to avert visual catastrophes.

Agents that inhibit metabolic enzymes, such as exogenous estrogen and cimetidine, reduce metabolic clearance of corticosteroids and increase the likelihood of toxicity. Reduction in corticosteroid dose may be possible in these circumstances if clinical end points are easy to access.

Potassium-wasting diuretics increase the kaliuretic effect of corticosteroids and hypokalemia may result. This is most likely to occur when corticosteroids are used in conjunction with agents such as thiazide or loop diuretics, but has also been reported with concurrent use of milder carbonic anhydrase inhibitors, such as acetazolamide.

CONTRAINDICATIONS AND PRECAUTIONS

Patients with chronic open angle glaucoma should avoid corticosteroids if possible. Although topical (ophthalmic) corticosteroids are more likely to increase intraocular pressure than oral agents, the latter should be avoided as well in patients at risk. If corticosteroids are absolutely essential, the primary care physician and ophthalmologist must work closely.

Because of the high risk of corticosteroid-induced osteoporosis in aged patients, preventive measures are indicated if prolonged or repeated treatment is anticipated. Agents that may be effective include calcium supplements, estrogen (in women), and thiazide diuretics, if there is no contraindication. Thiazides may reverse corticosteroid-induced urinary calcium loss and secondary hyperparathyroidism; however, they also enhance the hypokalemic effect of corticosteroids, so that serum potassium levels should be rigorously monitored. Vitamin D may be added in physiologic doses (no more than 400–800 units/day) in order to maximize calcium balance. These regimens may produce hypercalcemia in certain patients, so serum calcium levels should also be monitored and urinary calcium should be measured if practical. The use of sodium fluoride in corticosteroid-induced osteoporosis requires further study; its safety and efficacy in postmenopausal osteoporosis has been questioned (see Chap. 22).

Patients with active or recent peptic ulcer should take maximum antiulcer therapy while on corticosteroids. In patients with no known or unknown history of peptic ulcer, routine antiulcer prophylaxis is controversial. The convention of administering antacid routinely with corticosteroids is probably not necessary for younger, low-risk adult patients. However, until it has been shown that the elderly do not constitute a separate high-risk group for corticosteroid-related peptic ulcer, the common practice of administering a small dose of antacid is probably warranted.

Because of the high prevalence of remote exposure to tuberculosis in the older population, tuberculin skin testing with anergy profile should be done in elderly patients who are about to be treated with a course of systemic corticosteroids. Patients with positive skin tests should receive chemoprophylaxis against tuberculosis (see Chap. 31).

INDICATIONS

The chief geriatric indications for systemic corticosteroids are temporal arteritis, polymyalgia rheumatica, bronchospastic disease that is refractory to bronchodilators, and as an alternative to colchicine and NSAIDs in the management of acute gouty arthritis. Corticosteroids are also used in cutaneous zoster to prevent postherpetic neuralgia, although there is some controversy as to their efficacy.

Small doses of corticosteroids may be quite effective in quelling disabling symptoms of rheumatoid arthritis that do not respond to other anti-inflammatory agents. Active rheumatoid arthritis is a relatively uncommon cause of rheumatologic symptoms in geriatric patients and systemic corticosteroids have no place in the management of the more common osteoarthritis or in inactive rheumatoid arthritis. However, intra-articular corticosteroid injections may provide significant relief in a variety of rheumatic disorders (see Gray et al.).

Severe autoimmune disease should be treated with corticosteroids in older individuals as in younger ones.

Use of Corticosteroids in Temporal Arteritis

Experts disagree on ideal dosing for temporal arteritis, recommendations ranging from 40 to 100 mg/day. Some investigators claim that the risk of complications from temporal arteritis is no greater with daily doses in the 20-mg range than with very high doses. This argument comes from a retrospective study, however, and requires prospective verification (see Delecoeuillerie et al.). In contrast, others cite cases of serious complications, particularly visual loss, occurring despite very high doses. The latter situation is uncommon, however, and it would be unwise to recommend extremely high doses in all cases because of the serious toxicity that can occur.

Another question is whether the dosage should be guided by recurrence of symptoms or the level of the erythrocyte sedimentation rate (ESR). Sometimes elevation of the ESR may be the first sign that serious symptoms are about to appear, making it important to use the blood test as a guide. However, if ESR alone guides dosing, it is more likely that the patient will develop corticosteroid toxicity. It is important to realize that many geriatric patients have elevated ESR in the absence of diseases such as temporal arteritis, which has led to the claim that the ESR increases "normally" with age. Thus, an effort to suppress the ESR to normal in certain patients may be in vain, whereas those who have demonstrated serious symptoms, such as blindness, may require aggressive suppression of ESR. The physician should keep an open mind when prescribing prednisone in this condition, being prepared to tailor the dose to specific circumstances.

DAILY VERSUS ALTERNATE-DAY DOSING

Once acute symptoms have subsided, certain disease can be controlled on an alternate-day regimen. The alternate-day regimen produces less adrenal suppression, and is less likely to produce important side effects such as diabetes, hypertension, obesity, and impaired immunity. This type of regimen has not been shown to reduce the incidence of osteoporosis, however.

During maintenance therapy of polymyalgia rheumatica, symptoms may be better controlled with daily therapy. In addition, there is some evidence that alternate-day therapy is less effective than daily dosing in the management of temporal arteritis, but this has not been firmly established.

DOSING

In Temporal Arteritis

Initial dose: 60–80 mg daily for 2 weeks or until symptoms are suppressed; then taper by reducing dose approximately 25% every 7–10 days if symptoms do not reappear. High-end initial doses should be used if visual symptoms are present. Alternate tapering schedules are commonly used.
Maintenance dose: 5 mg daily to complete an 8–12-month course, then taper and discontinue. If symptoms recur, the maximum dose (60–80 mg) should be resumed until symptoms are suppressed, followed by the previous tapering schedule.

In Polymyalgia Rheumatica

Initial dose: 15–20 mg daily for 2 weeks; then taper by 2.5 mg/week.
Maintenance dose: 5 mg daily. Further tapering may be possible, depending on symptoms, but treatment for 1–2 years or more may be required. Dose should be increased to maximum if symptoms recur.
Note: If symptoms suggestive of temporal arteritis appear, doses used for that condition should be initiated.

Short-Term Use in Rheumatoid Arthritis

Dose: 5–15 mg daily to suppress disabling symptoms.

Use of corticosteroids in gout, bronchial asthma, and shingles is discussed in Chapters 5, 29, and 33, respectively.

BIBLIOGRAPHY

Behrens, T.W., and Goodwin, J.S. Glucocorticoids. In D.J. McCarty (ed.), *Arthritis and allied conditions* (11th ed.). Philadelphia: Lea & Febiger, 1989. Pp. 604–621.
Delecoeuillerie, G., Joly, P., Cohen-de-Lara, A., et al. Polymyalgia

rheumatica and temporal arteritis: A retrospective analysis of prognostic features and different corticosteroid regimens (11 year survey of 210 patients). *Ann. Rheum. Dis.* 47:733–739, 1988.

Gallant, C., and Kenny, P. Oral glucocorticoids and their complications. *J. Amer. Acad. Dermatol.* 14:61–77, 1986.

Gray, R.G., Tenenbaum, J., and Gottlieb, N.L. Local corticosteroid injection treatment in rheumatic disorders. *Semin. Arthrit. Rheum.* 10: 231–254, 1981.

Lukert, B.P., and Raisz, L.G. Glucocorticoid-induced osteoporosis: pathogenesis and management. *Ann. Intern. Med.* 112:352–364, 1990.

Messer, J., Reitman, D., Sacks, H.S., Smith, H., and Chalmers, T.C. Association of adrenocorticosteroid therapy and peptic-ulcer disease. *N. Engl. J. Med.* 309:21–24, 1983.

Piper, J.M., Ray, W.A., Daugherty, J.R., et al. Corticosteroid use and peptic ulcer disease: role of nonsteroidal anti-inflammatory drugs. *Ann. Intern. Med.* 114:735–740, 1991.

Skalka, H.W., and Prchal, J.T. Effect of corticosteroids on cataract formation. *Arch. Ophthalmol.* 98:1773–1777, 1980.

Opioid Analgesics and Other Medications for Painful Conditions

Opioid ("narcotic") analgesics are useful adjuncts in the management of pain due to a variety of conditions. Although chronic use is generally reserved for the treatment of cancer pain, these drugs, particularly the weak opioids, can be highly useful in the management of pain of nonmalignant origin when other agents cannot be used or are ineffective. The side effects of opioids are well known, predictable, and almost always reversible. In contrast to NSAIDs, which may produce insidious and subtle effects in the elderly, opioid analgesics tend to produce toxicity that is easily recognizable and readily reversible. Although toxicity is likely to be enhanced in older individuals, cautious prescribing can minimize problems and can improve the patient's quality of life.

The management of pain is a complex issue and the approach to this problem can vary markedly, depending on the specific clinical setting. For example, potent opioids cannot necessarily be relied on to bring relief in all types of pain refractory to weaker analgesics. For detailed discussion of these topics, the reader is referred to the Bibliography (see Payne & Foley).

PHARMACOLOGIC CONSIDERATIONS

Mechanism of Action

Opioid analgesics are felt to act at the level of opioid receptors in the central nervous system by inhibiting the release of excitatory neurotransmitters and modulating neurotransmission in response to noxious stimuli, thus altering pain perception. Although they are effective in relieving somatic and visceral pain, in which the pain message is carried via generally intact neural pathways, opioids are less effective and often ineffective in relieving deafferentiation pain associated with damaged neural tissue. Thus, certain types of pain appear to be opioid-sensitive, whereas other types of pain are less sensitive, or insensitive, to these agents.

The analgesic effect of the opioids is believed to be mediated by specific receptors at specific loci, and thus occurs independently of other actions (see below). In actuality, however, currently available agents do not exhibit sufficient specificity to completely avoid side effects produced at extra-analgesic sites.

Although other analgesics exhibit a "ceiling effect," in which no further analgesia is produced beyond a certain dose, opioids produce additional analgesia when the dose is increased, as long as the pain is opioid-sensitive.

Other Actions

By modifying subtypes of opioid receptors or by acting at various sites in the central nervous system, individual agents can produce effects other than analgesia, including respiratory depression, sedation, cough suppression, vasodilation, alteration in gastrointestinal function, nausea and vomiting, miosis, and mood changes. Some effects may be related to secondary alterations in the activity of endogenous substances, such as histamine and acetylcholine. Although most of these actions can lead to undesirable side effects, others have important clinical applications. Certain opioids act selectively and are useful antidiarrheal agents or cough suppressants. Morphine has been used in the management of pulmonary edema, where it is thought to act by reducing the subjective sensation of dyspnea as well as by producing peripheral vasodilation, reducing left ventricular filling pressure. Its apparent ability to reduce dyspnea per se has been harnessed in the management of conscious dying patients who wish to have ventilatory support terminated. However, in the setting of terminal respiratory failure, it is difficult to know whether drug or carbon dioxide narcosis is responsible for symptom abatement.

Opioids are classified as agonists, mixed agonist-antagonists, partial agonists, and antagonists, depending on the receptor subtypes affected and whether the drug stimulates, fails to stimulate, or competitively inhibits the receptor. **True agonists,** (morphinelike) demonstrate activity at subtypes responsible for analgesia, respiratory depression, miosis, and a number of other effects detailed below. These are the drugs most commonly used in geriatric practice and will be considered here.

STRONG OPIOIDS

Morphine

Morphine is the prototypic opioid. Actions and side effects of this drug are generally seen with all opioid agonists discussed in this book. Exceptions will be noted in specific sections.

Pharmacokinetics

Morphine is absorbed orally and undergoes first-pass hepatic extraction, reducing its bioavailability as compared to parenteral drug. However, bioavailability may be increased with age, leading to higher plasma concentrations at any given dose. Morphine is metabolized to active and inactive metabolites, but metabolism does not appear to be significantly impaired in hepatic disease. One renally excreted metabolite, morphine-6-glucuronide, is much more potent than morphine and has a longer duration of action. Although quantitatively minor, this metabolite accumulates in renal failure and may be responsible for serious side effects in such patients. Because of its somewhat extended presence, this metabolite may also be responsible for the fact that relative efficacy of oral morphine compared to parenteral morphine increases with continued use, from a potency ratio of 1:6 with acute dosing to 1:3 or 1:2 with chronic administration.

The elimination half-life of morphine as parent drug in healthy nonelderly adults is approximately 2–3 hours but is probably longer in older and sick patients. Steady-state concentrations of immediate-release morphine preparations are achieved within 10–15 hours, allowing dose titrations to be made early and with relative safety. However, time to achieve steady state may be prolonged with age, especially when the presence of active metabolites is considered.

An age-associated increase in the sensitivity to morphine has been demonstrated. Clearance is reduced and, at a given dose, levels are higher in older as compared to younger adults. In addition, the duration of effect is prolonged and older patients may achieve adequate pain relief with a lower than expected dose, especially when treatment is first initiated. Pharmacokinetic alterations may not fully explain enhanced sensitivity, suggesting that pharmacodynamic factors may be operating. The contribution of morphine-6-glucuronide to enhanced morphine sensitivity in the elderly is not known, but the renal mode of clearance of this metabolite suggests that it may play a role. It is important to emphasize that studies demonstrating enhanced sensitivity in elderly patients have examined responses in patients with postoperative pain. Such patients tend to be "opioid naive," not having received such medications previously, and are likely to respond very differently than individuals who are being chronically treated and who will have developed tolerance (see below).

Side Effects

Morphine produces an array of central nervous system effects, including **sedation, dizziness, alterations in mental status,** and centrally mediated **nausea** and **vomiting.** Alterations in mood, such as **euphoria** and **apathy,** may occur. Many of these effects are dose-related, but there appears to be individual susceptibility to many of them. For example, only a minority of patients experience euphoria and not all patients experience opioid-induced nausea and vomiting. **Confusional states** are common in patients being treated with morphine, although in the presence of serious systemic disease or terminal malignancy it is not always certain whether confusion is due to drug or the disease itself. Both drug-induced and disease-related confusion are more common in older individuals.

Morphine decreases the brain stem respiratory center's response to hypercarbia, leading to **respiratory depression,** and although alterations in arterial blood gases can be demonstrated even at relatively low doses, clinical problems are most likely to occur in opioid-naive patients, at times when large dose increments are made, and in those with compromised ventilatory function. Respiratory rate and tidal volume may decrease and irregular breathing patterns may occur. By releasing histamine, morphine can produce bronchoconstriction, but the significance of this is uncertain.

Constipation is extremely common, necessitating the use of laxatives in most cases. Constipation is caused by delayed intestinal transit time and enhanced water reabsorption, and by direct reduction in peristalsis. **Fecal impaction** tends to occur readily in geriatric patients taking opioids, especially if they have limited mobility. Severe constipation poses a particular risk to the patient taking controlled-release formulations. Several doses may pile up in the intestine and absorption of large amounts of drug at once can occur as the blockage worsens; deaths from overdose have been reported under these circumstances.

By increasing biliary tone, morphine may produce **abdominal pain** or even **biliary colic** in susceptible individuals. By reducing gastroesophageal sphincter tone and prolonging gastroduodenal transit time, morphine may produce **gastroesophageal reflux.**

Opioid-induced **nausea and vomiting** are largely though not completely mediated by mechanisms outside the gastrointestinal system, namely, by stimulation of the chemoreceptor trigger zone of the medulla. There is individual variation in patient susceptibility to these effects, which are dose-related and tend to subside with continued use of the drug. Opioid-induced nausea appears to be less common in patients who are treated while recumbent than in those who are ambulatory.

By producing peripheral vasodilation, morphine can cause **hypotension.** Because there is an orthostatic component to this effect, it is less likely to be experienced by patients who are treated while supine, if they are hemodynamically stable, than by those who are ambulatory. Hypotension may be partly mediated by histamine release. **Pruritus** and **urticaria** may also occur, likewise mediated by histamine release.

Miosis occurs in virtually all patients and tends to subside little with continued use of the drug.

By increasing the tone of the bladder outlet, morphine may produce **urinary retention.** The drug also antagonizes centrally mediated inhibition of detrusor tone, resulting in **urinary urgency;** this could precipitate incontinence in patients with compromised bladder function due to detrusor hyperreflexia, a common condition in the elderly. Tolerance to these effects occurs rapidly, so they are less likely to be experienced by patients taking opioids chronically.

Abrupt discontinuation of morphine after continuous, though not necessarily prolonged, use may produce **withdrawal symptoms** consisting of sweating, nausea, vomiting, lacrimation, restlessness, and tremor. This physical dependence is a predictable phenomenon that can be controlled by gradual reduction in dosage. It is to be distinguished from true **addiction,** which is a psychological dependence characterized by continuous craving for the substance and typical behavioral patterns geared toward obtaining the drug, independent of the need to control pain. Probably fewer than 5% of patients treated with opioids crave the drug in this way once it is withdrawn, even if they are being treated for nonmalignant causes of pain. In most patients, desire for the drug is rather guided by the need to obtain pain relief. It is important to emphasize the rarity of true addiction in medical opioid use because there is abundant evidence that fear of addiction on the part of health professionals as well as some patients leads to undertreatment of pain and needless suffering. The exact prevalence of addiction related to nonmedical use of opioids in the geriatric population is not known but is believed to be low.

Toxic overdose of opioids can produce coma, respiratory depression, and death.

Side effects of opioids can be reversed by the opioid antagonist naloxone (Narcan) but this may also precipitate modified opioid withdrawal if dependence has developed. Excitatory symptoms of meperidine cannot be reversed in this way (see Meperidine below).

Tolerance

Tolerance to opioids develops rapidly with continuous use but tolerance to various effects develops at very different rates, presumably because of the different receptor subtypes involved. Tolerance to analgesia occurs more slowly than tolerance to most side effects, including respiratory suppression and nausea. In contrast, tolerance develops very slowly, if at all, to constipation. Tolerance to miosis also develops slowly and may be incomplete.

The rapidity with which analgesic tolerance develops is highly variable and is dependent not only on individual variations in pain perception and narcotic response, but, in the cancer patient, on the rapidity with which pain escalates. This has important implications for dosing. Some patients require increasing doses rapidly, whereas others are managed for prolonged periods on a stable dose. An unusual pattern of dose escalation should not bias the physician against increasing the dose if necessary.

Important Drug Interactions

Any agent with sedative-hypnotic effects may enhance the sedating effects of morphine.

Drugs that impair the action of hepatic microsomal enzymes may reduce the metabolism of morphine, increasing its effect. This mechanism has been implicated in one putative opioid interaction with monoamine oxidase inhibitors (MAOIs). Morphine does not produce the dangerous excitatory reaction reported when meperidine is used with MAOIs and is considered the appropriate alternative to meperidine when a short-term potent opioid is required; however, it should be instituted in such patients with great caution (see Meperidine below).

Metoclopramide has been reported to enhance the sedative effect of controlled-release morphine; this has been attributed to enhanced absorption of the opioid.

Contraindications

Morphine should not be used in patients with pain due to constipation or fecal impaction until the bowel problem has been alleviated. It should also not be used in patients with pain due to apparent biliary colic, in which case meperidine may be a suitable alternative opioid (see below).

Morphine should be used with caution in patients who have bronchospastic disease. Potent opioid analgesia in patients with respiratory failure should be reserved for extraordinary circumstances; ventilatory support and opioid antagonists should be available unless specifically refused by the patient or surrogate decision maker. Weak opioids may be better tolerated in such patients (see Weak Opioid Analgesics below).

Precautions

Constipation is such a common side effect that laxatives should be instituted early in the course of treatment. This is particularly important for the patient who is not ambulatory. Osmotic agents, irritant laxatives, or stool softeners should be used and adequate fluid replacement given (see Chap. 24). Bulk-forming agents should be avoided because they may increase the risk of constipation in seriously ill and immobilized patients. Bowel function should be carefully monitored and laxatives considered regardless of which opioid is given.

After continuous treatment with morphine and other opioids, the drug should be withdrawn gradually in order to prevent withdrawal symptoms.

Indications

Morphine is indicated in the management of moderate to severe pain that does not respond to nonnarcotic analgesics or to weaker opioids such as codeine or propoxyphene. It may be used in the management of nonmalignant as well as cancer pain. However, morphine and other opioids are generally **not** indicated in neuropathic pain, which may respond best to tricyclic antidepressants or anticonvulsants.

Dosage Forms

Oral morphine preparations are currently considered the treatment of choice for most patients with chronic cancer pain. Long-acting oral forms have been found to be as effective as equivalent doses of regular morphine given more frequently, are more convenient, allow nocturnal pain control, and produce side effects no more and possibly less often than shorter-acting agents.

Parenteral morphine is reserved for patients unable to take the drug by mouth, or if there is doubt about the status of gastrointestinal absorption. It may also be instituted in patients no longer achieving relief by the oral route. Intravenous drug can be given by bolus or continuous drip. The subject of continuous intravenous opioid administration is reviewed in the Bibliography references (see Payne et al.). Intrathecal and epidural delivery of opioids is also attempted in refractory cases although it is associated with high morbidity.

Dosing

Because elderly patients have increased sensitivity to opioids, dosages should be carefully titrated and initial doses should be somewhat lower than for younger adults, particularly if there is preexisting cognitive impairment. However, tolerance develops in older patients as it does in younger ones, so dose increments should be made as soon as the need arises. The correct dose is the one that gives pain relief short of producing unacceptable side effects.

In the management of chronic cancer pain, once appropriate dose titration has been achieved, the drug should be given on a regular schedule rather than as needed (prn). It has been clearly demonstrated that regular scheduled administration is more effective in reducing pain and ultimately leads to lower total doses. Importantly, regular administration avoids placing the patient in the role of supplicant and circumvents biased or uninformed judgments by nursing personnel and patients themselves that frequent narcotic use is "wrong" and likely to lead to addiction.

ORAL IMMEDIATE-RELEASE

Initial dose: 5 mg every 4–6 hours. Additional doses of 5–10 mg should be made available to patients with severe chronic pain to cover breakthrough pain until the appropriate dose has been determined.

Note: Higher initial doses are often required, especially for those who have been recently exposed to opioids. When patients recently on parenteral morphine are switched to oral drug, 2–3 times the previous parenteral dose should be given as an oral dose (Table 4–1). Suggested initial doses are low to account for the frailty of some sick elderly. The physician should be prepared to increase the dose as soon as it becomes apparent that more is required. This admonition applies to all potent opioids.

Usual effective dose range: Dose should be titrated according to the degree of pain relief short of producing serious toxicity. Total daily doses in nonelderly adult cancer patients chronically being treated with opioids average 240 mg; while this is a high dose, significantly higher doses are sometimes required.

48

Table 4-1. Strong Opioid Analgesics

Agent	Sample Brand	Peak Effect (hr)[a]	Elimination Half-Time (hr)	Duration of Analgesia (hr)	Equianalgesic PO[b]	Dose (mg) IM
Morphine	Many	1–1½	2–4	3–4	20–30	10
Controlled-release morphine (oral)	MS-Contin Roxanol-SR	4	3	12	20–30	—
Hydromorphone	Dilaudid	1 ½	2–3	2–3	7.5	1.5
Levorphanol	Levo-Dromoran	1–2	12–16	≤6	2–4	2
Methadone	Dolophine	½–2	15–36 or longer	≤8	10–20	10
Meperidine	Demerol	½ (after IM)	3–5	2–4	See text	75

Note: Properties based on data from nongeriatric adults. See text for discussion regarding older individuals.
[a] After oral administration unless otherwise noted.
[b] After chronic administration.

CONTROLLED-RELEASE ORAL (MS-CONTIN, ROXANOL-SR)

Initial dose: Total effective daily dose achieved by immediate-release morphine, given in 2 divided doses.

Note: Controlled-release preparations are available in tablets no smaller than 30 mg so that in opioid-naive geriatric patients it is generally advisable to first titrate the dose using immediate-release forms.

Usual effective dose range: As with regular-acting morphine, given in 2 to 3 divided doses.

Hydromorphone (Dilaudid)

Hydromorphone is a very potent, semisynthetic morphine analogue. It has a short half-life of 2–3 hours in nonelderly adults. With continuous administration a steady state is reached in less than 24 hours, as with morphine, allowing dose titrations to be made quickly and more safely than with longer-acting agents. This drug has not been specifically studied in geriatric patients, so that generalizations about its administration cannot be made. Because of its potency and the possibility that pharmacodynamic responses will be enhanced in the elderly, initial doses should be lower than for younger adults.

Indications

In patients with moderate to severe opioid-sensitive pain syndromes, hydromorphone is a suitable alternative to morphine in patients who cannot tolerate that drug. It occasionally brings relief to patients whose pain does not respond adequately to morphine.

Dosing

Initial oral dose: 1–2 mg every 4–6 hours.

Note: Higher initial doses are often needed, as with morphine.

Initial parenteral dose: 0.25 mg IM or SQ every 4–6 hours. The drug may also be given as an IV bolus but should be injected slowly over 3–4 minutes. Hydromorphone may also be given as a continuous drip.

Methadone (Dolophine)

This synthetic opioid is well absorbed orally and has very high bioavailability in most patients. It is metabolized by the liver but a significant amount is excreted unchanged in the urine. The average serum half-life is 15–24 hours, but is as long as 58 hours in some patients.

Because of the ultralong half-life seen in some patients, steady-state concentrations may not be reached for up to 10 days. This is an important disadvantage since the duration of analgesia is rarely longer than 8 hours, requiring relatively frequent dosing to provide relief until steady state is reached. Repeated dosing may lead to accumulation and delayed toxicity, including oversedation and respiratory depression. Deaths have been reported in elderly patients. Fixed doses of methadone designed to give continuous pain relief should generally be avoided by that age group unless alternative approaches are unsuitable.

Although it was once promoted as being preferable to short-acting opioids in cancer patients or was given as an adjunct to them, the availability of long-acting oral morphine has reduced the applicability of methadone.

Levorphanol (Levo-Dromoran)

The serum half-life of levorphanol is 12–16 hours but, like methadone, its duration of analgesic effect is approximately 8 hours. It is available for oral and parenteral use. Its long half-life leads to some of the same problems as methadone, and it should be avoided by the elderly unless alternative approaches are unsuitable.

Brompton Cocktail

Brompton cocktail, named for London's Brompton Hospital where it originated, is a combination of drugs that was designed for patients with cancer pain. Variations of the Brompton cocktail have contained combinations of a potent opioid (including heroin), cocaine, alcohol, or a phenothiazine. It has since been found that it is the opioid component of the combination that is responsible for relief of symptoms, and varieties of this cocktail have generally been abandoned in favor of opioid analgesics alone. When patients experience oversedation, nausea, or anxiety, adjunctive pharmacologic treatment can be prescribed as indicated.

Heroin itself has never been approved for therapeutic use in the United States and is unlikely to be in the future because of its widespread illicit use and because relief is believed to be available in the present pharmacopoeia. Heroin (diacetylmorphine) has been found to be a pro-drug that is first converted to morphine in the body before exerting its analgesic effect. Although its high lipid solubility causes rapid delivery into the central nervous system and a slightly more rapid onset of action than morphine, its duration of action is shorter, and it has no apparent advantages over rapidly acting and more potent hydromorphone when immediate relief is required. Moreover, once analgesia is obtained, continuous treatment with morphine eliminates the need for a rapidly acting agent. Morphine is equivalent in therapeutic efficacy and side effects to heroin.

Meperedine (Demerol)

Meperidine is a synthetic opioid that differs chemically from morphine. This difference has important clinical implications.

Orally administered meperidine undergoes extensive first-pass metabolism and is thus much less potent than parenteral drug, so that an ordinary dose of meperidine (approximately 50 mg) given orally has approximately the same analgesic potency as 650 mg of aspirin. In fact, 50 mg of parenteral meperidine does not exceed this potency by much either.

Meperidine is metabolized to normeperidine, which is cleared by the kidney. Clearance of meperidine itself declines with age, perhaps due to sluggish hepatic metabolism. Normeperidine outlasts the presence of parent drug in plasma and is responsible for excitatory side effects (see below). Metabolism of meperidine is reduced in hepatic disease, requiring dose reductions.

Adverse Effects

In addition to producing typical opioid side effects, meperidine also may produce **central nervous system excitation.** Tremulousness, myoclonus, agitation, and even seizures may occur. These symptoms are not reversed by naloxone, but have been attributed to normeperidine and are most likely to be produced in susceptible patients achieving critical levels of that metabolite, notably, after repeated dosing. Geriatric patients are at increased risk of this adverse effect on account of the renal mode of normeperidine elimination. Because of the high proportion of normeperidine to meperidine achieved when the drug is given orally, and because concentrations of normeperidine are likely to be higher in geriatric patients than in younger adults, oral meperidine should generally be avoided. However, clearance of normeperidine is prolonged with age after parenteral administration as well.

Meperidine is more likely than other potent opioid agonists to produce **dysphoria**.

Unlike morphine, meperidine does not increase biliary tone and has been used safely in patients with apparent biliary tract pain.

Important Drug Interactions

When given in conjunction with MAOIs, meperidine produces an **excitatory syndrome** that is more or less unique among opioids. This syndrome is characterized by agitation, alterations in blood pressure, hypertension, headache, tachycardia, hyperpyrexia, seizures, and muscle rigidity; it is felt to be due to the combined seritoninergic effects of MAOIs and meperidine. This syndrome has not been reported with other opioids, except perhaps dextromethorphan, a mild antitussive with a similar seritoninergic action to meperidine. A separate **depressive syndrome** may also occur and is characterized by respiratory depression, hypotension, and coma; this has been attributed to MAOI-induced inhibition of hepatic opioid metabolism, probably occurs with morphine, and should be considered a potential interaction with other opioids.

By accelerating the metabolism of meperidine, barbiturates and presumably other hepatic enzyme inducers may reduce the efficacy of meperidine while potentially increasing normeperidinelike toxicity.

Precautions

Meperidine should not be used in the management of **chronic** pain in the elderly because of the increased likelihood of toxic metabolite accumulation.

Indications

Meperidine is indicated for the short-term management of acute pain when a potent parenteral opioid is indicated, and in patients who cannot tolerate morphine. In contrast to morphine, meperidine is suitable for the management of pain in patients prone to biliary colic.

Dosing

Usual dose: 50–100 mg IM.

Ethical Issues in the Use of Strong Opioids

Although serious respiratory depression and hypotension may complicate the pain management of dying patients, these are actually very unusual complications of opioids in that clinical situation because of the development of tolerance. Importantly, fear of complications may deter the physician from prescribing enough opioid to give the patient adequate pain relief. This dilemma should be discussed openly with the patient or surrogate decision maker when appropriate so that they can be informed accurately of the risks and benefits of treatment. Although it is theoretically possible that potent opioids could hasten death by minutes or hours, there is a consensus among ethicists and health professionals that it is a morally acceptable risk for the patient who wants to avoid the alternative of a painful death (see Bibliography, President's Commission). This same ethical argument may be applied to the dying, respirator-dependent patient who has asked to have ventilatory support discontinued but who requires a sedative such as morphine in order to avoid the suffering that can occur before death.

Nursing personnel should be involved in discussions about these issues. They are often caught in the middle, required to follow the doctor's order but having serious personal misgivings about the ethical aspects of giving high doses of opioids to patients near death.

WEAK OPIOIDS

The following agents are classified as **weak opioids** because they produce intolerable side effects if given at the doses required to produce analgesia to the same extent as morphine. However, these agents are very useful in the treatment of pain syndromes in patients who are unable to tolerate or have an insufficient response to anti-inflammatory agents and other nonopioid analgesics.

Codeine

Codeine, the methyl ester of morphine, is a naturally occurring opium alkaloid but has less than 10% of the analgesic potency of morphine—a 30-mg dose of codeine may produce less analgesia than 650 mg of aspirin or acetaminophen. A small proportion is metabolized in the liver to morphine, the rest largely to inactive metabolites. The serum half-life is short at 2–3 hours in nonelderly adults. Although little drug is excreted unchanged in the urine, elimination is prolonged in renal failure. Codeine pharmacokinetics have not been specifically studied in geriatric patients.

Despite its relatively mild analgesic action, codeine is capable of producing typical opioid side effects, tolerance, and toxicity, depending on dose and individual susceptibility. It has been said that codeine has a somewhat higher likelihood of producing nausea than other weak opioids, but there are no comparative studies to substantiate this.

The analgesic efficacy of codeine may be enhanced somewhat by nonopioid analgesics, presumably because they have a different mechanism of action. This enhanced efficacy is most likely to occur if the dose of nonopioid is not lower than the equivalent of 650 mg of aspirin. Codeine is available in a number of combination preparations with aspirin and acetaminophen.

Codeine is a potent cough suppressant and is widely used for this purpose.

Indications

Codeine is indicated in mild to moderately severe, opioid-sensitive pain syndromes that fail to respond to nonopioid analgesics. Codeine-acetaminophen combination agents (Tylenol #2, others) may be particularly useful in patients with osteoarthritis and related musculoskeletal pain syndromes who are unable to tolerate nonsteroidal anti-inflammatory agents (NSAIDs).

Dosing

Initial dose: 30 mg in combination with equivalent of 650 mg aspirin or acetaminophen (e.g., 2 tablets of Tylenol #2). If a smaller initial dose of codeine is desired, it can be administered in combination with a nonopioid at a dose equivalent to 650 mg aspirin.

Oxycodone

This agent is a semisynthetic opioid with an analgesic potency that is less than that of morphine but greater than that of codeine. Like codeine, its analgesic potency may be enhanced by nonopioid analgesics and it is commonly prescribed in combination with aspirin (Percodan) or acetaminophen (Percocet, Tylox). Thus, oxycodone in combination with acetaminophen is useful in patients who are unable to tolerate or do not achieve relief from NSAIDs, and it may provide additional pain control in patients who do not respond to codeine.

Oxycodone is felt to have an addiction potential that is significantly greater than codeine, perhaps because it has a higher likelihood of producing euphoria.

Dosing

Initial dose: 2.5–5.0 mg alone or in combination with acetaminophen or aspirin bid-qid.

Propoxyphene (Darvon)

Pharmacologic Considerations

MECHANISM OF ACTION. Propoxyphene is structurally related to methadone, but has only a fraction of methadone's analgesic potency. It binds to opioid receptors in the CNS, producing analgesia. When used alone, the analgesic efficacy of propoxyphene is comparable to codeine, aspirin, or acetaminophen. Although propoxyphene is marketed in combination with aspirin or acetaminophen, there is disagreement over whether these combinations produce better analgesia than the analgesics given alone.

Propoxyphene is available as a soluble hydrochloride salt (Darvon, others) and as a less soluble napsylate compound (Darvon-N, others). The former catalyzes the degradation of aspirin, necessitating specialized formulations when combinations are used; certain generic preparations of these combinations have been associated with aspirin instability. This problem does not arise in the napsylate compound, which has no effect on aspirin degradation.

PHARMACOKINETICS. Propoxyphene is well absorbed, the hydrochloride achieving peak plasma levels (1–2 hours) somewhat more rapidly than the napsylate (3–4 hours) when tablets are given. The drug undergoes extensive first-pass metabolism to norpropoxyphene, a metabolite that does not produce central nervous system or respiratory depression, but which is able to depress cardiac conduction. This does not seem to be clinically important in humans at ordinary doses. The half-life of propoxyphene is approximately 12 hours, but that of norpropoxyphene ranges from 22 to 36 hours. Propoxyphene is excreted largely in bile.

Although propoxyphene pharmacokinetics have not been studied in the elderly, it is known that both parent drug and renally excreted norpropoxyphene accumulate in renal failure. The significance of this for geriatric patients is not known.

Adverse Effects

The chief disadvantage of propoxyphene is its tendency to produce opioidlike side effects in the central nervous system, such as **confusion, hallucinations,** and **dizziness.** In high doses, propoxyphene may produce **respiratory depression,** and although it is less likely to do this than codeine and other opioids, death from overdose and respiratory failure is not uncommon. **Cardiac arrhythmias** and **conduction disturbances** may also occur in the setting of **toxic overdose.**

Propoxyphene is subject to abuse because of its ability to produce a "high," but produces fewer pleasant sensations than other opioids and is probably abused far less for this reason. Physical dependence after ordinary use of this drug is not major. However, **abrupt withdrawal** after several months of use **may produce minor gastrointestinal symptoms** in some patients. It is prudent to dispense this agent with the same caution observed for narcotic analgesics and to discontinue the drug gradually.

Important Drug Interactions

Like other opioids, propoxyphene used concurrently with other centrally acting agents, including alcohol, may lead to central nervous system toxicity, including respiratory depression.

Indications

Propoxyphene is indicated as adjunctive treatment for mild to moderate pain syndromes when other analgesics cannot be used. It should be particularly suitable for musculoskeletal problems, including osteoarthritis, in patients who cannot tolerate anti-inflammatory agents or codeine. However, propoxyphene should not be expected to produce greater analgesia than acetaminophen alone.

Dosing

Usual dose:
Propoxyphene hydrochloride: 65 mg every 4–6 hours as needed to a maximum daily dose of 260 mg.
Propoxyphene napsylate: 100 mg every 4–6 hours as needed to a maximum daily dose of 400 mg.

OTHER AGENTS USED FOR PAIN

Tricyclic Antidepressants

The tricyclic antidepressants (TCAs), in particular those with strong seritoninergic properties, exert analgesic action in certain pain syndromes. This is believed to be at least partly independent of the antidepressant action, and may be related to the ability of these agents to inhibit the enzymatic degradation of enkephalin and to enhance serotonin at the synaptic cleft. Enhancement of serotonin and enkephalin is thought to block the afferent pain message.

Conditions that sometimes respond include diabetic neuropathy, facial pain, arthritis, cervical and low back pain, headache, and postherpetic neuralgia. Cancer pain is less likely to respond. Analgesia may be obtained with doses lower than those used in depression, and generally with only a short delay. The seritoninergic agents amitriptyline, doxepin, and imipramine are the best-studied and possibly most effective TCAs for this indication, but since they tend to be less well tolerated in elderly patients, other agents of this class are sometimes used.

Tricyclic antidepressants are discussed in detail in Chap. 8.

Anticonvulsants

Anticonvulsants are sometimes used for chronic pain syndromes, particularly when the pain is neuropathic in origin. Phenytoin, carbamazepine, and the benzodiazepine clonazepam are the anticonvulsants most commonly used for these indications. Carbamazepine is structurally related to TCAs; it is particularly useful in the management of trigeminal neuralgia, but the mechanism of analgesic action is not known, and in other forms of neuropathic pain its efficacy is less predictable. For example, carbamazepine is less effective in the management of postherpetic neuralgia than the TCA amitriptyline. The efficacy of phenytoin in pain syndromes is likewise unpredictable. Clonazepam produces considerable sedation, making its efficacy difficult to assess. This sedation also limits its suitability for the geriatric patient.

Anticonvulsants used in geriatric practice are discussed more thoroughly in Chap. 11.

CENTRALLY ACTING SKELETAL MUSCLE RELAXANTS

Skeletal muscle spasm, which may occur as a result of traumatic muscle strain, often contributes to pain experienced in joint disease or soft tissue rheumatism. Secondary muscle contraction occurs as a compensatory mechanism to make up for the loss of function brought about by the primary problem, and painful spasm may result. This in essence extends the original problem and may produce a vicious cycle. In the case of arthritis and soft tissue injury, additional stress may be imposed on the involved area and the inflammatory condition may itself worsen. Skeletal muscle relaxants are often employed to break this cycle or to alleviate the pain itself.

Skeletal muscle relaxants are less toxic to the gastrointestinal tract than NSAIDs and do not possess most of the problems associated with opioids. However, they produce their own range of toxicities and must be used cautiously.

Pharmacologic Considerations

Mechanism of Action

Skeletal muscle relaxants are chemically dissimilar from one another. They are grouped together because of their putative muscle relaxant properties and because they are thought to act at least in part through the central nervous system.

The pathophysiology of skeletal muscle spasm is complex and incompletely understood and the precise mechanism of action of skeletal muscle relaxants is not known. A proposed mechanism is that these drugs affect the reflex arcs that synapse in the spinal cord and elsewhere in the central nervous system, altering involuntary motor pathways that affect the muscle spindle. Alternatively, relief may be brought about by sedation, which leads to subjective improvement or which enforces rest. In fact, it has been observed that the degree of drowsiness may correlate with the degree of relief. A direct central action on pain control centers has also been reported but this has not been substantiated fully.

It has been difficult for investigators to determine the comparative efficacy of the various agents in use, and to define precise indications. These agents do appear to be more effective than placebo in relieving muscle spasm from a variety of musculoskeletal ailments, but are more likely to produce relief in acute muscle spasm than in chronic conditions.

The centrally acting skeletal muscle relaxants are not effective in relieving the chronic spasticity of neurological disorders, such as stroke or Parkinson's disease. For a discussion of chronic spasticity, the reader is referred to the Bibliography (see Katz).

Pharmacokinetics

These drugs are metabolized in the liver, largely to inactive metabolites. There is no specific pharmacokinetic data for the elderly. Profiles of individual agents are summarized in Table 4-2. Dose recommendations are also given and are adjusted downward based on the enhanced susceptibility of geriatric patients to drug-induced confusional states and certain other side effects.

Drug Interactions

Centrally acting skeletal muscle relaxants have the potential of interacting pharmacodynamically with unrelated centrally acting agents that have either depressant or excitatory effects, so combined use should be avoided if possible. It is noteworthy that some agents are available in fixed combinations with codeine or caffeine, albeit in smaller doses.

Those muscle relaxants possessing anticholinergic activity (i.e., orphenadrine, cyclobenzaprine, and, to a lesser extent, carisoprodol) may produce additive toxicity when used with other anticholinergic agents.

The specific interactions of the tricyclic cyclobenzaprine are discussed below.

Indications

Centrally acting skeletal muscle relaxants may be used sparingly as adjunctive treatment in acute muscle spasm associated with trauma or rheumatic conditions. However, they should be used only when nonpharmacologic approaches or topical agents do not provide relief, or when ordinary analgesics are ineffective or cannot be used.

Dosing

There are no data on which to base dosing guidelines for these agents in the elderly. Thus, the smallest available dose should be given as a trial before the patient is advised to take the drug as part of a regular regimen.

Specific Agents

Methocarbamol (Robaxin, Others)

Methocarbamol has a shorter serum half-life and duration of action than most of the other agents and is thus potentially one of the safer agents of this class for older patients. However, **drowsiness** and **light-headedness** are common side effects, and **overstimulation** and **confusion** may also occur. In addition, **blurred vision** has been reported.

Table 4–2. Centrally Acting Skeletal Muscle Relaxants

Agent	Sample Brand[a]	Duration of Action (hr)[b]	Serum Half-Life (hr)	Trial Dose (mg)	Usual Dose Frequency
Methocarbamol	Robaxin	2	2	500	bid-qid
Chlorzoxazone	Paraflex Parafon Forte	3–4	1	250–500	bid-qid
Metaxalone	Skelaxin	4–6	2–3	400	bid-qid
Carisoprodol	Soma	4–6	8	[c]	—
Orphenadrine	Norflex	4–6	14	[c]	—
Cyclobenzaprine	Flexeril	12–24	Up to 3 days	[c]	—

[a]For skeletal muscle relaxant alone. Combination agents may contain other ingredients, such as aspirin, acetaminophen, codeine, or caffeine.
[b]In nongeriatric patients. There is inadequate data on which to draw conclusion about older individuals.
[c]Best avoided because of side effect profile.

Chlorzoxazone (Paraflex, Parafon Forte)

In addition to the side effects listed above for methocarbamol, **hepatitis** has occasionally been reported in patients while on chlorzoxazone, although it is not clear if these cases were directly related to the drug. Mild **gastrointestinal upset** may also occur. Chlorzoxazone may produce **orange discoloration of the urine** in some patients, but this is thought to be without clinical importance. Patients should be advised of this in advance.

This drug has a relatively short half-life and is probably one of the safer of this class of agents for the elderly.

Metaxalone (Skelaxin)

In addition to **central nervous system effects,** metaxalone has been reported to produce **hemolytic anemia** and **hepatitis.** It produces a false-positive reaction for glucose with the copper reduction test (Clinitest).

Carisoprodol (Soma, Others)

Carisoprodol is chemically related to the well-known sedative meprobamate. In addition to the central nervous system effects discussed above, **ataxia** and **depression** have been reported with this drug. It has weak anticholinergic action and therefore has the potential, though probably slight, of producing acute glaucoma, urinary retention, and other **atropinelike symptoms.** A reversible but severe idiosyncratic reaction consisting of **quadriplegia, visual loss,** and **confusion** has been reported. **Other hypersensitivity reactions** have occurred as well.

Orphenadrine Citrate (Norflex, Others)

Orphenadrine citrate is structurally similar to the sedating histamine-1 blocker diphenhydramine. Orphenadrine has anticholinergic action and a related agent, orphenadrine hydrochloride (Disipal), has in fact occasionally been used in the treatment of Parkinson's disease. This is mentioned for clarification only, since orphenadrine citrate is not used in that disorder.

Because of its anticholinergic action, orphenadrine may produce **dry mouth, acute glaucoma, urinary retention, tachycardia,** and other atropinelike effects. As expected, **drowsiness, confusion,** and **other central effects may occur.** Death from overdose has been reported.

Cyclobenzaprine Hydrochloride (Flexeril)

Cyclobenzaprine is structurally related to the tricyclic antidepressants, and shares many of their side effects. It has potent anticholinergic activity, effects on the cardiac conducting system, and ganglionic blocking action. **Atropinelike effects, heart block,** and **orthostatic hypotension** may occur, in addition to **central nervous system effects** reported in other agents discussed in this section. These troubling effects may be prolonged because the drug is slowly eliminated.

ADDITIONAL DRUG INTERACTIONS. Cyclobenzaprine may produce hypertensive crisis when used with monoamine oxidase inhibitors. It may also interact pharmacodynamically with drugs that affect the cardiac conducting system or with those possessing anticholinergic action. Like other drugs discussed in this section, it may also potentiate the effects of central nervous system depressants.

Diazepam (Valium) as a Skeletal Muscle Relaxant

Diazepam is sometimes used for its muscle relaxant properties, which may be directly related to sedation. Physicians may be more familiar with the spectrum of effects of diazepam, and the drug may be better tolerated than certain of the muscle relaxants discussed above. However, its efficacy is controversial and it must be used cautiously in the elderly because of its tendency to accumulate in the central nervous system. Diazepam is discussed more fully in Chap. 7.

NONPHARMACOLOGIC AND OTHER MODALITIES

Skeletal muscle spasm and other pain syndromes can also be relieved by rest, massage, moist heat, hydrotherapy and diathermy. Transcutaneous electrical nerve stimulation (TENS) is used by specialists in pain management for a number of pain syndromes with varying success, but its efficacy has not uniformly been demonstrated in controlled studies. Local injections of saline or anesthetics into "trigger points" may provide temporary and sometimes lasting relief to patients with musculoskeletal pain. Vapocoolants, such as ethyl chloride spray, are applied topically, and are often used in conjunction with passive stretching or massage.

Specialized modalities should be used by physicians and therapists experienced in their application. TENS is contraindicated in patients with cardiac pacemakers. Ethyl chloride spray should be used conservatively, not near an open flame, and should not be inhaled.

Rehabilitation units and specialized pain clinics often utilize a multidisciplinary approach that can be successful in patients with acute and chronic pain syndromes.

BIBLIOGRAPHY

Elenbaas, J.K. Centrally acting oral skeletal muscle relaxants. *Am. J. Hosp. Pharm.* 37: 1313–1323, 1980.

Foley, K.M. Analgesic drug therapy in cancer pain: principles and practice. *Med. Clin. N. Amer.* 71:207–232, 1987.

Katz, R.T. Management of spasticity. *Am. J. Phys. Med. Rehabil.* 67:108–116, 1988.

Payne, R., and Foley, K.M. Cancer pain. *Med. Clin. N. Amer.* 71:153–352, 1987.

Portenoy, R.K., and Farkash, A. Practical management of non-malignant pain in the elderly. *Geriatrics* 43:29–47, 1988.

President's Commission for the Study of Ethical Problems in Medicine and Biomedical and Behavioral Research. *Deciding to forego life-sustaining treatment.* Washington, D.C., 1983.

Medications for Gout

Gout is commonly mistreated. Since gout is not a fatal illness but misuse of powerful agents used to treat it may cause fatalities, it is important that hypouricemic agents and colchicine be given only when the diagnosis is certain. This admonition is particularly important in the geriatric patient, for whom these medications may be particularly toxic.

Treatment of uric acid disease is only an emergency in the rare case of tumor lysis, where large amounts of urate may suddenly pass through the kidney and produce urate nephropathy. In painful arthritis, symptomatic treatment can be given while the etiology is explored.

In geriatric practice, common errors in treating gout include pharmacologic treatment of asymptomatic hyperuricemia, treatment of hyperuricemia that is associated with nongouty arthritis, failure to substitute less toxic medications in patients with a poor medical prognosis, and overdosing.

Many conditions can produce hyperuricemia, but prolonged exposure—perhaps as long as 15–20 years—to high uric acid levels are required before gout actually occurs. In addition, a minimum of two additional years without treatment must go by after the first episode of gout before significant joint destruction begins to occur. This time span must be compared to the projected lifespan of the patient when treatment options are being considered.

Perhaps the most common cause of hyperuricemia in the elderly is diuretic use. The risk-benefit ratio of hypouricemic agents does not warrant treatment of hyperuricemia in the absence of gouty symptoms. The physician should rather consider discontinuing the offending agent, or, if this is not possible, should avoid treatment of hyperuricemia unless an acute attack of gout does occur.

Hyperuricemia may coincidentally be present in patients who have other forms of arthritis, soft tissue rheumatism, chronic pain syndromes, or a painful bunion. Psoriasis, which may cause arthritis, is also commonly associated with hyperuricemia. In these conditions, if there is no evidence of gout, these associations should be approached as if they were asymptomatic hyperuricemia and should not be treated as though they were gout. In practice, it may be difficult to confirm the diagnosis with absolute certainty. The definitive diagnosis of gout rests on demonstration of negatively birefringent, needle-shaped crystals under polarized light in fluid aspirated from a joint or tophus. In the absence of this, there must be a history that is utterly classic of gout, or X-ray changes considered pathognomonic.

Symptomatic gout in very old, debilitated patients is not an absolute indication for hypouricemic agents or colchicine. The toxicity of these agents is particularly high in sick elderly, and prophylaxis against recurrent gout, a nonfatal illness, is generally ill advised in a patient whose medical prognosis is poor. Moreover, today's pharmacopoeia contains a wide selection of nonsteroidal anti-inflammatory agents, most if not all of which are effective in the treatment of acute gout and which are sufficiently well tolerated on the short term (see Chap. 2). Oral indomethacin sometimes brings dramatic relief almost as rapidly as intravenous colchicine. Systemic or intraarticular corticosteroids may also be used when other agents are contraindicated.

Finally, when colchicine or hypouricemic agents are indicated, they must be properly used. Dose adjustments are generally required in the patient over 70.

HYPOURICEMIC AGENTS

When Should Hypouricemic Agents Be Prescribed?

The purpose of prescribing a hypouricemic agent is to lower the uric acid and prevent recurrent attacks of gout in patients with a history of at least one proven attack of gout. These agents will also lower the total uric acid pool and may dissolve existing tophi.

Asymptomatic hyperuricemia should not be treated with medication, except in the setting of acute hyperuricemia of tumor lysis when massive kidney urate loading is expected. In this case, allopurinol and not probenecid should be used.

There is no evidence that treatment of asymptomatic hyperuricemia prevents the development of urate nephropathy, a slowly progressive and probably mild form of renal insufficiency, associated with, but perhaps not caused by, the deposition of urate in the renal interstitium. In the case of kidney stones, most rheumatologists would argue against treating uncomplicated hyperuricemia associated with a kidney stone of unknown composition, since it is unusual for a true uric acid stone to occur in patients who have not yet experienced gouty arthritis. Moreover, they argue, uric acid stones cause fewer deaths than does allopurinol.

Pharmacologic intervention for chronic hyperuricemia should be undertaken only in the following situations:

1. If there is acute gouty arthritis, after the second attack has occurred, or if the first attack is associated with subcutaneous tophi or proven uric acid stone.
2. If there is a proven uric acid stone.
3. In symptomatic diuretic-related hyperuricemia, only if the diuretic cannot be discontinued.
4. If there is no contraindication.

Allopurinol

Pharmacologic Considerations

MECHANISM OF ACTION. Allopurinol reduces the production of uric acid. The last two steps in uric acid synthesis involve the conversion of hypoxanthine to uric acid under the direction of the enzyme xanthine oxidase. Allopurinol, which is structurally related to hypoxanthine, inhibits this enzyme and lowers both serum levels and urinary excretion of uric acid. When serum uric acid levels are reduced to approximately 6.5 mg/dl or less, uric acid remains soluble in serum and crystal formation does not occur.

PHARMACOKINETICS. Allopurinol is well absorbed with peak plasma levels occurring in 30–60 minutes. It is metabolized in the liver under the direction of xanthine oxidase to oxypurinol, which is also an inhibitor of xanthine oxidase. After one dose, only small amounts of drug are excreted unchanged in the urine, but, since allopurinol inhibits the enzyme that directs its metabolism, less is converted with chronic ingestion, and the proportion of renally excreted drug increases to 30%. Oxypurinol is eliminated primarily through the kidneys. The serum half-life of allopurinol is 2–3 hours, whereas the half-life of active oxypurinol is 14–30 hours. The half-lives of both allopurinol and oxypurinol are increased in renal insufficiency, and, although no geriatric data are available, one would predict a prolonged half-life of active drug and metabolite in this age group. In renal insufficiency, the half-life of oxypurinol may be as long as a week or more.

Allopurinol is not bound to serum proteins.

Adverse Effects

Skin rashes occur commonly with allopurinol. Serious reactions consisting of **nephritis, hepatitis,** and **desquamative dermatitis** may occur, and can be fatal. **Toxic epidermal necrolysis, fever,** and **eosinophilia** may be part of this syndrome. These serious reactions are thought to be hypersensitivity phenomena, usually occurring within the first few weeks of treatment. However, they are seen most commonly in patients with renal insufficiency, in which "ordinary doses" may be inappropriately high. It has been suggested that prolonged circulation of oxypurinol or other metabolites may play a role in this syndrome. Thus, the elderly are theoretically more susceptible.

Any agent that acutely lowers serum uric acid **may precipitate an acute attack of gout** in a patient prone to gouty arthritis. This happens because the solubility of uric acid is increased and urate crystals or microcrystals become destabilized. Small pieces of formed urate crystals may break off and become phagocytized, inciting the inflammatory reaction that is gout. When hypouricemic therapy is first instituted, prophylaxis against acute gout is usually recommended.

Important Drug Interactions

The renal clearance of allopurinol and oxypurinol is increased by probenecid. This drug combination does not seem to reduce the hypouricemic effect and may enhance it.

Allopurinol inhibits hepatic microsomal enzymes, reducing the metabolism of phenytoin, warfarin, and possibly theophylline. Although clinical interactions are not inevitable, concurrent administration of allopurinol may require reduction in dosage of these drugs. Likewise, if allopurinol is discontinued, dosage adjustments may be required. A similar interaction occurs with certain chemotherapeutic agents with which allopurinol is often prescribed. Caution is advised. An interaction occurs with azathioprine and its active metabolite 6-mercaptopurine, which are metabolized by xanthine oxidase; azothioprine toxicity may occur.

Contraindications

Allopurinol is contraindicated in patients with a known history of allopurinol hypersensitivity.

Precautions

During the first few months of allopurinol therapy, patients should be observed for the development of skin rash and changes in renal or hepatic function, since early detection of the hypersensitivity syndrome may improve prognosis.

Because rapid lowering of uric acid can precipitate acute gout, medication to prevent interval gout should be prescribed during the first 3 months of treatment (e.g., colchicine 0.6 mg/day).

The Place of Allopurinol in Therapy
In general, it is recommended that allopurinol be given only if probenecid cannot, such as in the patient with acute tumor lysis. In practice, geriatric patients often have concurrent medical problems and practical limitations proscribing probenecid, so that allopurinol is more commonly used.

Dosing
Allopurinol should be given at the lowest daily dose that normalizes the serum uric acid.
Initial dose: 100 mg/day. Increase in increments of 50 mg after 2 weeks, or until uric-acid level normalizes. Lower doses are required in renal failure.
Usual maintenance dose: 100–200 mg/day. Higher doses may be required in certain patients, but 300 mg/day should generally not be exceeded in geriatric patients.

Probenecid
Pharmacologic Considerations
MECHANISM OF ACTION. Probenecid is an organic acid that acts by competitively inhibiting the tubular reabsorption of uric acid, thereby enhancing its excretion. As with other uricosuric agents, probenecid inhibits reabsorption of some compounds while inhibiting secretion of others. This is because transport of endogenous and exogenous substances across the tubular membrane is affected by a complex interplay of factors, such as urine pH and the chemical nature and dose of the transported compounds. Probenecid is most likely to compete with other organic acids but may also interfere with transport of other substances.

Probenecid is ineffective when glomerular filtration rate is lower than roughly 30–60 ml/min. Normal serum creatinine in geriatric patients often masks a creatinine clearance that is low enough to diminish the drug's efficacy. The ability of probenecid to lower uric acid in this group has not been specifically studied.

PHARMACOKINETICS. Probenecid is well absorbed, with peak plasma concentrations being reached within 2–4 hours. It is metabolized in the liver to inactive and active uricosuric metabolites. The half-life in plasma of a standard uricosuric dose (approximately 500 mg) is roughly 5 hours in nonelderly adults. Higher doses are reabsorbed by back diffusion in the renal tubule, prolonging the half-life. Probenecid is highly protein-bound.

Adverse Effects
By enhancing the excretion of uric acid, probenecid increases the urate load to the kidney and may increase the risk of **uric acid stones** in susceptible individuals, e.g., those with hyperuricosuria. The urate load also poses a potential risk of **worsening renal insufficiency** in patients with impaired renal function. Precipitation of urate in the kidney can be prevented by high fluid intake and ingestion of alkalinizing agents.

Gastrointestinal symptoms occur in a dose-dependent fashion but are not common and not severe. **Skin rash** and **fever** have been reported.

Important Drug Interactions

Probenecid competes for active transport in the renal tubule with a variety of other agents that have acidic properties. Its interactions with other compounds may be via different mechanisms. Probenecid increases the serum concentration or half-life of penicillins, cephalosporins, thiazide diuretics, furosemide, chlorpropamide, and a number of NSAIDs. This type of interaction has been exploited in the treatment of certain infections in which probenecid is given to increase serum levels of the penicillins. However, the addition of probenecid is probably superfluous in elderly patients with uncomplicated infections (see below).

Salicylates antagonize the uricosuric effect of probenecid and should not be given concurrently.

The Place of Probenecid in Therapy

Probenecid is effective in lowering serum uric acid in patients with normal renal function. Because it is relatively nontoxic, it is preferred over allopurinol, except in patients with hyperuricosuria. It may be less effective than allopurinol in chronic tophaceous gout, in which the total uric acid pool may be too large to be adequately diminished by a uricosuric agent.

Unfortunately, probenecid is ineffective when creatinine clearance is low, which is often the case in geriatric patients despite normal serum creatinine levels.

Measures to alkalinize the urine with agents such as sodium bicarbonate are often recommended when probenecid is being given, especially on initiation of therapy when renal precipitation of urate is most likely. This is not only impractical for many patients but inadvisable for those whose medical condition will not tolerate the sodium load. This may further limit the use of probenecid in the geriatric age group.

Probenecid is sometimes used in situations in which high and prolonged blood levels of penicillin or ampicillin are desired. However, the addition of probenecid to such regimens is redundant in geriatric patients with uncomplicated infections because the half-life of penicillins without probenecid in older patients is nearly that in younger adults who receive penicillins with probenecid.

Contraindications

Probenecid is contraindicated in the presence of kidney stones if the possibility exists that they are composed of urate. Because the exact composition of kidney stones is difficult to prove, probenecid should not be used to treat hyperuricemia in any patient with a history of kidney stones.

Probenecid is also contraindicated in the presence of renal insufficiency. It should also not be given in the presence of hyperuricosuria (800–1000 mg or more of urate in 24 hours).

Precautions

Because rapid lowering of uric acid can precipitate acute gout, medication to prevent interval gout should be given during the first 3 months of probenecid therapy, as in the case of allopurinol.

Dosing

Initial dose: 250 mg bid. Increase in increments of 250 mg/day until uric acid normalizes.
Maximum dose: 500 mg bid. Some patients may require a dose as high as 1 g bid.

Alternative Uricosuric Agent: Sulfinpyrazone

Sulfinpyrazone (Anturane) is sometimes used in the management of gout as an alternative to probenecid. It is a more potent uricosuric agent than probenecid but is not as well tolerated. In particular, it has a high incidence of **gastrointestinal side effects**. It is also a potent platelet antiaggregant and may produce **bleeding**. Sulfinpyrazone is structurally related to phenylbutazone, and experimentally has been shown to suppress erythropoeisis, but clinical bone marrow depression has not been reported. **Hypersensitivity reactions** may occur, and are usually manifested as rash and fever. As a weak prostaglandin inhibitor, cross-reactions in aspirin-sensitive individuals are theoretically possible.

Sulfinpyrazone can enhance the anticoagulant action of warfarin, possibly because of a protein displacement interaction. Other drug interactions have less consistently been described on this basis.

This drug should only be used when other means of lowering uric acid are unavailable or not tolerated.

Dosing

Initial dose: 100 mg once a day.
Maximum dose: 200 mg/day in divided doses.

COLCHICINE

Colchicine is an anti-inflammatory agent derived from the plant Colchicum autumnale. Its anti-inflammatory action is limited to crystal-induced inflammation.

Oral and intravenous colchicine are very different in the nature of their toxicity and in their indications. For this reason, they should be viewed as though they were different agents.

Long considered the first-line treatment for acute gout, colchicine is losing favor to NSAIDs, which may be equally effective and less toxic.

Pharmacologic Considerations

Mechanism of Action

Colchicine binds to and disrupts microtubules of neutrophils and a number of other cells in the body. Its action on neutrophils is believed to inhibit the production of a chemotactic factor that is released in response to crystal ingestion by the white cell. Thus, colchicine is active in gout and pseudogout, which are produced by uric acid crystals and by calcium pyrophosphate or basic calcium phosphate crystals, respectively. It is not effective in other forms of arthritis.

Colchicine has no analgesic activity apart from its anti-inflammatory actions, and has no effect on uric acid metabolism. As such, it does not raise or lower serum or urine uric acid. It is ineffective in arthritis that is not crystal-induced. It is ineffective when symptoms of an acute attack of gouty arthritis have been present for more than 5 to 7 days.

Pharmacokinetics

Oral colchicine is absorbed from the jejunum and ileum. Some drug binds to microtubules in intestinal cells, which is probably a factor in colchicine-related intestinal toxicity.

After oral intake, peak plasma levels occur within $\frac{1}{2}$ to 2 hours. The drug is metabolized in the liver, and excreted in bile and urine. Circulating bile most likely presents colchicine once again to the intestinal cell, where it can be bound. If hepatic function is normal, only 20% of ingested colchicine is excreted in the kidney. However, while colchicine disappears from plasma relatively quickly, a single dose is retained in neutrophils and other cells for up to 10 days, and renal excretion occurs throughout this period. Thus, the tissue half-life of colchicine is prolonged.

The disappearance rate of colchicine is further prolonged in patients with renal insufficiency, and it is thus likely that elimination is prolonged with age.

Intravenous colchicine has a plasma half-life of roughly 20 minutes, but, as with oral colchicine, tissue concentrations are maintained for days. Although intestinal mucosal concentrations of intravenously administered drug are lower than those achieved by oral colchicine, some uptake occurs and gastrointestinal symptoms may result. Severe gastrointestinal symptoms often occur in a delayed fashion with intravenous colchicine, reflecting accumulation to toxic levels.

Adverse Effects

Intravenous colchicine may produce **venous inflammation** at the injection site, and extravasation can cause **tissue necrosis**.

Oral colchicine may produce **abdominal cramping, diarrhea, nausea, and vomiting**. Gastrointestinal symptoms most often occur in the setting of full doses given in acute attacks of gout, where they are very common, and are relatively uncommon at low prophylactic oral doses. Gastrointestinal symptoms occur much less commonly with short-term intravenous administration alone.

Colchicine may produce leukocytosis, but chronic treatment has been reported to produce **bone marrow suppression.**

Severe colchicine toxicity may manifest as disseminated intravascular coagulation, bone marrow aplasia, hepatic failure, myopathy, alopecia, and seizures. A full-blown **choleralike syndrome** may occur, leading to shock and death.

Colchicine produces relatively few systemic side effects at low doses. Serious toxicity occurs when inappropriately high doses are used. Toxic levels are most likely to be attained in elderly patients with renal or hepatobiliary dysfunction. Reported deaths from colchicine have generally occurred in such settings. Toxicity is expected to occur more readily in elderly patients because of reduced renal elimination.

Drug-Nutrient Interaction

Colchicine may impair intestinal absorption of vitamin B_{12}.

Contraindications

Colchicine is contraindicated in patients with renal, liver, or gastrointestinal disease, and in biliary obstruction.

Precautions

Great caution should be observed when administering intravenous colchicine to ensure that extravasation does not occur.

In contrast to oral colchicine, intravenous colchicine is not associated early on with dose-related gastrointestinal symptoms to serve as a warning that doses are approaching the toxic range. Thus, the physician should determine the total maximum dose to be administered in advance rather than on the basis of the patient's ability to tolerate the initial dose.

Once a course of intravenous colchicine is completed, oral colchicine should not be started for at least 7 days to 3 weeks, in order to avoid toxic accumulation. If gout recurs in this interval, alternative anti-inflammatory therapy should be used. Likewise, if a patient has been taking oral prophylactic colchicine at the time an acute attack occurs, the acute attack should be treated with an agent other than colchicine. Suggested alternative treatments are indomethacin, other nonsteroidal anti-inflammatory agents (NSAIDs), or corticosteroids.

Consideration should be given to treating gout with agents other than colchicine.

Indications

Intravenous colchicine is indicated in the treatment of acute gout if the attack has not been present for more than 5 to 7 days.

In a fresh attack of gout, colchicine may be used diagnostically, when other diagnostic methods are not available. Relief of symptoms typically occurs in 6–12 hours or less. Diagnostic use of colchicine is highly sensitive, but will not distinguish between gout and pseudogout.

Oral colchicine is indicated for prophylaxis of acute attacks when instituting a hypouricemic agent. It is also indicated for the prevention of interval gout when hypouricemic agents cannot be given. Oral colchicine should not generally be used in the treatment of acute gout because it may be poorly tolerated and works no more rapidly than potent NSAIDs such as indomethacin.

Dosing

The relative milligram dose of intravenous colchicine is estimated to be roughly half that of oral colchicine.

Intravenous

ACUTE GOUTY ARTHRITIS. 1 mg given over 30–60 min, followed by 0.5 to 1.0 mg every 4–6 hours, to a maximum total dose of 2 mg.

Oral

ACUTE GOUTY ARTHRITIS. 1.2 mg. Repeat in 12 hours if needed.
PREVENTION OF INTERVAL GOUT. 0.6 mg daily to bid.
PROPHYLAXIS OF ACUTE GOUTY ARTHRITIS WHEN INSTITUTING HYPOURICEMIC AGENT. 0.6 mg daily to bid for 3 months.

Table 5-1. Time to Anti-Gout Effect (hr)

Intravenous colchicine	6–12
Systemic corticosteroids	12
Oral colchicine	12–48
NSAIDs	24–48

ALTERNATE TREATMENT

If hypouricemic medications are contraindicated, interval gout can be treated as needed.

In acute gout, if colchicine is contraindicated or if the attack has been established for several days, NSAIDs or corticosteroids can be given. It is increasingly argued that NSAIDs may be preferable to colchicine even if there is no absolute contraindication to the latter, although relief may be more prompt with colchicine (Table 5-1). Corticosteroids are particularly applicable to the patient with renal insufficiency.

Acute Gout

Indomethacin: 50–100 mg followed by 25–50 mg every 6 hours until attack has subsided.

Naproxen: 500–750 mg followed by 250 mg every 8–12 hours until attack has subsided.

Note: Successful treatment has been reported with most NSAIDs. They differ from other approaches only in their rapidity of effect (see Table 15–1). NSAIDs are discussed in more detail in Chap. 2.

Prednisone: 20 mg followed by 5 mg every 8 hours until the attack has subsided (usually within 3 days). Intra-articular corticosteroids may also be effective.

Prophylaxis for Interval Gout

Indomethacin: 25 mg daily. Higher doses may sometimes be required.

Prednisone: 5 mg daily, or the lowest dose to suppress attacks. Attempt should always be made to taper and discontinue this medication.

BIBLIOGRAPHY

German, D.C., and Holmes, E.W. Hyperuricemia and gout. *Med. Clin. Nor. Amer.* 70:419–436, 1986.

Groff, G.D., Franck, W.A., and Raddatz, D.A. Systemic steroid therapy for acute gout: a clinical trial and review of the literature. *Semin. Arthrit. Rheum.* 19:329–336, 1990.

Hande, K.R., Noone, R.M., and Stone, W.J. Severe allopurinol toxicity. *Am. J. Med.* 76:47–56, 1984.

Roberts, W.N., Liang, M.H., and Stern, S.H. Colchicine in acute gout; reassessment of risks and benefits. *JAMA* 257:1920–1922, 1987.

Wallace, S.L., and Singer, J.Z. Review: systemic toxicity associated with the intravenous administration of colchicine—guidelines for use. *J. Rheumatol.* 15:495–499, 1988.

Drugs Used in Dementia

Dementia, a decline in memory and higher intellectual function, is not a part of normal aging, but it affects 5% to 15% of people over age 65 and the prevalence increases with age. Dementia in the elderly is sometimes referred to as "senile dementia". In the geriatric age group, at least 80% of cases are irreversible. Irreversible dementia in the elderly is due to Alzheimer's disease in 50% to 70% of cases, vascular ("multi-infarct") dementia in 20%, and a combination of the two in an additional 20%. The remainder of cases are due to Parkinson's disease and a variety of neurodegenerative conditions. Potentially reversible conditions are primary causes of dementia in fewer than 20% of affected elderly, but individuals with established dementia often suffer reversible deterioration in cognition from superimposed illness or drugs. Reversible dementia is treated by removal of the underlying cause.

Alzheimer's disease is a degenerative process of unknown etiology that affects the brain, resulting in deficits of central neurotransmitters, defective cerebral carbohydrate metabolism, and neuronal loss. Acetylcholine deficiency is a consistent finding and is proportional to the degree of dementia. Deficiencies in serotonin, norepinephrine, and dopamine also occur to a certain extent, but their role in the clinical syndrome is less well established.

Brain damage from a major vascular insult may result in dementia, but classic multi-infarct dementia is thought to be due to a series of small, generally unnoticed lacular infarcts that produce progressive cognitive decline. There is no evidence that chronic ischemia from cerebral arteriosclerosis (traditionally, "hardening of the arteries") results in senile dementia.

Patients with dementia often exhibit agitation, depression, or paranoia. In the absence of the reversible factors noted above, these so-called secondary features may be treated with medications such as neuroleptics, benzodiazepines, or antidepressants. There remains no satisfactory treatment for the cognitive deficits themselves, but a number of agents are available and are frequently, though inappropriately, prescribed. Others are taken by patients without prescription. This chapter will review these agents in an effort to put them in a realistic perspective.

Distraught family members and frustrated physicians often seek any hope available and medications of debatable efficacy are often prescribed for that reason. They generally offer little more than psychological benefit, and that probably more to the family than the patient, but they may "buy time" for the family to accept the reality of the patient's condition. One agent, ergoloid mesylates (Hydergine) may have some demonstrable benefit in early dementia, but this is highly controversial.

Some agents have no theoretical or clinical effect whatsoever. Patients may "swear by" these agents and by the doctors and paraprofessionals that recommend them. However, not all the agents are innocuous, and it is the physician's responsibility to advise the patient of any possible harmful effects that may occur.

CONTROVERSIAL AGENT: ERGOLOID MESYLATES (HYDERGINE)

Pharmacologic Considerations

Hydergine is a mixture of semisynthetic dihydrogenated derivatives of ergot alkaloid methanesulfonates (mesylates) that exist in a natural fixed ratio. These hydrogenated forms are far less potent pharmacologically than their parent compounds, but exert a variety of effects related to their interactions with several neurotransmitter systems in the central nervous system (CNS). The drug is a metabolic enhancer with some noradrenergic, dopaminergic, and serotoninergic agonist activity. Hence, its effect is nonspecific, but also of theoretic benefit in Alzheimer's disease. It is not a cerebral vasodilator as was once thought, and it seems to lack vasoconstrictor action seen with other ergot alkaloids.

A recent American study (see Thompson et al.) demonstrated no beneficial effect in a group of patients with Alzheimer's disease treated with Hydergine 3 mg/day. There were only 39 patients in the treatment group and the dose used was lower than that recommended by investigators who have reported benefit with higher doses (6–12 mg/day). Although the formulation used (Hydergine-LC) is said to have greater bioavailability than standard preparations, this difference is slight. For these reasons the study cannot yet be taken as definitive, although it was methodologically satisfactory.

The drug is rapidly absorbed from the gastrointestinal tract with peak plasma levels attained within 1½–3 hours. It undergoes extensive first-pass metabolism in the liver with less than 50% of the active drug reaching the circulation. Half-life of the unmetabolized compound is 2½–5 hours, but that of its metabolites, not all of which are inactive, may last up to 13 hours.

Adverse Effects

Mild transient nausea may occur but is unusual. Bradycardia has been reported but the significance of this is not known. Although this drug is used to treat hypertension in some countries, hypotension has not been an important adverse effect in clinical trials of dementia.

The Place of Ergoloid Mesylates in the Management of Dementia

Hydergine is the only substance currently available that has any effect in altering behavior in senile dementia, and even this effect is inconstant, short-lived, and of questionable practical significance. The effects that have been reported include improved mood and social behavior, improved physical function and performance of activities of daily living, decreased somatic complaints, and increases in intellect, all of which could be attributed to an antidepressant effect. There is no evidence that the drug prevents cognitive decline, and it has no effect in advanced dementia.

Although there is no established rationale for its use in reversing the symptoms of vascular dementia, Hydergine's effect is most likely a nonspecific one. Moreover, many affected patients have combined Alzheimer's and vascular dementia so that a trial may be warranted in a spectrum of patients with dementia. In all cases, reversible conditions should be thoroughly ruled out or treated before use of the drug is considered.

Since the efficacy of Hydergine is disputed, the use of this agent is decried in some circles. However, it has a wide margin of safety even in very elderly individuals and may be worth trying in a condition that has so few therapeutic options. Another factor in favor of this drug is that by buying time it provides psychological support to caregivers, who are so important in the management of the patient and who require time to adjust to the new and difficult situation.

When prescribing this agent it is important to make it clear to the family that a cure or dramatic improvement cannot be expected.

Dosing
Minimum dose: 1 mg tid.
Maximum dose: 4 mg tid.
Note: Although the approved dose is 1 mg tid, geriatricians generally recommend a starting dose of 2 mg tid. If no effect has been noted after a 6-month trial, the drug should be discontinued.

AGENTS NO LONGER IN FAVOR

Vasodilators
The agents categorized as vasodilators have long been prescribed for senile dementia on the notion, now disproved, that senile cognitive decline is due to chronic ischemia from progressive cerebral arteriosclerosis and that pharmacological manipulations to increase cerebral blood flow can alleviate symptoms. Diminished cerebral blood flow occurs in several forms of dementia but this is probably a result of the disease state, rather than the cause. The vasodilator agents produce varying degrees of cerebral vasodilation but they produce systemic vasodilation as well, an effect that theoretically could impair cerebral blood flow. In fact, they have not been shown to increase cerebral blood flow significantly. Their action, though limited, may be related to their effects on central neurotransmitter systems. None are particularly effective in dementia.

Papaverine (Pavabid; Others)
Papaverine is a naturally occurring alkaloid derivative of opium that is devoid of narcotic properties. As a smooth muscle relaxant, it increases cerebral blood flow, but it also has some dopamine receptor blocking action. Although it is more effective than placebo in improving cognitive measures in various dementias, improvement is inconsistent and its clinical usefulness is highly questionable. It has been shown to be less effective than ergoloid mesylates in several comparative studies, and has more reported side effects, including nausea, headache, vertigo, constipation, and hepatic disturbances. There is little rationale for its use in dementia.

Cyclandelate (Cyclospasmol; Others)
Cyclandelate is structurally related to papaverine but is pharmacologically more potent and less toxic. The drug has not been consistently demonstrated to improve cognitive function in dementia.

Isoxsuprine (Vasodilan; Others)
Isoxsuprine is a derivative of epinephrine with alpha antagonist and beta agonist activity. There is no evidence that it produces signifi-

cant clinical improvement in dementia. Its vasodilating properties may result in systemic hypotension and flushing. Moreover, since it is a sympathomimetic agent, it can produce tremulousness, palpitations, tachyarrhythmias, and other untoward cardiac effects. Thus, it should not be used for dementia in elderly patients.

Nylidrin (Arlidin; Adrin; Others)

This agent is structurally similar to isoxsuprine. As such, there is no evidence that it is particularly effective in dementia. Like isoxsuprine, it is not innocuous.

Other Agents

Choline, a metabolic precursor of acetylcholine, and **lecithin,** a natural source of choline as phosphatidylcholine, enhance brain levels of acetylcholine. Under experimental conditions, they may have subtle memory-enhancing effects in normal adults, but are ineffective in producing clinical benefit in Alzheimer's disease. In addition, there is no evidence that they prevent age-related cognitive decline. Unabsorbed choline is metabolized by intestinal bacteria to trimethylamine, which has the odor of decayed fish and is thus unacceptable to many patients. Commercially available lecithin contains only small amounts of phosphatidylcholine and any theoretical benefit that could be achieved would be limited by dose-related gastrointestinal symptoms such as bloating and anorexia.

Nicotinic acid (niacin) is a water-soluble vitamin for which the official recommended daily allowance is 13-16 mg. It acts as a vascular smooth muscle relaxant at doses greater than 3 gm/day. These actions are not related to its vital actions in intermediary metabolism, and, in fact, high doses saturate the capacity of the liver to convert further nicotinic acid to its nutrient form, nicotinamide. Nicotinic acid is ineffective in dementia, does not increase cerebral blood flow, and is potentially toxic at vasodilating doses. Nonetheless, nicotinic acid and its derivatives continue to be used, alone or in combination with other putative cognitive enhancers. Its use as a lipid-lowering agent is discussed in Chap. 17.

Gerovital, once a popular European "anti-aging" remedy, is a 2% solution of the local anesthetic procaine hydrochloride. It is combined with benzoic acid, potassium metabisulfite, and disodium phosphate, a formulation that is claimed, apparently incorrectly, to increase the half-life of rapidly hydrolyzed procaine. It can be given orally but is generally given as an intramuscular injection.

The proponents and users of Gerovital claim that it confers a wide range of cognitive and physical benefits. Procaine does have some monoamine oxidase inhibitor activity and one of its metabolites can produce euphoria, so theoretically it could benefit individuals whose apathy and cognitive impairment are due to depression. However, double-blind studies have not demonstrated clinical benefit in dementia. Nonetheless, the producers of these agents have many satisfied followers. Gerovital is available in Nevada but not elsewhere in the United States. It is mentioned here because of patient inquiries.

INVESTIGATIONAL AGENTS

Tetrahydroaminoacridine (THA; Tacrine) is a cholinesterase inhibitor that increases cerebral levels of acetylcholine. It has recently been under investigation for the management of Alzheimer's disease and has received a significant amount of publicity. Improvements in memory and function have been reported in a few patients but the importance of these reports has been questioned. It is expected that improvements would be short-lived, since cholinergic enhancement is ultimately dependent on intact neuronal function. THA, further-more, may produce hepatotoxicity and cholinergic side effects. The drug has not received FDA approval for general use. Several long-term studies are now in progress.

Other investigational agents are currently undergoing active in-vestigation. This topic is discussed in detail by Davidson and Stern (see Bibliography).

NONPHARMACOLOGIC TREATMENT

Although there is presently no effective medical treatment for cogni-tive symptoms of dementia, certain things must be done. Acute con-fusional states superimposed on the chronic dementing disease must be diagnosed and treated in order to maximize cognitive function. Secondary features such as agitation, nocturnal wandering, inconti-nence, and depression should be treated. Contact with the real world should be maintained with conversation, touching, and involvement of the patient in social activities when feasible. Social and commu-nity supports should be maximized so the patient can stay in the familiar home environment as long as possible. Families can be coun-seled by trained psychotherapists and social workers, and can be ad-vised to join local self-help groups or to contact local Alzheimer's disease resource centers.

Vigilance is essential so that the patient does not experience in-jury. Patients with advanced dementia usually cannot feed them-selves and may lose the ability to swallow. Oral feeding should be maintained as long as possible, even if amounts are small. Feeding exclusively by tube lacks a sensory component and prevents the pa-tient from appreciating the pleasurable aspects of food. If tube feed-ing is instituted, it should be supplemented by oral feeding if at all possible. Enteral feeding is discussed in Chap. 25.

Institutionalization may become necessary if family, home, and social supports are exhausted. In far advanced dementia, nontreat-ment of serious intercurrent illness, such as infection, is thought to be morally justified in certain circumstances, and is legally con-doned, provided this approach is consistent with the patient's ap-parent wishes.

MAJOR TRANQUILIZERS

Major tranquilizers (also referred to as **neuroleptics** or **antipsychot-ics**) include phenothiazines and phenothiazinelike drugs. They differ from other CNS depressants in that they have comparatively less global, sedating effect and more prominent specific effects on psy-chotic symptoms and behavior. Compared to other CNS depres-sants, such as the benzodiazepine anxiolytics, the neuroleptics have little or no addictive potential, are not associated with excitatory withdrawal syndromes, and do not appear to produce tolerance. However, they produce a different spectrum of problematic adverse effects, to which geriatric patients are particularly susceptible.

Although they are primarily intended for use in the management of delusions, hallucinations, aggressive behavior, and other features of the psychoses, in geriatric practice these agents are usually used in the management of secondary features of dementia. **Neuroleptics**

are not appropriate for all symptoms of dementia. They may be helpful if used selectively for symptoms such as restlessness, emotional outbursts, assaultive behavior, agitation, hallucinations, or paranoia, when these symptoms are discomfiting to the patient or endanger the welfare of the patient or caregiver. When symptoms do not pose imminent danger, sedation is best avoided. However, caregivers, many being elderly themselves, are frequently so exhausted by the patient's behaviors that they cannot cope. In such cases, cautious pharmacologic treatment may provide significant relief, actually improve care of the patient, and may sometimes be the only way to prevent institutionalization.

Other secondary symptoms of dementia, such as wandering and poor self-care, do not respond well to pharmacologic approaches and are best handled with interpersonal methods in a protected environment. Neuroleptics have no ameliorative effect on the primary features of dementia, such as memory loss and impaired intellectual function, and in fact may worsen cognition.

Another application of neuroleptic medication in the geriatric age group is chronic schizophrenia that has persisted into late life. Nowadays, schizophrenia does not necessarily shorten life span, and many patients with long-standing disease now reside in nursing homes. Typically, however, elderly patients with schizophrenia have less florid symptomatology than younger patients, and will require lower doses of neuroleptics than they may have required at a younger age. Many will require no sedation at all.

Before making the decision to prescribe a neuroleptic, it is important that potentially reversible problems are diagnosed and treated. Although most dementing disorders are not reversible, established dementia can be exacerbated by medical disease or medications. Recent change of behavior in a patient with dementia should prompt a careful search for intercurrent illness.

It is also important to point out that the use of psychotropics for behavioral control in long-term-care institutions is under increasing scrutiny by governmental regulatory agencies. Among the new regulations is that psychiatric consultation and family permission generally be obtained before these treatment strategies are employed.

Pharmacologic Considerations

Mechanism of Action

As a group, neuroleptic agents are thought to act by blocking dopamine at receptor sites in the brain that specifically mediate psychotic symptoms. Dopamine blockade in the limbic system and frontal cortex supposedly results in antipsychotic symptom control, whereas dopamine blockade in the basal ganglia results in largely unwanted extrapyramidal symptoms.

Neuroleptics have a variety of other pharmacologic effects. The phenothiazines, chlorpromazine and thioridazine, possess potent alpha$_1$ adrenergic blocking activity and a quinidinelike effect that is both antiarrhythmic and potentially arrhythmogenic. All neuroleptic agents posses some anticholinergic action because of competitive blockade of muscarinic receptors. Those with the greatest anticholinergic action are thioridazine and chlorpromazine.

Central dopamine antagonists have varying amounts of antiemetic effects because of dopamine blockade in the chemoreceptor trigger zone. Many neuroleptics posses significant histamine-blocking activity, but other potent actions make most unsuitable to use as antihistamines.

Important pharmacologic actions of the neuroleptics are summarized in Table 6-1. These should help the physician select an agent that will be best tolerated by a particular patient.

Pharmacokinetics

The pharmacokinetic properties of neuroleptics are complex and not well defined. Oral absorption is erratic, and can be modified by food, antacids, and genetic factors. Liquid preparations are probably absorbed more rapidly, but their chief advantage is that they can be given with greater ease to patients with paranoia or those with swallowing difficulties.

All neuroleptics are extensively metabolized in the liver and have a long duration of action, which is partly due to the production of active metabolites. Although these processes are most likely prolonged in older patients, complex metabolism and genetic variables make it difficult to predict a patient's response from a given dose. In geriatric patients, it is prudent to assume that clearance could be prolonged and tissue sensitivity enhanced.

An important feature of these agents is the fact that they are very lipophilic and membrane-bound. Their levels in the brain tend to be far higher and last much longer than their levels in plasma, another factor that accounts for their prolonged duration of action. Since lipophilic drugs have a higher volume of distribution in late life, steady-state levels of neuroleptics are achieved very slowly, probably after a week at the very least, and if dose adjustments are made too quickly problems may arise. A common situation is that a patient does not respond in the first few days, higher doses are given, and sometime later the patient becomes severely withdrawn, overly sedated, or severely parkinsonian. Because of the tendency for drug to accumulate, side effects may then be very prolonged, lasting days or weeks after the drug is withdrawn. In the case of extrapyramidal reactions, symptoms may also persist because of dopamine receptor hypersensitivity.

Adverse Effects

There is variation in the tendency of these agents to cause particular adverse effects (see Table 6-1). The following discussion focuses on the general adverse effects.

Major tranquilizers may produce **cognitive deterioration** in elderly patients with dementia. This may be due partly to the anticholinergic properties of these agents superimposed on the central cholinergic deficits of Alzheimer's disease, and due partly to sedation. **Oversedation** may occur; this can produce functional deterioration and increases the risk of aspiration pneumonia.

Neuroleptics with potent dopamine blocking activity have a tendency to produce a range of **extrapyramidal symptoms,** including parkinsonism, tardive dyskinesia, akathesia, and dystonia.

Drug-induced parkinsonism is an extremely common concomitant of neuroleptic treatment and the risk appears to be greatly increased in late life. It may be clinically indistinguishable from idiopathic Parkinson's disease, but more often tremor is absent. The predominant features are slow initiation of motor activity (bradykinesia), gait problems, rigidity, and typical "masklike" fascies. Drooling may not occur if anticholinergic effects are prominent. These

Table 6-1. Properties of Some Major Tranquilizers

Agent	Sample Brand	Sedative	Anticholinergic	Cardiac-hemodynamic	Extra-pyramidal
Thioridazine	Mellaril	3+	3+	3+	1+
Haloperidol	Haldol	1+	1+	1+	4+
Thiothixene	Navane	1 to 2+	1+	1+	3+
Chlorpromazine	Thorazine	3+	3+	3+	2+
Fluphenazine	Prolixin	1+	1+	1+	4+

1+ = mild
2+ = moderate
3+ = strong
4+ = marked

symptoms are generally, though not always, reversible on discontinuation of the offending agent. It is important to emphasize that the symptoms may appear in the first few days of treatment or may present in a delayed fashion and sometimes persist for days to weeks after the drug is discontinued. This may represent hypersensitivity of dopamine receptors produced by drug withdrawal or the persistence of drug in the tissues for extended periods of time. Occasionally, symptoms do not resolve.

Drug-induced parkinsonism can impair gait and **increase the risk of falls** and fracture. Elderly patients living at home or those living in understaffed institutions may be at greater risk of this problem because there may be an incentive for harassed caregivers to give doses that produce such heavy sedation that the patient becomes incapable of moving about.

Anticholinergic agents, such as benztropine (Cogentin) or trihexyphenidyl (Artane) have been used to minimize neuroleptic-induced parkinsonism, but routine use of these drugs is not warranted. They often fail to reduce parkinsonian symptoms, may increase the risk of tardive dyskinesia, and produce a separate spectrum of side effects. Amantadine (Symmetrel), a dopaminergic agent that is mildly anticholinergic, has been used with varying benefit.

Although drug-induced parkinsonism occurs frequently, individual susceptibility varies widely. Some patients may be exquisitely sensitive and develop profound symptoms within a short time. Advanced age and a history of stroke may be important risk factors but it is not generally possible to predict who will be affected. Virtually all major tranquilizers can produce parkinsonism, although thioridazine in low doses may have a lower tendency to do this. Clozapine, a newly released "atypical" neuroleptic, is very safe in this regard but is associated with other problems (see below).

Another important reaction is **tardive dyskinesia.** It consists of involuntary movements of the lips, mouth, and tongue, and less often the trunk and extremities. Although this disorder may present during neuroleptic treatment, it often develops after the offending agent has been discontinued, or when the dose has been lowered. Tardive dyskinesia is thought to occur when prolonged dopamine antagonism produces hypersensitivity of dopamine receptors. It is very common, particularly in women, and the risk increases steadily with age. In fact, neuroleptic-induced tardive dyskinesia occurs with a markedly greater frequency among demented elderly treated chronically for agitation than among younger patients treated for schizophrenia. This has been attributed to age-related changes in the number or sensitivity of dopamine receptors, and to the fact that older patients have a higher neuroleptic burden than younger patients at any given dose. It is also possible that dementia itself increases the risk of tardive dyskinesia because of neurologic and neurohormonal alterations.

Patients themselves seem less distressed by the symptoms of tardive dyskinesia than do their family members or caregivers. This is fortunate because there does not appear to be a reliable way of preventing this complication. Thioridazine may be somewhat less likely than other agents to produce tardive dyskinesia, but, with the possible exception of the atypical neuroleptic clozapine (see below), no specific class of neuroleptic eliminates the risk. Use of the offending agent probably masks the development of the pathologic process because it keeps the dopamine receptors at bay. Although reinstituting the offending agent or increasing the dose may suppress the symptoms, this approach runs the risk of exacerbating the underlying problem. Prophylaxis with anticholinergic agents does not protect against the development of tardive dyskinesia and may actually increase the risk by disrupting the physiologic balance between dopaminergic and cholinergic systems. The risk of tardive dyskinesia may be decreased if the smallest possible dose is used for the shortest period of time, and if the neuroleptic is reserved only for that subset of patients who have target symptoms that are likely to be neuroleptic-responsive. Since dementia patients often require treatment for prolonged periods, the need for continued medication should be reevaluated at periodic intervals.

Akathesia is a symptom that is frequently not recognized. It consists of a feeling of restlessness, tension, or frank anxiety, and may be mistaken for the underlying condition. Misdiagnosis often leads to an increase rather in the dosage of the neuroleptic, making the symptoms worse rather than better.

The **neuroleptic malignant syndrome** is an unusual but extremely serious condition, which may be more common in elderly patients than previously recognized. Among its many features are hyperpyrexia, hypotension, delirium, muscular rigidity, and myoglobinuria. Death may occur. This syndrome can occur at any time during treatment with agents possessing potent antidopaminergic properties. It is thought to result from dopamine antagonist effects on thermoregulatory mechanisms, but it affects few patients and does not always recur on rechallenge. Early recognition is essential since the elderly probably have a higher risk of mortality or long-term sequelae. The syndrome may respond well to early symptomatic treatment and to the dopamine agonist bromocriptine.

Another effect that may result from impairment of thermoregulation is **hypothermia.** The risk of neuroleptic-associated hypothermia increases with age and in the presence of hypothyroidism.

Acute dystonic reactions appear early on and may be life-threatening, but are relatively uncommon in elderly patients. Patients who develop mild dystonic reactions occasionally continue to use the offending agent and tolerance may develop over time. Parenteral diphenhydramine (Benadryl) may reverse dystonia and should be given if the reaction is severe.

Stimulation of dopamine receptors blocks the secretion of prolactin. Therefore, dopamine antagonists may produce **hyperprolactinemia.** The consequences of this in elderly patients are probably more pronounced in men than in women, manifesting as gynecomastia and erectile dysfunction.

Neuroleptics with significant anticholinergic effect, such as chlorpromazine and thioridazine, may produce **urinary retention, blurred vision, dry mouth, constipation,** or **acute angle closure glaucoma.** Because of underlying pathology, elderly patients are at increased risk of developing these effects, which may be easily missed in those with dementia. It should be emphasized that chronic, open angle glaucoma, which accounts for more than 95% of glaucoma cases in older patients, does not represent a contraindication to the use of these drugs.

Neuroleptics with alpha$_1$ adrenergic blocking action may produce **supine or orthostatic hypotension.** Chlorpromazine and thioridazine are more likely than the other agents to lower blood pressure. Frank hypotension is more common when medication is given parenterally and is unusual with the oral doses recommended here.

Cardiac arrhythmias may occur, particularly with thioridazine, somewhat less so with chlorpromazine. These agents have a quinidinelike effect on the myocardium and the conducting system. However, this is potentially an *anti*arrhythmic effect, and, in fact, the arrhythmogenic potential of the phenothiazines is probably slight when low doses are given and dose increments made cautiously. Nonspecific T-wave changes are very common, and are considered benign, but widening of the QT interval may predispose to ventricular arrhythmias. In addition, these agents may enhance the release of catecholamines, and a variety of ventricular arrhythmias and occasional supraventricular conduction disturbances have been reported. Thioridazine is the agent most often implicated in the production of arrhythmias, but it is important to emphasize that even thioridazine-induced arrhythmias are infrequent in the absence of underlying factors, such as hypokalemia or concurrent use of cardiac drugs (see Important Drug Interactions below).

Cholestatic jaundice is a relatively uncommon side effect. It is thought to be a hypersensitivity phenomenon and usually occurs within the first few weeks of treatment. The agent most often implicated in this problem is chlorpromazine, but it has been reported with a number of other phenothiazines. **Agranulocytosis**, though rare, probably occurs most often in older patients; it is usually reversible when the drug is withdrawn. **Skin rash** and **photosensitivity** occur occasionally, and have been reported most commonly with chlorpromazine. **Pigmentary retinopathy** has been reported with thioridazine; however, this is generally seen with higher doses than would be used in this setting.

Important Drug Interactions

The sedative, dopamine-blocking, and anticholinergic effects can all be exacerbated by drugs possessing similar properties and concurrent use of such agents should be avoided unless the clinical situation specifically calls for them.

Neuroleptics may lower the seizure threshold in patients with epilepsy, reducing the efficacy of anticonvulsants. However, phenothiazines have been reported to increase as well as decrease serum levels of anticonvulsants. Thus, patients with seizure disorders who are taking these agents require careful monitoring.

Agents used for idiopathic Parkinson's disease, such as levodopa, counteract the antidopaminergic action of neuroleptics and may reduce their efficacy. Conversely, the dopamine-blocking action of neuroleptics may counteract the efficacy of antiparkinsonian agents.

Major tranquilizers with potent alpha$_1$ blocking activity, namely, thioridazine and chlorpromazine, may potentiate the hypotensive effect of prazosin and many other antihypertensive agents. Alpha blockade may also lead to hypotension when epinephrine is used because uninhibited beta stimulation results. Neuroleptics may decrease the antihypertensive action of guanethidine by blocking its uptake at the site of action.

The quinidinelike effect of the phenothiazines can be accentuated by tricyclic antidepressants (TCAs) and antiarrhythmic agents, resulting in arrhythmias and conduction disturbances. TCAs also possess potent anticholinergic effects and can interact at this level.

The effect of neuroleptics may be altered by drugs that affect the hepatic microsomal enzyme system, such as rifampin, barbiturates, and phenytoin.

For a complete review of the many drug interactions that have been reported to occur with these agents, the reader is referred to the Bibliography. (See Rizack & Hillman.)

Indications and Nonindications

Major tranquilizers are indicated for the management of psychotic symptoms and severe behavioral problems in patients with chronic dementia if nonpharmacologic measures are ineffective or inappropriate. The symptoms that respond the best to neuroleptics include agitation, restlessness, hallucinations, and emotional lability. Neuroleptics are **not a substitute** for personal assistance, vigilance, and other nonpharmacologic measures of modifying behavior and ensuring safety.

Major tranquilizers are also indicated in the management of "positive" symptoms of the functional psychoses. In the geriatric age group, the syndrome most often seen is chronic schizophrenia that has persisted into late life. Specialized use of neuroleptics is beyond the scope of this book. Interested readers are referred to the Bibliography (see Arana & Hyman).

Neuroleptics should not be used for nonaggressive features of dementia such as wandering, apathy, and neglect of personal habits, which do not respond well to these drugs, nor for social withdrawal, depression, or memory loss, which may be worsened by them.

In patients without psychosis or dementia, anxiety disorders should be treated with minor tranquilizers, in most cases the benzodiazepines. Occasionally, satisfactory management of the agitation of dementia can be obtained with the use of these agents.

Selection of Agent

Information on patient response to neuroleptics comes from clinical experience rather than from well-controlled studies. It is unclear if individuals who fail to respond to one neuroleptic respond better to an agent from a different class. Patients appear to vary widely in their clinical response so it is best to select the agent on the basis of avoiding adverse effects. For example, haloperidol is sometimes selected over thioridazine on the belief that is is less likely to worsen cognition, whereas thioridazine may be preferred because it is less likely to produce extrapyramidal symptoms.

Although some neuroleptics are more potent than others, this potency is determined on a per-weight basis. Thus, "potent" haloperidol 1 mg is roughly equivalent to 50 mg of "less potent" chlorpromazine in its ability to control unwanted symptoms.

Specific features of neuroleptics commonly used in geriatrics are summarized on Table 6-1.

Dosing

The neuroleptic dose for elderly patients with dementia is far lower than that for the nonelderly adult with schizophrenia. As a rule of thumb, the **initial dose should be only 20% to 25%** of the usual adult dose.

These drugs all have a long duration of action, and in some cases total daily dose can be given all at once. However, until the patient's peculiar neurologic and hemodynamic response can be assessed, the total daily dose should be divided.

Dose increments should be made very slowly. As discussed above, steady-state levels are not reached for at least a week.

Although these medications are often prescribed and used by care-givers on an as-needed (prn) basis, there is less pharmacologic ratio-nale for this than is supposed. Additional sedation can be provided relatively quickly when an extra dose is given, but this sort of erratic administration should only be undertaken in a highly structured set-ting, where the total number of doses is recorded. The reason for this is that erratic, prn administration will contribute to the total amount of drug stored in the system, and if side effects occur it will be difficult to assess what maintenance dose was responsible for this. For short-term management of insomnia or agitation, a small dose of a short-acting benzodiazepine may be a useful adjunct.

Specific Agents

Thioridazine (Mellaril)

Thioridazine is one of the most widely used agents in the manage-ment of dementia. It is less likely than other neuroleptics to produce extrapyramidal symptoms. It is moderately **sedating**, a feature that may be problematic but that can also be harnessed when patients require extra sedation at night.

The cardiotoxic potential of thioridazine is not high in the doses generally required in elderly dementia patients. In fact, unless other drugs affecting cardiac conduction are given, the incidence of ar-rhythmias is extremely low. However, **changes on the resting EKG** (nonspecific T wave changes) occur with a very high frequency in daily doses of 100 mg or more. Although these changes are probably benign, prolongation of the QT interval may predispose to poten-tially dangerous **ventricular arrhythmias.**

A potential disadvantage of thioridazine is that it has relatively prominent **anticholinergic effects.**

CONTRAINDICATIONS. Thioridazine is contraindicated in patients with unstable cardiac arrhythmias, hepatic disease, and blood dys-crasias.

PRECAUTIONS. Baseline EKG should be performed. Periodic EKG should be performed to document "benign" T wave changes that might be due to the medication, so that if the patient were to have an unrelated ischemic episode there would be no confusion as to the eti-ology. Patients taking more than 100 mg per day should have EKG performed if further dose increases are made.

INDICATIONS. Unless contraindicated, thioridazine is a first-line oral drug in the management of agitative symptoms associated with dementia.

DOSING
Initial dose: 10 to 25 mg.
Usual daily dose range: 30–100 mg in 2 to 4 divided doses. Some patients may require up to 200 mg/day.

Haloperidol (Haldol)

The nonphenothiazine haloperidol is widely used in geriatrics. Its popularity is derived not only from its efficacy but from its virtual lack of cardiotoxicity in ordinary doses and the fact that it is some-what less sedating and has fewer anticholinergic effects than thioridazine. It has a greater tendency to produce extrapyramidal syndromes, however, and some geriatricians prefer to prescribe thioridazine unless unstable cardiac disease is present. Haloperidol should be considered a first-line drug when parenteral administration is required.

DOSING
Initial dose: 0.25 to 0.5 mg.
Usual daily dose range: 1–4 mg in 2 to 3 divided doses. Some patients may require total daily doses of up to 8 mg.
Intramuscular use: Parenteral dose may be relatively equivalent to the oral dose but this should be adjusted carefully according to the patient's needs.

Thiothixene (Navane)

Thiothixene is fairly well tolerated by elderly patients. It has a low tendency to produce cardiotoxicity and hemodynamic compromise, is relatively nonsedating, and has less anticholinergic effect than thioridazine. It has a greater tendency than thioridazine to produce **extrapyramidal syndromes.** Thiothixene closely resembles haloperidol in its spectrum of action, although the two drugs are chemically unrelated. It has been claimed that thiothixene is less likely than haloperidol to produce extrapyramidal syndromes, but this has been disputed. Like haloperidol, thiothixene can be given parenterally.

DOSING
Initial dose: 1 mg.
Usual daily dose range: 3–12 mg in 2 to 3 divided doses.
Intramuscular use: Parenteral dose may be slightly smaller or relatively equivalent to the oral dose but this should be adjusted carefully according to the individual patient's needs.

Chlorpromazine (Thorazine)

Chlorpromazine is pharmacologically very similar to thioridazine and shares its potent anticholinergic properties and its cardiovascular effects. Like other phenothiazines, its metabolism is complex and the pharmacokinetics and dose-response are unpredictable.

ADVERSE EFFECTS. Chlorpromazine has been implicated more than other neuroleptics in the production of **hepatic cholestasis.** It is also more likely to produce **photosensitivity reactions** and has been implicated more often in **extrapyramidal syndromes** than thioridazine. However, the two drugs have not been compared in elderly patients with dementia in carefully controlled studies.

The ability of oral chlorpromazine to produce **cardiotoxicity** is roughly comparable to or slightly less than that of thioridazine. However, its potent central and peripheral alpha$_1$ adrenergic blocking activity makes it somewhat more likely to produce **supine and orthostatic hypotension.** This propensity is markedly accentuated when the parenteral route is used.

Chlorpromazine is not commonly used in elderly patients with dementia. Its use has been eclipsed by thioridazine, which has a very similar spectrum of action but which may be somewhat safer. Because of its tendency to produce hypotension, chlorpromazine should not be offered to elderly dementia patients as a parenteral alternative to thioridazine, which is available only orally. If parenteral medication is required, haloperidol or thiothixene should be used instead.

Fluphenazine Decanoate (Prolixin Injection)

This drug is available orally, but it is probably best known for its availability in its injectable depot form (fluphenazine decanoate). The duration of action of this preparation may be as long as 2–3 weeks in nonelderly adults. The metabolism and clearance of fluphenazine, as with other neuroleptics, may well be further prolonged in elderly patients.

Fluphenazine is associated with a high incidence of extrapyramidal symptoms, which may occur within the first few days of treatment and which obviously cannot be managed by simple withdrawal of the drug when the depot form is used. Fluphenazine is not frequently associated with hemodynamic compromise, but the long duration of action would produce obvious problems if hypotension or cardiac problems were to occur.

This preparation is designed for use in younger adults when shorter-acting agents cannot be properly administered because appropriate caregivers are not available. It should **not** be used in this fashion in the elderly because the risk of **falls and impaired mobility** outweigh the benefits. A **depot form of haloperidol** is also available and should generally be avoided for the same reasons.

Clozapine (Clozaril)

Clozapine is an atypical neuroleptic that affects the dopaminergic as well as many other neurotransmitter systems. The drug has been found to be very effective in the management of schizophrenia. In addition, it is increasingly being used for patients with idiopathic (but **not** neuroleptic-induced) Parkinson's disease who develop psychotic symptoms from levodopa. However, clozapine has only received FDA approval for schizophrenia, and only in cases unresponsive to other agents.

An important feature of clozapine is that it exhibits relative dopamine$_1$ selective blocking action, so that it is associated with a much lower incidence of parkinsonian side effects than other neuroleptic agents. As such, it would be a useful alternative to older neuroleptics. Unfortunately, a number of cases of **agranulocytosis** have been reported and current recommendations are that its use be highly restricted.

Other side effects of clozapine could be particularly troublesome to geriatric patients. The drug may produce **hypersalivation, tachycardia,** and **orthostatic hypotension.** Hypersalivation is particularly troublesome at night and could pose problems to neurologically impaired patients who are at risk for aspiration pneumonia. There is also an increased risk of **seizures** at high doses and the drug can produce **delirium.**

In short, aside from its risk of producing agranulocytosis, a risk that does not appear to increase with age, there may be a high risk-to-benefit ratio overall in elderly patients. Until there is further experience with this drug in the geriatric age group, it cannot be recommended for routine use.

ADJUNCTIVE TREATMENT—PSYCHOSTIMULANTS

Stimulants, such as methylphenidate and amphetamines, have been prescribed for elderly patients with dementia. Although they have no consistent or lasting effect in improving cognition, they may have some utility as adjunctive therapy in highly selected patients with dementia who are apathetic or withdrawn. In such patients, cautious use of psychostimulants may increase alertness and motivation. This subject is explored more fully in Chap. 8.

MINOR TRANQUILIZERS

In general, the minor tranquilizers, such as the benzodiazepines, are probably less effective in the management of dementia than are the major tranquilizers. Compared to the latter, the minor tranquilizers are less likely to control agitated behavior in such patients and the doses required would be likely to produce oversedation, increased confusion, dizziness, and ataxia. These doses may significantly increase the risk of falls in the patient with dementia who does not live in a well-supervised environment. Another disadvantage of the minor tranquilizers is that tolerance to the sedating effects occurs rapidly.

An important advantage of minor tranquilizers is that in general they lack cardiovascular and extrapyramidal toxicity.

Benzodiazepines

Benzodiazepines are used widely for the management of anxiety in patients without cognitive impairment. Although their spectrum of action makes them somewhat less suitable for the management of dementia than the neuroleptics, their pharmacokinetics and dose-response are more predictable. In addition, they are specifically useful for insomnia and, if used cautiously, can be given as adjunctive therapy in the management of dementia patients with sleeplessness. They may also be used to control agitative symptoms in these patients if they cannot tolerate neuroleptics, and are sometimes used as first-line agents in patients with mild to moderate dementia who have milder behavioral symptoms.

An important difference between benzodiazepines and neuroleptics is that tolerance to sedation develops rapidly to the former but not to the latter. This may be an advantage but only for patients in whom the anxiolytic action is sufficient to control their symptoms. An important disadvantage of the benzodiazepines is that withdrawal syndromes may occur when the drug is discontinued abruptly.

Benzodiazepines and other sedative-hypnotics are discussed further in Chap. 7 in connection with the management of insomnia.

Specific Benzodiazepines

LORAZEPAM (ATIVAN). Lorazepam has an intermediate duration of action. It is degraded in the liver to inactive metabolites and does not progressively accumulate in elderly patients. Lorazepam tends to be well tolerated and is probably one of the better-suited non-neuroleptic anxiolytics to use in patients with dementia. Despite this, cognitively impaired patients are very sensitive to all benzodiazepines and lorazepam must be used cautiously, in a well-supervised environment.

Dosing

Initial dose: 0.5 mg once daily.
Maximum dose: 1–2 mg every 8–12 hours.

OXAZEPAM (SERAX). Oxazepam is one of the active metabolites of diazepam but is itself degraded in the liver to inactive metabolites. It closely resembles lorazepam in its spectrum of action but is slowly absorbed and therefore may have a delayed onset of action. There is currently no particular advantage to using this agent in patients with dementia when lorazepam is available. However, the slower onset of action may be useful in patients without dementia who are abuse prone, since an immediate effect will be less noticeable.

Dosing
Initial dose: 10–15 mg once or twice a day.
Maximum dose: 30 mg tid.

ALPRAZOLAM (XANAX). Alprazolam is structurally related to the hypnotic agent triazolam but is said to be somewhat less sedating than other benzodiazepines. It is rapidly absorbed and peak levels are achieved within an hour. The drug is metabolized by hepatic microsomal enzymes to inactive metabolites that are excreted in the kidney, with about 20% of the parent drug being excreted unchanged. The elimination half-life is approximately 10 hours in nongeriatric adults but may be longer in older individuals. Levels of alprazolam are increased with concurrent use of drugs that inhibit hepatic microsomal enzymes, such as cimetidine.

This agent has gained popularity because of the impression, though controversial, that it has antidepressant activity. The drug has also been used in the management of panic disorders. Although a useful anxiolytic in neurologically normal elderly, alprazolam should be used cautiously in those with dementia because paradoxical reactions have occasionally been reported. The incidence of such reactions may be no greater than that seen with other benzodiazepines, however.

Dosing
Initial dose: 0.25 mg once.
Usual dose range: 0.25–0.5 mg bid–tid.

Other Benzodiazepines

Diazepam (Valium), chlordiazepoxide (Librium), and other benzodiazepines have been widely used for the treatment of anxiety. Although they may be highly effective, these agents and their active metabolites have durations of action that are unacceptably long for routine use in the elderly. Long-acting benzodiazepines are particularly likely to produce lethargy and to worsen confusion in patients with dementia and should be avoided entirely.

The benzodiazepines are summarized on Table 7–2 in Chap. 7.

Buspirone (BusPar)

Buspirone is chemically unrelated to other anxiolytics. It has provoked interest because it has little or no sedative effect and, unlike other tranquilizers, it does not appear to worsen cognitive or motor function. This property would make it particularly useful in elderly patients with dementia. However, its use in the treatment of anxiety is modified by the fact that clinical efficacy may not be attained for up to 2–4 weeks of continuous use.

Pharmacologic Considerations

MECHANISM OF ACTION. The exact mechanism of action of buspirone is not known. It does not bind to benzodiazepine receptors but is thought to exert its mechanism of action through a subtype of serotonin receptor. Its effects on serotoninergic systems could be responsible for its anxiolytic action. Although excitatory withdrawal syndromes do not appear to occur with buspirone, its different site of action makes it inappropriate to use for benzodiazepine withdrawal. Buspirone has also been found to have dopamine blocking action.

Buspirone has been found to be equally or somewhat less effective than benzodiazepines in the management of anxiety. Patients self-administering the drug might be more likely to discontinue it before efficacy has been achieved, a factor that could modify assessments of its effectiveness. Its efficacy in the setting of dementia is not known.

PHARMACOKINETICS. Buspirone is well absorbed and undergoes extensive first-pass metabolism. It is partly metabolized by microsomal enzymes. Limited study indicates that its average 2–3 hour half-life is not prolonged with age and dose adjustments have not been recommended by investigators, but the drug has not been well studied in nursing home patients. Elimination is prolonged in hepatic cirrhosis and somewhat in renal insufficiency so that it is possible that the pharmacokinetic profile would be altered in debilitated elderly.

Adverse Effects

Sedation has been reported but the incidence may be no greater than that associated with placebo. Other central effects, such as **headache, dizziness,** and **nervousness,** may occur, and **excitation** has been reported. Nonspecific **gastrointestinal symptoms** are additional recognized side effects.

Extrapyramidal symptoms have been reported and attributed to the drug's mild dopamine blocking action. However, there were confounding factors in these reports so that the contribution made by buspirone is unclear. The long-term effects of buspirone on extrapyramidal and other systems are not known.

No withdrawal syndromes of an excitatory nature have yet been reported. It is too soon to know if other withdrawal symptoms, such as movement disorders or depression, might emerge after long-term use.

Drug Interactions

Buspirone does not appear to potentiate the depressant effects of alcohol or other agents that depress the central nervous system. It has been reported to reduce the elimination of digoxin but does not yet appear to participate in interactions with other drugs, despite the fact that it is highly protein-bound.

Applications

Buspirone may be useful in the management of anxiety in the elderly. Although it has not been adequately studied in the setting of dementia, scattered reports of behavioral improvement in such patients suggest that the drug might have a useful role in treating symptoms such as aggressiveness and hostility as well as anxiety. It is important to emphasize that clinical improvement occurs in a delayed fashion, sometimes after 2 to 4 weeks have elapsed. This could limit its use in patients with severe behavioral problems, but it could also cause the drug to be dismissed as ineffective.

Buspirone cannot be relied upon to suppress withdrawal symptoms in patients on long-term benzodiazepine therapy because it has a different mechanism and site of action. Patients being switched from benzodiazepines to buspirone should be withdrawn from the former slowly while buspirone is being instituted. In this regard, it is important to point out that buspirone has not been found to be particularly effective in patients failing to respond to benzodiazepines.

Dosing
Initial dose: 2.5 mg bid–tid.
Usual dose range: 5–30 mg/day in divided doses.
Note: Because of the delay in clinical effect, 2 to 3 weeks should elapse before dose increments are made.

ANTIHISTAMINES (HYDROXYZINE AND DIPHENHYDRAMINE)
Hydroxyzine (Atarax; Vistaril) and diphenhydramine (Benadryl) are sedating antihistamines that have been used in the treatment of insomnia and anxiety. Their anxiolytic effect is lower and less predictable than that achieved by the benzodiazepines and tolerance to sedation develops fairly rapidly, but withdrawal syndromes do not occur. Unlike neuroleptics, they are devoid of adverse cardiac effects at ordinary doses and rarely produce extrapyramidal syndromes. Like neuroleptics, however, antihistamines do possess anticholinergic action and may produce dry mouth, urinary retention, confusion, and acute angle glaucoma. For a complete discussion of antihistamines and their adverse effects, the reader is referred to Chap. 30.

Indications
Hydroxyzine and diphenhydramine may be used for short-term management of agitation when other agents cannot be used or when symptoms are very mild.

Dosing
Hydroxyzine: 10–25 mg once to 4 times daily.
Diphenhydramine: 10–50 mg once to 3 times daily.

BARBITURATES
Barbiturates are still occasionally used in the management of anxiety. Their disadvantages are outlined in Chap. 7. They have no particular advantages over the benzodiazepines and many disadvantages, notable among them being their ability to participate in many drug interactions. There is little rationale for their use as anxiolytics in geriatrics today.

MEPROBAMATE (EQUANIL, MILTOWN)
This once fashionable drug has been supplanted by the benzodiazepines but is still used religiously by some patients, most of them elderly. It has no particular advantages over the benzodiazepines and has several disadvantages, including its participation in drug-drug interactions. Meprobamate should not be instituted for the management of anxiety. Patients willing to discontinue the drug should be withdrawn slowly because withdrawal syndromes may occur with abrupt discontinuation. Meprobamate is discussed in greater detail in Chap. 7.

SPECIAL CONSIDERATIONS
Neuroleptics and other anxiolytics occasionally worsen cognition and increase agitation. Improvement may occur if the dose is low-

ered rather than increased. If dose adjustments do not improve symptoms, a neuroleptic from a different class may be effective. Occasionally, major tranquilizers may have to be abandoned entirely and a minor tranquilizer used, or vice versa.

Dementia of the Alzheimer type is generally progressive. Thus, agitation and related symptoms may wane with time, and a patient with dementia may "outgrow" the need for a tranquilizer. It is important to periodically reevaluate the need for these agents by giving the patient a drug holiday.

NONPHARMACOLOGIC MANAGEMENT

Potentially reversible deterioration in cognitive function should be managed by recognition and treatment of underlying problems, such as drug toxicity, infection, or other medical illness. Whenever possible, problems such as wandering, leaving the oven on, and misplacing property should be managed by vigilance, with close interpersonal interaction between patient and caregiver. The use of physical restraints must be reserved for exceptional circumstances, since they lead to immobility and its attendant consequences, may cause injury, and often increase the patient's agitation.

OTHER PSYCHIATRIC DISORDERS IN THE ELDERLY

Geriatric patients may be afflicted with a number of psychiatric disorders, including acute schizophrenia, mania, and classic panic attacks. These problems are less commonly encountered than dementia and depression in general geriatric practice and their management is beyond the scope of this book. Interested readers are referred to the Bibliography (see Arana & Hyman; Jeste & Zisook). Depression is discussed in Chap. 8.

BIBLIOGRAPHY

Addonizio, G. Neuroleptic malignant syndrome in elderly patients. *J. Amer. Geriatr. Soc.* 35:1011–1012, 1987.

Arana, G.W., and Hyman, S.E. *Handbook of Psychiatric Drug Therapy* (2nd ed.). Boston: Little, Brown, 1991.

Baldessarini, R.J., and Frankenburg, F.R. Clozapine. *N. Engl. J. Med.* 324: 746–754, 1991.

Besdine, R.W. Dementia and Delirium. In J.W. Rowe and R.W. Besdine, *Geriatric Medicine* (2nd ed.). Boston: Little, Brown, 1988, pp. 375–401.

Black, J.L., Richelson E., and Richardson, J.W. Antipsychotic agents: a clinical update. *Mayo Clin. Proc.* 60:777–789, 1985.

Davidson, M., and Stern, R.G. The treatment of cognitive impairment in Alzheimer's disease: beyond the cholinergic approach. *Psychiatr. Clin. N. Amer.* 14:461–479, 1991.

Elkayam, R., and Frishman, W. Cardiovascular effects of phenothiazines. *Am. Heart. J.* 100:397–401, 1980.

Funck-Brentano, C. Topics in clinical pharmacology: buspirone: a new nonbenzodiazepine anxiolytic agent. *Amer. J. Med. Sci.* 297:49–52, 1989.

Hartshorn, E.A. Interactions of CNS drugs: Psychotherapeutic agents—the antipsychotic drugs. *Drug Intell. Clin. Pharm.* 9:536–550, 1975.

Hollister, L.E. Alzheimer's disease. Is it worth treating? *Drugs* 29:483–488, 1985.

Hollister, L.E., and Yesavage, J. Ergoloid mesylates for senile dementia. *Ann. Intern. Med.* 100:894, 1984.

Horowitz, G.R. What is a complete work-up for dementia? *Clin. Geriatr. Med.* 4:163–180,1988.

Jahnigen, D.W., and Schrier, R.W., eds. Ethical issues in the care of the elderly. *Clin. Geriatr. Med.* 2(3):457–637, 1986.

Jeste, D.V., and Zisook, S. (eds.). Psychosis and depression in the elderly. *Psychiatr. Clin. Nor. Amer.* 11(1), 1988.

Kane, J.M., and Smith, J.M. Tardive dyskinesia: prevalence and risk factors, 1959–1979. *Arch. Gen. Psychiatr.* 39:473–481, 1982.

Klawans, H.L., and Genovese, N. Pharmacology of dementia, *Neurol. Clin.* 4:459, 1986.

Lathers, C.M., and Lipka, L.J. Cardiac arrhythmia, sudden death, and psychoactive agents. *J. Clin. Pharmacol.* 27:1–14, 1987.

Neshkes, R.E., and Jarvik, L.F. The Central Nervous System—Dementia and Delirium in Old Age. In J.C. Brocklehurst (ed.), *Textbook of Geriatric Medicine and Gerontology* (3rd ed.). New York: Churchill Livingstone, 1985, pp. 309–327.

Risse, S.C., and Barnes, R. Pharmacologic treatment of agitation associated with dementia. *J. Amer. Geriatr. Soc.* 34:368–376, 1986.

Rizack, M.A., and Hillman, C.D.M. *The Medical Letter Handbook of Adverse Drug Interactions.* New Rochelle, NY: The Medical Letter, 1989.

Task Force on Late Neurological Effects of Antipsychotic Drugs. Tardive dyskinesia: summary of a task force report of the American Psychiatric Association. *Am J. Psychiatr.* 137:1163–1172, 1980.

Thompson, T.L., Filley, C.M., Mitchell, W.D. et al. Lack of efficacy of hydergine in patients with Alzheimer's disease. *N. Engl. J. Med.* 323:445–448, 1990.

Wragg, R.E., and Jeste, D.V. Neuroleptics and alternative treatments. Management of behavioral symptoms and psychosis in Alzheimer's disease and related conditions. *Psychiatr. Clin. N. Amer.* 11:195–213, 1988.

Sedative-Hypnotics

MANAGEMENT OF INSOMNIA IN THE ELDERLY

Insomnia is a symptom complex that may include difficulty falling asleep, difficulty obtaining deep and refreshing sleep, difficulty in maintaining sleep throughout the night, or early morning awakening. Complaints of insomnia and chronic use of hypnotic medications are far more common in the elderly than in younger adults. What is the source of these complaints and how can use of these potentially harmful medications be curtailed?

Sleep patterns tend to change progressively from infancy to old age. Throughout adulthood, little or no electrophysiological change occurs in REM sleep (rapid eye movement or "dream" sleep) until extreme old age, but significant alterations occur in all four stages of non-REM sleep. With aging there is a reduction in the proportion of time spent in deep sleep (stages 3 and 4), and an increase in light sleep (stages 1 and 2). There is also an increase in the number of microawakenings, which are periods of electrophysiologic alertness not noticed by the subject. Sleep may become fragmented with the patient complaining of disordered sleep and daytime drowsiness. There is often a tendency to "phase advance" with age—the individual becomes drowsy earlier in the evening and awakens earlier in the morning. Napping often increases, but this is often accompanied by a decrease in nocturnal sleep time, so that total 24-hour sleep time can remain the same.

Although the proportion of time spent in REM sleep does not change significantly, the absolute amount of REM sleep may decrease with age. This happens because the distribution of REM sleep changes, becoming more evenly spread throughout the night so that it is more likely to be disrupted by the many arousals that occur. The significance of this is not known.

There is no evidence that any of these changes is pathological, even if they are upsetting to the patient. There is furthermore no evidence that the amount of sleep needed changes with age. Finally, there is immense variation in sleep patterns and age-related changes among elderly individuals.

Some geriatric patients who complain of insomnia may be having difficulty adjusting their life-style or long-held opinions to these sleep changes. Others may be truly suffering from primary sleep disorders or from disordered sleep due to medical or extrinsic factors. The physician should make a concerted effort to uncover the cause of the sleep complaint before prescribing hypnotic agents.

Medical, psychological, and environmental factors that cause insomnia are summarized in Table 7-1. In general, any cause of physical or psychic discomfort can result in disordered sleep. Most of these factors are more common in the elderly; some are specific to geriatric patients.

Sleep is often seriously disordered in dementia. Patients with dementia also may become agitated at night or wander and get into trouble. This can be frightening to the patient and a serious management problem for caregivers. The patient may forget that a hypnotic was given and may repeatedly ask for a pill, becoming increasingly agitated in the process.

Table 7–1. Causes of Insomnia in the Elderly

Anxiety
Fear of burglary
Fear of sleeplessness
Hospitalization
Noise, light, excessive cold or heat in bedroom
Uncomfortable bed
Depression
Dementia
Boredom
Imposition of caregiver sleep schedule
Medical causes
    Nocturia
    Bladder disturbances
    Pain or discomfort
    Diarrhea
    Dyspnea
    Pruritus
    Drug or alcohol withdrawal
Medications
    Stimulants
    Bronchodilators
    Thyroid hormone
    Centrally acting antihypertensives
    Corticosteroids
    Alcohol
    Caffeine
Primary sleep disorders
    Sleep apnea
    Restless leg syndrome
    Nocturnal myoclonus (periodic leg movement)
    Advanced or delayed sleep phase

Institutionalized elderly have an in-bed cycle dictated by the needs of the institution. Shift schedules and inadequate staffing impose unnatural in-bed demands that are too long or out of phase with patients' intrinsic and often disordered sleep patterns. On top of this, patients are less able to adjust the internal sleep clock to external cues. They generally lack adequate physical activity during the day to contribute to restful sleep at night, and often suffer from medical problems that disrupt sleep. Agitated patients are likely to disturb other light sleepers nearby unless sedated. Caffeine may be a regular staple in the nursing home diet.

Boredom may cause a patient to complain of insomnia in a context that is so troublesome that hypnotic dependence occurs. Geriatric patients often suffer from social isolation and consequent inactivity in the evening. Resourceful individuals may spend the time reading, doing needlework, watching television, and so on, but there are few alternatives for the elderly patient with low vision, impaired manual dexterity, or inadequate financial resources. Such individuals often go to bed at an inappropriately early hour for lack of anything else to do and complain that they cannot sleep until morning.

USE AND RISKS OF HYPNOTICS IN THE ELDERLY

The elderly are more sensitive to agents from all classes of hypnotics, probably independent of any pharmacokinetic changes that may occur. For this reason, both therapeutic and adverse effects may be achieved with lower doses than in younger adults. Oversedation can result in cognitive and motor impairment, falls, fractures, and aspiration pneumonia. Respiratory suppression can occur and sleep apnea can worsen. Antihistamines given for sleep pose special problems in the elderly (see below). Whenever possible, nonpharmacologic measures should be used to treat complaints of insomnia. When hypnotic agents are used, the starting dose should be only 50%–75% of the usual adult dose.

Tolerance develops to the hypnotic effect of all agents over time. This presents a danger that patients will self-administer higher and higher doses, leading to habituation and addiction, a probably underrecognized situation in the elderly. Chronic hypnotic use actually results in disordered sleep, which resolves on gradual withdrawal. Hypnotics should be given with extreme caution to patients with chronic insomnia. Unfortunately, it is extremely difficult for physicians and their elderly patients to adhere to this advice, in view of the extreme distress that insomnia causes the patient requesting the sleeping pill. An elderly patient may be viewed as having "few pleasures" and hence deserving endless prescription refills, and a physician who rightly or wrongly refuses to prescribe the sleeping pill may be viewed as cruel or unsympathetic. Habituated patients usually shop until they are able to find a physician who will prescribe something.

CONTRAINDICATIONS AND PRECAUTIONS

Hypnotics are contraindicated in sleep apnea, respiratory depression, and in patients with recurrent aspiration pneumonia. They are contraindicated in delirium that is not due to drug withdrawal. They should not be given to patients at risk of falling or to those with dementia, unless the patient is in a protected environment.

Certain hypnotics may produce paradoxical excitation, particularly in elderly patients. If this occurs, a hypnotic of a different chemical class should be given.

Hypnotics should never be prescribed to be taken every night. Shorter-acting agents should be restricted to a maximum of 3 nights in 7. Patients should be advised not to take long-acting hypnotics, but those who resist this advice should be told to restrict their use to once a week.

BENZODIAZEPINES

Compared to older hypnotic agents, the benzodiazepines are less addicting, produce less severe withdrawal syndromes, and participate in fewer pharmacokinetic drug interactions. They have a very wide therapeutic index so that deaths from overdose rarely occur unless the drug is combined with another sedating agent. While, as a group, the benzodiazepines are preferred to other agents for treating insomnia in the elderly, only certain members of this group should be prescribed.

Although individual benzodiazepines are approved or marketed for specific indications, differences between agents are probably not qualitative but rather depend on differences in pharmacokinetic properties. Four benzodiazepines—temazepam, flurazepam, triazolam, and most recently quazepam—are officially approved for use in insomnia, but the other agents are effective hypnotics and some are commonly used for that purpose.

The benzodiazepines are sometimes grouped into two major categories—short- and long-acting. Short-acting benzodiazepines, such as triazolam, oxazepam, temazepam, and lorazepam, are metabolized to inactive compounds and do not tend to accumulate in the body. There is considerable interindividual variability on their duration of action, and when used as hypnotic agents all may produce next-day sedation in specific individuals. Well-known long-acting benzodiazepines include diazepam, chlordiazepoxide, and flurazepam. These agents are metabolized to active compounds that themselves have a long half-life and drug accumulation occurs with regular use, so that side effects may occur in a delayed fashion.

The individual benzodiazepines are summarized in Table 7-2.

Adverse Effects

The most important side effects of the benzodiazepines are related to their **central depressant effect,** a property common to all sedative hypnotics. **Excitatory withdrawal syndromes** may occur with prolonged use. The nature and onset of withdrawal syndromes vary according to the pharmacokinetics of the specific agent. In general, they are less severe and less likely to occur than with other hypnotic agents.

Benzodiazepines may produce **paradoxical excitation;** if this occurs, a non-benzodiazepine hypnotic should be given instead.

Drug Interactions

The most important benzodiazepine drug interactions are on a pharmacodynamic level. When administered with any CNS depressant, the risk of cognitive impairment, lethargy, ataxia, and falls is increased.

The importance of pharmacokinetic interactions is less well defined. The clearance of benzodiazepines can be altered by drugs that interfere with hepatic metabolism. Thus, agents such as beta blockers and cimetidine can increase their effects and agents such as rifampin can reduce them. Beta blockers and cimetidine, in addition, may themselves produce confusional states. Long-term use of diazepam and chlordiazepoxide have been found to increase hepatic microsomal enzyme activity. The importance of this observation is not known.

A complete list of reported drug interactions can be found in the references in the Bibliography (see Rizack & Hillman).

Specific Agents

Temazepam (Restoril, Others)

Temazepam is 80% absorbed after an oral dose. However, the formulation available in the United States is a hard capsule that impairs absorption, delaying the onset of action for up to 2 hours after ingestion. Absorption may be further delayed by food. The drug is conjugated in the liver primarily to inactive metabolites that are excreted

Table 7-2. The Benzodiazepines

Drug (Sample Brand)	Onset[a]	Rate of Elimination[b]	Use
Short- to Intermediate-Acting			
Temazepam (Restoril)	Slow	Int	Nocturnal & early AM awakening
Triazolam (Halcion)	Fast	Prompt	Prolonged sleep latency
Lorazepam (Ativan)	Fast–Int	Int	Anxiety; nocturnal & early AM awakening
Oxazepam (Serax)	Int–Slow	Prompt–Int	Anxiety; nocturnal awakening
Alprazolam (Xanax)	Int	Int	Anxiety; anxiety associated with depression; panic
Intermediate- to long-acting[c]			
Diazepam (Valium)	Very fast	Prolonged	Anxiety; prolonged sleep latency; muscle spasm
Flurazepam (Dalmane)	Fast	Prolonged	Prolonged sleep latency; nocturnal & early AM awakening
Quazepam (Doral)	Fast	Prolonged	Prolonged sleep latency; nocturnal & early AM awakening
Chlordizepoxide (Librium)	Int	Int–Slow	Anxiety
Clorazepate (Tranxene)	Fast	Prolonged	Anxiety
Halazepam (Paxipam)	Int–Slow	Slow	Anxiety
Prazepam (Centrax)	Slow	Slow–Prolonged	Anxiety
Clonazepam (Klonipen)	Int	Slow–Prolonged	Seizures; panic; restless leg

[a]Onset
Fast = < 30 min
Int = 1–2 hr
Slow = 2 hr

[b]Rate of Elimination (nongeriatric)
Prompt = < 8 hr
Int = 8–12 hr
Slow = 12–24 hr
Prolonged = > 24 hr; may be more than 100 hr

[c]Not generally recommended for geriatric patients.

in the kidney. The duration of action averages about 8 hours. Elimination is not significantly impaired with age.

Temazepam has a variable effect on sleep latency, probably because of its delayed absorption in the hard-capsule form. However, the drug decreases the number of arousals and increases the quality of sleep. Its intermediate duration of action minimizes the likelihood of accumulation and next-day sedation while being more likely than shorter-acting agents to promote a full night of sleep.

USE. Temazepam is suitable for use in insomnia but may appear to be ineffective in sleep latency disorders because of its delayed onset of action. This drug appears to be relatively safe for older individuals as compared to other benzodiazepine hypnotics. However, studies directly comparing it with popular triazolam are lacking in this age group.

DOSING

Initial dose: 15 mg.

Maximum dose: 30 mg.

Note: Temazepam should be administered on an empty stomach at least 1 hour before bedtime.

Triazolam (Halcion)

Triazolam is well absorbed orally, with peak levels occurring roughly 1⅓ hours after ingestion. There is no change in absorption or volume of distribution with aging. Pharmacologically active metabolites of triazolam are produced by hepatic oxidation, but these are rapidly converted to inactive conjugates so the clinical significance of their presence may be minimal. The average elimination half-life of triazolam is 2 to 3 hours in nongeriatric adults. Any age-related increase in half-life of this short-acting agent would not lead to important accumulation. However, duration of action may be unexpectedly prolonged in some patients.

In addition, triazolam is cleared more slowly in late life, owing to reduced hepatic extraction. This leads to higher serum concentrations and greater sedation at a given dose than that seen in younger adults. Recent study also suggests that older individuals may be unaware of the higher degree of sedation conferred by increasing dose (see Greenblatt et al.).

The drug may begin to act within 15 to 30 minutes of ingestion. Sleep latency is decreased, arousals decreased, and total sleep time increased. The short duration of action of triazolam minimizes but does not eliminate the risk of next-day sedation. Some patients actually report increased alertness and functioning, presumably because they have obtained refreshing sleep without a hangover. The short action of triazolam also has its down side. **Rebound insomnia** and **intense withdrawal syndromes** have occurred. **Paradoxical reactions** have been reported, and may represent an end-of-dose withdrawal phenomenon or may be directly related to the chemical properties of the drug itself. In elderly patients, doses as low as 0.125 mg have been associated with **delirium** and **severe psychological reactions** such as paranoia, anxiety, depersonalization, and antegrade amnesia. Intense reactions or antegrade amnesia are more likely to occur when the drug is combined with alcohol.

USE. Triazolam is appropriate for patients with difficulty falling asleep but is less suitable for those whose main problem is early morning awakening. It should be avoided in frail or cognitively impaired patients who do not reside in a well-supervised setting.

DOSING
Initial dose: 0.0625 to 0.125 mg.
Maximum dose: 0.25 mg.
Note: If next-day sedation occurs, the dose should be reduced by 50%.

Flurazepam (Dalmane, Others)

Flurazepam is very rapidly absorbed, more so than triazolam, and is highly effective in sleep latency insomnia. This is due to the early production of active metabolites that are eliminated after a few hours. However, one metabolite, N-desalkylflurazepam, has an ultralong half-life. Elimination may be markedly prolonged in the elderly, with drug activity being present for up to 2 weeks in some patients. For this reason the drug accumulates after repeated dosage, with peak plasma concentrations more than quadrupling after 2 weeks of use. Accumulation is much greater in the elderly than in younger adults. As expected, flurazepam is associated with **next-day sedation** and the **delayed appearance of cognitive and motor impairment.** These effects are far more common with a nightly dose of 30 mg than with the 15 mg dose.

It is important to emphasize that lack of sedation after long-term flurazepam use represents the development of tolerance.

Withdrawal symptoms are less severe than with shorter-acting agents, and are generally seen only when high doses are given for prolonged periods. However, the appearance of withdrawal symptoms may be very delayed.

USE. Although flurazepam has been used safely in elderly individuals, patients with insomnia cannot always be relied upon to use this agent judiciously. This drug should generally be avoided in elderly patients.

DOSING
15 mg.

Quazepam (Doral)

This agent, like flurazepam, has a rapid onset of action but a very long half-life. It is metabolized in the liver to active substances, one of which is identical to the flurazepam metabolite, N-desalkylflurazepam. This metabolite has a half-life twice as long as that of the parent drug and its half-life may be doubled in geriatric patients. Quazepam has no apparent advantages over flurazepam, and until further information is available it should generally be avoided by geriatric patients.

DOSING
7.5 mg.

Lorazepam (Ativan)

Lorazepam is an intermediate-acting benzodiazepine that is not officially approved for use in insomnia but is marketed primarily as an anxiolytic and for use in insomnia due to "anxiety states." Nonetheless, like all benzodiazepines, it will induce sleep and is suitable for this purpose in certain situations.

Lorazepam is slowly absorbed. Peak plasma levels are attained within 3 hours but pharmacological effect may exist after 30 minutes. It is conjugated in the liver to an inactive metabolite. The mean elimination half-life of 8 hours is not prolonged in the elderly, but significant blood levels may be maintained for several hours more in many patients. In addition, this relatively nonlipophilic benzodiazepine may egress from the brain slowly, extending its sedative effect. Although a prolonged effect is of benefit in the patient being treated for anxiety, the insomnia patient might complain of a "hangover" or a dizzy or "peculiar" sensation the next morning.

As with all sedative-hypnotics, the elderly may be ultrasensitive to the central effects of this agent. In general, when problems such as cognitive and motor impairment occur, they present within the first days of therapy rather than in a delayed manner.

USE. Lorazepam is suitable for patients who are troubled by nocturnal arousal or early morning awakening. It has not been officially approved for use in insomnia.

DOSING
Initial dose: 0.5 mg.
Maximum dose: 2 mg.

Oxazepam (Serax)

Oxazepam differs from lorazepam mainly in its slower (2 to 3 hour) onset of action and its generally shorter duration of action. The delayed onset makes oxazepam less suitable than lorazepam as a hypnotic agent, but it does not differ much in this regard from temazepam.

USE. As a hypnotic, oxazepam has few if any advantages over temazepam, but it may be a suitable alternative in some patients who experience next-day sedation with other agents and who cannot tolerate triazolam.

Like lorazepam, oxazepam has not been officially approved for use in insomnia.

DOSING
Initial dose: 10–15 mg.
Maximum dose: 30 mg.

Diazepam (Valium, Others)

Diazepam is the most quickly absorbed of the benzodiazepines and has a very rapid onset of action. Because of its significant lipophilicity it is quickly distributed to inactive lipid storage sites and its immediate duration of action may be relatively brief in many individuals. However, it is oxidized in the liver to desmethyldiazepam, an active metabolite with a long duration of action that may persist in the circulation for more than a week in some elderly.

Diazepam must be used cautiously in geriatric patients. Its rapid onset of action not only gives it abuse potential, but in susceptible individuals it may produce **acute confusion, dizziness,** and **falls.** Diazepam and its metabolites accumulate over time, causing **delayed sedation and cognitive and motor impairment.**

Addiction has been reported. However, intense withdrawal states probably occur only with long-term use of very high doses.

USE. Diazepam has not been officially approved for use in insomnia and is promoted primarily as an anxiolytic and muscle relaxant. However, its rapid onset of action makes it a popular hypnotic in sleep latency insomnia. Its use in general has declined in recent years, possibly because of adverse publicity following a decade of overenthusiasm, overuse, and abuse. It is not considered a first-line agent in geriatrics either for the management of insomnia or anxiety, but it is often requested by patients who have used it in the past.

DOSING
Initial dose: 1–2 mg.
Maximum dose: 10 mg.

Other Benzodiazepines

A number of other benzodiazepines are available. Their pharmacokinetic profile makes them primarily useful for conditions other than insomnia (see Table 7–2). Alprazolam is discussed in Chaps. 6 and 8.

CHLORAL HYDRATE

Pharmacological Considerations

Chloral hydrate is well absorbed with onset of action at roughly 30 minutes. It is rapidly converted in the liver under the direction of the enzyme alcohol dehydrogenase to trichloroethanol (TCE), which exerts the sedative action. This reaction is accelerated by ethanol. TCE is lipid-soluble and rapidly distributes into the brain and other tissues. Peak plasma levels of TCE are reached in 20 to 60 minutes, and the plasma half-life averages 8 hours with a range of 4 to 12 hours. Chloral hydrate is also converted to trichloroacetic acid (TCA), which is inactive but highly protein-bound and has a half-life of 4 days.

Chloral hydrate reduces sleep latency, and decreases the number of awakenings. There is a slight decrease in slow wave sleep but probably no decrease in REM sleep and a variable effect on total sleep time. These effects on sleep probably last for only 2 weeks of continued dosing, after which tolerance occurs.

TCE and TCA undergo glucuronidation in the liver to inactive metabolites that are excreted primarily by the kidney along with a small amount of parent drug. The elimination half-life of chloral hydrate does not increase with age.

Like chloral hydrate, triclofos sodium is a chloral derivative and for all practical purposes is identical to chloral hydrate in its pharmacokinetics and spectrum of action. It is somewhat more likely to produce gastrointestinal irritation.

Adverse Effects

In addition to CNS depressant effects, chloral hydrate may produce **gastrointestinal symptoms** such as nausea, epigastric discomfort, and flatus.

Toxic overdose can produce hypotension, respiratory depression, impaired cardiac contractility, and gastric necrosis. Sudden withdrawal can precipitate **rebound insomnia** as well as **severe withdrawal symptoms** such as excitability, seizures, tremor, hallucinations, and even death.

Important Drug Interactions

The complex action of chloral hydrate on warfarin sensitivity can lead to dangerous over- or underestimation of anticoagulant dose. The drug stimulates the hepatic microsomal enzyme system, increasing the metabolism of agents such as warfarin. However, it may increase warfarin sensitivity acutely when its protein-bound metabolite displaces the anticoagulant from binding sites.

Ethanol accelerates the conversion of chloral hydrate to active TCE and TCE in turn competes with alcohol for the metabolic enzyme alcohol dehydrogenase, thus increasing blood levels of alcohol.

This interaction enhances the usual additive effect that alcohol has on CNS depressants. The combination of chloral hydrate and alcohol constitutes the legendary "Mickey Finn."

Contraindications
The chloral derivatives are contraindicated in liver disease, renal insufficiency, active peptic ulcer, alcoholism, and severe cardiac or respiratory decompensation.

Precautions
Because tolerance can develop rapidly, this agent can be habituating in individuals severely troubled by chronic insomnia who may self-administer increasing doses and become dependent. The importance of this is enhanced by the drug's relatively narrow therapeutic index. The lethal dose is approximately 10 g in nonelderly adults; however, fatalities have been reported with amounts as low as 4 g.

Use
Chloral hydrate is suitable for patients with sleep latency insomnia. Its intermediate duration of action minimizes next-day sedation. This combination of properties makes it advantageous over most benzodiazepines. However, it should not be prescribed to patients who are unreliable, because of its relatively narrow therapeutic index, ability to participate in drug interactions, and potential for severe withdrawal syndromes.

Dosing
Initial dose: 250 mg.
Maximum dose: 1 g.

ANTIHISTAMINES
The unwanted central depressant effect of certain antihistamines (histamine$_1$ receptor antagonists) can be exploited in order to induce sleep. The sedating antihistamines enter the brain where they bind to H_1 receptors, although it is not known exactly how they exert their central depressant effect.

The antihistamines are often prescribed for sleep in the elderly because they are thought to be mild agents. This concept is reinforced by the fact that antihistamines are the hypnotic ingredients in over-the-counter sleep aids. They do cause less confusion than other sedating agents, and although tolerance develops to their sedating effects, they are nonaddicting and have not been associated with withdrawal syndromes. However, they have anticholinergic (atropinelike) activity and on this basis may produce **urinary retention, constipation,** and, at higher doses, **reversible dementia.** They have a tendency to cause **dry mouth,** which can be a particular problem in geriatric patients, especially those who wear dentures. The anticholinergic effects are sometimes harnessed in patients with Parkinson's disease (see Chap. 10). Antihistamines are contraindicated in **narrow angle glaucoma** and in symptomatic prostatic hyperplasia.

Because tolerance to the sedative effects develops, some patients may self-administer increasing doses of antihistamines over time in order to induce sleep. **Tolerance does not develop to the anticholinergic effects, so with increasing doses side effects are likely to** emerge. This potential problem is worsened by the fact that antihistamines are available over the counter. Their atropinelike action makes their margin of safety narrower for geriatric patients than for younger adults.

Not all antihistamines have sedating activity, and some, such as cyproheptadine, may produce stimulant effects in an occasional patient.

Diphenhydramine (Benadryl, Nytol, Sominex, Others)

Diphenhydramine has an onset of action at 30 minutes, and a duration of action of 4 to 6 hours. It is available by prescription or over the counter, depending on the product labeling.

Like all sedating antihistamines, this one does not produce somnolence in all patients. It is frequently prescribed for this purpose, however, because it has a shorter duration of action than most other sedating antihistamines.

Dosing

10–25 mg at bedtime.
Note: Liquid formulations contain up to 14% alcohol.

Pyrilamine (Dormarex, Others)

Except for occasional gastrointestinal irritation, this agent is tolerated about as well as diphenhydramine. The usual dose is 25 mg at bedtime. It is available without prescription.

Hydroxyzine (Atarax, Others)

Hydroxyzine produces sedation but its duration of action is 20 hours in nonelderly adults, making it unsuitable as a hypnotic agent for many patients. It is sometimes prescribed as an anxiolytic.

Antihistamines are discussed in detail in Chap. 30.

OTHER SEDATIVE-HYPNOTICS

Meprobamate (Miltown, Equanil, Others)

Meprobamate is an intermediate-acting sedative-hypnotic that gained popularity in the late 1950s when it was promoted as a safer, less-sedating alternative to barbiturates. It was considered to be well tolerated in geriatric patients, causing less daytime sedation when used as a hypnotic and fewer overall side effects when used for sedation. The drug had a tendency to cause hypotension in elderly patients and was occasionally used in the treatment of hypertension, as well as for a variety of other conditions in which a state of calm was thought to be helpful. Its efficacy has been disputed by clinical investigators while being praised by patients. It was soon found to be as addictive as barbiturates and prone to important drug-drug interactions, while having a therapeutic index that was not much safer. Like the barbiturates, it was eventually supplanted by the benzodiazepines.

There is little indication for meprobamate today, but because of its history of use in geriatrics it is not uncommon to encounter elderly people who still use this drug. Meprobamate continues to be officially approved for use in anxiety, but not for insomnia.

Meprobamate is well absorbed, peak plasma levels being achieved within 1–3 hours. It does not bind greatly to plasma proteins. More than 80% is metabolized in the liver by both oxidation and conjugation. Roughly 10%–15% is excreted unchanged in the urine. The elimination half-life of meprobamate is approximately 6–17 hours but may be up to 48 hours after chronic administration. The pharmacokinetics have not been studied specifically in geriatric populations.

Meprobamate decreases stage-1 sleep, increases stage-2 sleep and REM sleep, and has no effect on stages 3 and 4.

Adverse Effects

Meprobamate occasionally produces **hypotension** in elderly patients. **Hypersensitivity reactions** consisting of rash or of systemic symptoms such as fever, shaking chills, or syncope occur in a small proportion of patients. It also has been rarely associated with **blood dyscrasias**, including aplastic anemia. It stimulates delta-ALA synthetase and is contraindicated in **porphyria.**

Like any central depressant, meprobamate may produce unwanted sedation, confusion, and motor incoordination. Tolerance occurs fairly rapidly and addiction may occur at relatively low doses. **Lethal overdose** has been reported with doses as low as 12 g (usual sedative-hypnotic dose 200–400 mg). After several weeks of continuous treatment, **severe withdrawal reactions** may occur soon after the drug is discontinued; this tends to happen in patients who have been taking high doses. Tremor, delirium, seizure, and even death have been reported in these situations.

Drug-Drug Interactions

Hepatic microsomal enzyme induction is produced by meprobamate and at high doses the drug accelerates warfarin metabolism. Specific drug interactions have not been elucidated, but care should be taken when chronic users of meprobamate require drugs metabolized by hepatic oxidation, such as theophylline and warfarin, or when patients ingesting such drugs discontinue meprobamate.

Use

Meprobamate is not recommended for general use. It is probably less effective than the benzodiazepines and is not as safe, and withdrawal can be difficult. In patients who have been taking the drug for prolonged periods, an attempt should be made to withdraw it gradually over several weeks.

Barbiturates

The barbiturates, though popular hypnotics for decades, are now rarely indicated for the treatment of insomnia. Tolerance to hypnotic and sedative effects—but not to toxic effects—develops very early and continues to increase with continued use. Barbiturates are highly addicting, have a very narrow therapeutic-to-toxic ratio, and are subject to many drug interactions. As hypnotics, they depress REM sleep as well as stages 3 and 4 of non-REM sleep, so that rebound phenomena may include not only insomnia but also excessive dreaming and nightmares.

Adverse Effects

Barbiturates have a tendency to produce **hyperalgesia,** which could pose a problem for elderly insomniacs, many of whom suffer from chronic pain syndromes. **Paradoxical reactions**—consisting of disinhibition, agitation, or socially inappropriate behavior—and agitation may occur. As expected, the elderly are more likely to develop states of **delirium** and **cognitive and motor impairment** from barbiturates. Many of these nervous system effects are common to other sedative-hypnotics.

Barbiturates stimulate delta-aminolevulinic acid, increasing the production of porphyrins, and so are contraindicated in **porphyria.**

Drug and Nutrient Interactions

Barbiturates are potent inducers of the hepatic microsomal enzymes. This is thought to enhance the degradation of vitamin D and chronic administration may produce vitamin D deficiency. This problem has been characterized primarily in conjunction with long-term use of the anticonvulsant phenobarbital (see Chap. 11).

A more clearly characterized consequence of enzyme induction is the problem of drug interactions. Barbiturates accelerate the degradation of many important drugs, including warfarin, theophylline, and quinidine. Discontinuation of barbiturates results in return of prior efficacy of these drugs at unpredictable times; thus, it is risky to administer barbiturates not only at the same time but even within 2 weeks or more. Pharmacokinetic interactions related to enzyme induction are summarized in Table 7-3.

The pharmacodynamic interactions of barbiturates are also important, as with other sedative hypnotics. Particularly important is the interaction with alcohol, which also acutely impairs the metabolism of barbiturates; this can produce serious CNS depression. For a complete overview of potential interactions, the reader is referred to the Bibliography (see Rizack & Hillman).

Despite the disadvantages of the barbiturates, occasional long-term users of barbiturates, mostly elderly, are still encountered. The most commonly used barbiturate hypnotics are secobarbital (Seconal) and pentobarbital (Nembutal).

Table 7-3. Some Important Drug Interactions with Barbiturates

Agents Whose Effect Is Reduced by Barbiturates

Warfarin
Theophylline
Tricyclic antidepressants
Quinidine
Digitoxin
Acetaminophen
Corticosteroids
Metronidazole
Chloramphenicol
Vitamin D
Beta blockers
Anticonvulsants*

*Effect on anticonvulsants is variable.

USE OF SEDATIVE-HYPNOTICS IN THE MANAGEMENT OF ANXIETY

Many of the agents discussed in this chapter have been employed in the management of anxiety. They are discussed briefly in Chap. 6 in connection with control of selected symptoms in dementia, for which they should be used sparingly. For patients without dementia or psychosis, the benzodiazepines are currently the preferred anxiolytics, with the newer agent buspirone finding its place in therapy. Pharmacologic aspects and adverse effects of the benzodiazepines as discussed in Chap. 6 are also pertinent to geriatric patients without dementia. For a complete discussion of this topic, the reader is referred to the Bibliography (see Salzman; Arana & Hyman).

Anxiety frequently responds to psychotherapy without the addition of medications. Whenever possible, interpersonal, nonpharmacologic methods, including psychotherapy, should be instituted first. Psychiatric consultation should be obtained whenever there is doubt as to the best management strategy.

OTHER AGENTS

Major tranquilizers (neuroleptics) with sedating properties, such as thioridazine, are often used in the management of nocturnal agitation of patients with dementia. Even less sedating agents, such as haloperidol, may promote sleep because of their calming effect. However, these agents are likely to produce rigidity and other parkinsonian symptoms, which can increase the risk of falling in these patients, who are already prone to accidental injuries. It is best to manage sleep in these patients by altering the environment. Major tranquilizers are discussed in detail in Chap. 6.

Sedating **tricyclic antidepressants** (TCAs) are often prescribed at bedtime to depressed patients whose depression is complicated by insomnia. Because the TCAs are structurally related to the phenothiazines, the quality of sedation differs from that produced by the benzodiazepines and other sedative-hypnotics. Consequently, the TCAs may actually produce dysphoria in nondepressed patients. This attribute, combined with their long duration of action, lead to an unpleasant "hangover" in many patients, making them inappropriate for general use in insomnia. TCAs are discussed further in Chap. 8.

NONPHARMACOLOGIC MANAGEMENT

In long-term treatment of insomnia, hypnotics should be given intermittently, rather than nightly, or as adjunctive therapy. For example, if chronic pain, depression, or dementia cause insomnia, hypnotics should be given as adjuncts to preferred treatment with analgesics, antidepressants, or major tranquilizers. Whenever possible, treatment should concentrate on the underlying condition, an attempt should be made to limit hypnotics to non-nightly use, and nonpharmacologic measures should be instituted.

Reassurance is an important tool in managing the elderly patient with insomnia, who may not realize that alterations in the sleep pattern can be normal and not harmful. An effort should be made to identify problems that may be disturbing sleep, such as anxiety, depression, urinary disturbances (often due to diuretic ingestion), nocturnal dyspnea, chronic pain syndromes, or other medical problems. Drugs that might disturb sleep, such as diuretics, certain antihypertensive agents, caffeine, bronchodilators, decongestants, and antiparkinsonian agents, should be discontinued or given early in the day if possible. Long-acting thiazide diuretics can sometimes be replaced by early-morning doses of shorter-acting furosemide. Patients should be encouraged to establish regular sleep patterns, however odd they may seem, and to maintain them. They should be encouraged to have regular exercise and may be helped by a late evening bath or snack. The sleeping environment, including lights, noise, ambient temperature, and bed, should be conducive to sleep. The bed should be used when the patient is sleepy; tossing and turning should take place somewhere else.

Patients who cannot sleep at night should be discouraged from taking hypnotics because they are bored but should be encouraged to adopt nighttime activities. They may be soothed by late night television, radio, or music. Those with visual disorders should have a complete ophthalmologic exam with low-vision evaluation if necessary. Large-print and "talking" books are widely available and may be very helpful to the anguished insomniac who might otherwise not be able to read himself to sleep.

In the nursing home, massage, warm bath, or traditional remedies such as hot milk, carbohydrate snack, and even placebo are safer alternatives than addicting drugs. Chronic low-dose hypnotic therapy often exerts a placebo effect on patients, and an actual placebo is probably safer and hence justified in carefully selected patients. Commonly, patients with dementia forget that they have already received their hypnotic, may stubbornly reject assurances to the contrary, and may be soothed by the administration of a placebo.

The patient with dementia is at high risk for falls and other complications of nocturnal sedatives. Whenever possible, the environment should be adjusted to fit the needs of the patient. Sleep-disturbed patients who require 24-hour home care are best managed by split-shift personnel, so that a night-shift caregiver can be awake to attend to the patient's needs. This is far better for the patient than the administration of a hypnotic so that the caregiver can sleep. In nursing homes, the staffing should be maximized and the schedule designed for the patients' waking hours. Unfortunately, fiscal realities make sufficient staffing difficult in many cases, but when making choices about treatment, it is important to ask whether the pharmacologic management is directed towards the patient or the caregiver.

BIBLIOGRAPHY

Arana, G.W., and Hyman, S.E. *Handbook of Psychiatric Drug Therapy.* (2nd ed.) Boston: Little, Brown, 1991.

Greenblatt, D.J., Harmatz, J.S., Shapiro, L., et al. Sensitivity to triazolam in the elderly. *N. Engl. J. Med.* 324:1691-1698, 1991.

Greenblatt, D.J., Shader, R.I., and Abernethy, D.R. Current status of benzodiazepines. *N. Engl. J. Med.* 309:354,410, 1983.

Howard, G.F. Management of chronic sleep disorders in the elderly. *Comp. Ther.* 13:3, 1987.

National Institute of Mental Health. Drugs and insomnia: The use of medications to promote sleep. *J.A.M.A.* 251:2410, 1984.

Patterson, J. Triazolam syndrome in the elderly. *South. Med. J.* 80:1425–1426, 1987.

Rizack, M.A., and Hillman, C.D.M. *The Medical Letter Handbook of Adverse Drug Interactions.* New Rochelle, N.Y.: The Medical Letter, 1989.

Salzman C. *Clinical Geriatric Psychopharmacology,* New York: McGraw Hill, 1984, pp. 132–170.

Sleep Disorders Classification Committee. Diagnostic classification of sleep and arousal disorders. *Sleep* 2:1, 1979–1980.

Antidepressants

DEPRESSION IN THE ELDERLY

The incidence of depression is very high in the elderly, and the consequences of untreated depression may include serious illness, inanition, institutionalization, and suicide. It is not always appreciated that the highest risk of suicide in the United States is in white men over the age of 60.

Antidepressant medication is one effective approach to treating depression in the elderly, although adverse effects develop more often in this age group and the consequences are potentially more severe. For this reason, it is important that depression be accurately diagnosed before the medication is prescribed. On the one hand, transient depression and sadness due to uncomplicated bereavement may respond to nonpharmacologic treatment such as supportive psychotherapy, and in most cases antidepressants need not be prescribed unless there are clear signs of major depression. These include "vegetative" symptoms such as weight loss, insomnia, impaired concentration, and psychomotor retardation.

On the other hand, depression in the elderly is often missed because it is masked, presenting as cognitive dysfunction or somatic symptoms such as chronic pain, gastrointestinal difficulties, or fatigue. Elderly patients tend to deny depressive symptoms more often than do younger people, and either do not seek treatment or continue to be depressed while they visit their primary care physician for physical ills. Major depression in the elderly may manifest as a dementialike illness sometimes referred to as *pseudodementia*, which can be tragically untreated if misdiagnosed. Not uncommonly, major depression in the elderly is accompanied by paranoia, delusions, and other "psychotic symptoms" that may confound the diagnosis. Finally, there are medical causes of depression that, if treated, may sometimes alleviate depressive symptoms (Table 8–1).

Supportive therapy can often be given successfully by the primary care physician, and antidepressant medication prescribed and monitored skillfully. However, if major depression or prolonged grief reaction is suspected, if depressive symptoms are complicated by suicidal thinking or psychotic symptoms, or if there is any doubt as to the diagnosis or the indication for pharmacotherapy, psychiatric consultation should be obtained. Hospitalization, vigorous psychopharmacological intervention, or intensive psychotherapy may be required for seriously impaired patients and electroconvulsive therapy may be required in patients who do not respond to these measures or in whom medical therapy is contraindicated.

The main purpose of this chapter is to familiarize the primary care physician with antidepressant medications in order to facilitate the identification of adverse effects and drug interactions.

ANTIDEPRESSANT MEDICATION

The tricyclic antidepressants (TCAs), monoamine oxidase inhibitors, (MAOIs), and newer antidepressants are thought to act by enhancing the action of the biogenic monoamines norepinephrine, serotonin, or dopamine. Since a minimum of 2 weeks must transpire before clinical effects are observed and up to 8 weeks before optimal

Table 8-1. Medical Causes of Depression

Medications
  Reserpine
  Methyldopa
  Beta blockers
  Clonidine
  Corticosteroids
  Anxiolytics
  Neuroleptics
Illnesses
  Hyper- or hypothyroidism
  Electrolyte disorders
  Uremia
  Cancer (pancreatic; brain; lung; other?)
  Stroke*
  Pernicious anemia
  Cerebral vasculitis
  Parkinson's disease*
  Congestive heart failure

*Though a medical cause of depression, generally requires treatment directed at the depression itself.

effect occurs, enhancement of these neurotransmitters is only one factor in the antidepressant action; however, this may initiate a cascade of events culminating in a delayed clinical effect. It is currently felt that an alteration in sensitivity of neurohormonal receptors occurs with time, resulting in an apparent normalization in the relationship between presynaptic release-inactivation processes and postsynaptic neurotransmission. It has also been suggested that repletion of deficient neurotransmitters such as serotonin takes place as a result of pharmacotherapy, and that this repletion takes several weeks to occur.

Psychostimulants such as the amphetamines exert their effect acutely and seem to have antidepressantlike effect. Although not considered standard antidepressant therapy, these agents are sometimes used in very old and debilitated individuals because of their relative safety and rapid onset of action.

SPECIFIC AGENTS

Tricyclic Antidepressants

Pharmacologic Considerations

MECHANISM OF ACTION. The tricyclic antidepressants (TCAs) are so named because of their three-ringed structure and antidepressant activity. One agent, maprotiline, has a four-ringed structure but is otherwise similar and is generally classified in this group. These agents are felt to exert antidepressant effect by increasing the availability of neurotransmitters such as norepinephrine, serotonin, and dopamine in the synaptic cleft, with a probable effect on postsynaptic neurotransmission as well. They also have potent central and peripheral anticholinergic (antimuscarinic) activity, and antagonize central H_1 and H_2 receptors, but it is not known to what extent these actions affect mood.

The TCAs, in particular those with strong seritoninergic properties, exert analgesic action in certain pain syndromes. This is believed to be at least partly independent of the antidepressant action, and may be related to the ability of these agents to inhibit the enzymatic degradation of enkephalin and to enhance serotonin at the synaptic cleft. Enhancement of serotonin and enkephalin is thought to block the afferent pain message.

PHARMACOKINETICS. All TCAs are well absorbed orally and are highly protein-bound. They undergo extensive hepatic extraction and are degraded in the liver by oxidative processes to active metabolites. In fact, imipramine is degraded to desmethylimipramine (desipramine) and amitriptyline to nortriptyline, both themselves clinically useful TCAs. Ultimately these metabolites are conjugated to inactive glucuronides and excreted by the kidney. The elimination half-lives of these agents approach or exceed 24 hours in nonelderly and may be as long as 4 days in elderly patients, possibly because of sluggish oxidative metabolism. At a given dose, plasma levels tend to be higher in older patients and steady state may not be reached for 20 days. At all ages, there is marked interindividual variation in plasma levels achieved at a given dose, which is probably a reflection of genetic variability in metabolic processes. This variability is further enhanced in older age groups.

Adverse Effects

Orthostatic hypotension occurs commonly with these agents, probably as a result of alpha adrenergic receptor blockade. Many elderly have baseline orthostatic hypotension due to factors such as venous insufficiency, and any additional compromise of this autoregulatory system could have significant consequences. Patients with impaired left ventricular function probably have an enhanced risk of developing orthostatic hypotension from TCAs.

The risk of orthostatic hypotension is greatest at night and the consequences in geriatric patients are potentially severe. These include falls, fractures, and ischemic events. It is important to educate all patients on precautionary maneuvers, which are most important when the patient gets out of bed in the middle of the night or in the morning. Orthostatic hypotension only occurs in a subgroup of patients and is probably not dose-related, but may occur even at low doses. The risk of this problem varies, depending on the agent used (see Table 8–2).

The importance of **other cardiovascular side effects** must be put in perspective. The TCAs have a quinidinelike action that results in slowed conduction through the electrical system, and suppression of ventricular and atrial ectopy. Heart block may occur in patients with underlying conduction abnormalities. However, ventricular and atrial arrhythmias are sometimes ameliorated at therapeutic doses. Although the literature alludes to sudden death from TCAs, and although tricyclic overdose can lead to dangerous arrhythmias, the potential for these agents to produce arrhythmias has probably been overstated. Judicious dosing and careful patient selection should minimize these problems (see Precautions).

Table 8-2. Characteristics of Commonly Used Antidepressants

Agent	Brand	Sedative	Anticholinergic	Orthostasis	Initial Dose (mg)
Tricyclic Antidepressants					
Amitriptyline	Elavil	3	3	2	10–25
Doxepin	Sinequan	3	2	2	10–25
Imipramine	Tofranil	2	2	3	10–25
Desipramine	Norpramin	1	1	1	10–25
Nortriptyline	Pamelor	2	1	1	10–25
Newer Antidepressants					
Maprotiline	Ludiomil	2	2	1	12.5–25
Amoxapine	Asendin	2	2	3	12.5–25
Trazodone	Desyrel	3	<1	1	25–50
Fluoxetine	Prozac	1	<1	1	5–10*
Bupropion	Wellbutrin	<1	<1	<1	100 bid
Monoamine Oxidase Inhibitors					
Phenelzine	Nardil	2	1	1	15
Tranylcypromine	Parnate	–	<1	–	10

<1 = Negligible
1 = Low
2 = Moderate
3 = High
*Currently available as 20-mg capsule and liquid; see text.

There is no evidence that TCAs worsen myocardial function when given in therapeutic doses.

Increased sinus heart rate may occur, particularly with strongly anticholinergic agents such as amitriptyline. Heart rate usually remains in the normal range, and is less likely to increase at all in the elderly, who tend to be less sensitive to the cardiac effects of atropine. However, this effect is of potential importance in the patient with ischemic heart disease.

Treatment with TCAs may be associated with nonspecific ST-T wave changes in the electrocardiogram.

Anticholinergic effects, partly mediated through blockade of receptors at muscarinic sites, are more common and potentially more severe in the elderly. These effects include constipation, urinary retention, dry mouth (xerostomia), and confusion. Xerostomia can increase the risk of dental caries, and, in the elderly who wear dentures, it can lead to gingival ulceration. Blurred vision due to impairment of accommodation is probably less noticeable in older individuals who already lack the ability to accommodate to close vision. However, acute angle closure glaucoma can occur in susceptible people.

If anticholinergic effects are mild they need not necessitate drug withdrawal. However, particularly troublesome effects such as gingival ulcers or fecal impaction require prompt and ongoing attention. If the drug produces urinary retention, dementia, or angle closure glaucoma, it must be discontinued.

Other side effects that may occur with TCAs include sedation, sleep disturbance, fatigue, visual hallucinations, sexual dysfunction, fine tremor, and weight gain. Since these symptoms can occur as a result of depression itself, a baseline delineation of symptoms is essential. TCAs can lower the seizure threshold and cause exacerbation of seizure disorders. Tinnitus and rash have also been reported.

TCA **overdose** may occur with lower-than-expected doses in the elderly. Symptoms of overdose include hypotension, delirium, hallucinations, fever, dry mucous membranes, dilated and poorly reactive pupils, tachy- and bradyarrhythmias, heart block, respiratory failure, cardiac failure, seizures, coma, and death. Moderate overdose may present with accentuation of anticholinergic effects discussed above. Treatment consists of appropriate supportive measures. Anticholinergic symptoms, delirium, and coma can be reversed with intravenous physostigmine. Great care must be observed when intravenous physostigmine is given to elderly patients because of its tendency to produce bradyarrhythmias.

Therapeutic Blood Monitoring

Most laboratories now perform serum or plasma levels of TCAs for clinical therapeutic monitoring. With the exception of nortriptyline, however, the utility of laboratory determinations is limited by the fact that there is inexact correlation between blood levels and clinical response. The TCAs are highly lipid-soluble and readily leave the plasma compartment, so that blood levels are often a poor reflection of tissue levels. In addition, blood levels are best measured after steady state has been attained. In older patients, this occurs later than for younger adults. A therapeutic level for one patient may be subtherapeutic or toxic for another. Also, there may be a significant inter-assay variability since these agents are present in extremely small concentrations in the blood. Certain drugs cross-react with the assays, yielding falsely high values for TCAs. Therapeutic monitoring has not been well studied at all in the elderly, and therapeutic ranges for these agents have not yet been determined.

Because of these difficulties, blood monitoring is not routinely performed, but is reserved for specific situations such as suspected overdose or noncompliance, to differentiate between symptoms of an underlying disorder versus a drug side effect, or to determine if an adequate trial has been given to a nonresponder before terminating treatment. In addition, patients with heart failure, renal disease, and hepatic insufficiency, or those taking potentially interacting drugs, may benefit from therapeutic drug monitoring. It is best to interpret blood levels with the assistance of the psychiatry consultant.

Important Drug Interactions

The TCAs may interact at the pharmacodynamic level with any agent that shares their effects, namely, sedative-hypnotics, anticholinergic agents, drugs that slow cardiac conduction, and myocardial depressants. The interaction with sedating barbiturates is more complicated, since these agents induce hepatic microsomal enzymes and accelerate the degradation of TCAs. Other enzyme inducers, such as anticonvulsants and rifampin, may have the same result. Agents that inhibit hepatic microsomal enzymes, such as estrogen and cimetidine, may precipitate TCA toxicity.

TCAs reverse the antihypertensive effect of guanethidine by blocking the amine pump responsible for its uptake. TCAs can also reverse the antihypertensive effect of clonidine and may do so on a central level. However, TCAs can potentiate the hypotensive effect of other antihypertensive agents, presumably by an additive effect.

By blocking the uptake of norepinephrine, TCAs markedly potentiate the hypertensive effects of sympathomimetic agents. They may also potentiate the adrenergiclike actions of thyroid hormone.

Although TCAs are rarely given together with MAOIs, an important drug interaction may occur for a week or more after MAOIs are discontinued; the syndrome resembles the adrenergic crisis that occurs when MAOIs are used with sympathomimetic agents (see below). The combination of TCAs and lithium has been reported to increase mania and tremor.

Contraindications

TCAs are contraindicated in states of urinary retention, angle closure glaucoma, and untreated high-degree atrioventricular block.

Precautions

Supine and upright blood pressure and heart rate should be monitored and EKG performed at baseline and 1–3 weeks after each dose increment. Conduction disease in the elderly is not always overt and conduction abnormalities may only occur periodically, so a normal baseline examination does not eliminate the need for these precautions. If a decision is made to administer TCAs to patients with pre-existing conduction system disease, no more than half the usual starting dose should be given initially and more frequent monitoring should be performed.

Indications

The TCAs are effective in major depressive illness, reducing dysphoria and vegetative symptoms. They may be indicated for the treatment of prolonged grief reactions (adjustment disorder or bereavement with depressive symptoms) unresponsive to psychotherapy, especially if suicidal thinking or severe vegetative symptoms are present. They are less effective if used alone in the management of depression complicated by psychotic symptoms (delusional depression); in this situation, TCAs are often given in conjunction with antipsychotic agents.

Sedating antidepressants given at night may ameliorate insomnia that is due to depression, and the insomnia itself improves as the drug begins to ameliorate the underlying depression, regardless of whether the drug is sedating. However, TCAs are not indicated in the treatment of uncomplicated insomnia. Their duration of action is inappropriately long for this indication, and their sedative effect is qualitatively similar to that provided by the phenothiazines, to which the TCAs are structurally related. This sedating action is perceived as unpleasant to nondepressed patients, and is commonly experienced the following day as an unpleasant "hangover."

Other Uses

TCAs are used in the treatment of panic disorder and other psychiatric syndromes, where they have been used effectively in geriatric patients. For further discussion of these specialized applications, the reader is referred to the Bibliography readings (see Arana & Hyman).

Certain chronic pain syndromes, with or without depression, may respond to TCAs. Conditions that sometimes respond include diabetic neuropathy, facial pain, arthritis, cervical and low back pain, headache, and postherpetic neuralgia. Cancer pain is less likely to respond. Analgesia may be obtained with doses lower than those used in depression, and generally with only a short delay. The seritoninergic agents amitriptyline, doxepin, and imipramine are the best studied and possibly most effective TCAs for this indication, but since they tend to be less well tolerated in elderly patients, other agents of this class are sometimes used.

Imipramine has been used for the management of urinary incontinence (see Chap. 23). Its efficacy has not been compared to other TCAs.

Selection of Specific Agent

The various TCAs differ qualitatively and quantitatively from one another in terms of seritoninergic, adrenergic, and cholinergic actions. However, the clinical application of these differences to various types of depression has not been precisely worked out and all TCAs seem to have equivalent antidepressant efficacy in adults of all ages. Thus, at the present time, selection of TCA is based on the need to treat secondary features or the need to avoid specific adverse effects. If the decision is made to use a TCA, it is generally prudent to avoid agents likely to produce anticholinergic effects or orthostatic hypotension (amitriptyline, imipramine) and initiate treatment with agents such as desipramine or nortriptyline. The presence of agitation or insomnia may call for a sedating agent, such as amitriptyline or the non-TCA trazodone, while the presence of a chronic pain syndrome might call for imipramine, doxepin, or amitriptyline. Protriptyline has an ultralong elimination half-life and should be avoided in this age group since any serious effects would disappear too slowly.

If there is no response after an adequate trial of desipramine or nortriptyline, which are considered relatively adrenergic, patients sometimes respond to agents that are qualitatively different, such as doxepin, maprotiline, or trazodone, or newer agents such as fluoxetine or bupropion.

Qualitative differences among the antidepressants are summarized in Table 8–2.

Dosing

Usual doses of antidepressants are summarized in Table 8–2.

Newer Agents

Since the advent of the classic TCAs, new agents have been developed that have attempted to minimize adverse effects that sometimes limit the use of their predecessors. These agents resemble the TCAs in some ways but differ in others. Some may be particularly applicable to geriatric patients while others add little.

Trazodone (Desyrel)

Trazodone differs structurally from the TCAs. It is a highly selective inhibitor of serotonin uptake in vitro and has minimal anticholinergic action.

Trazodone is rapidly absorbed when given without food and undergoes phase I metabolism in the liver to active and inactive products that are ultimately excreted in the kidney. The drug has an overall elimination half-life of 6–11 hours in nonelderly subjects, which is shorter than that of the TCAs, but which is perhaps twice as long in elderly individuals.

ADVERSE EFFECTS. Trazodone is **very sedating.** While oversedation may produce confusion in geriatric patients, this drug is otherwise less likely to produce dementia, hallucinations, and other adverse CNS effects than TCAs, perhaps because of its lack of anticholinergic action.

There are scattered reports of **cardiac arrhythmias** with trazodone use, including atrioventricular block, ventricular ectopy, and bradyarrhythmias. The significance of these reports, most of which are in older individuals, is not known. Overall, the drug is believed to be less cardiotoxic than TCAs. However, **hypotension** may occur with trazodone.

Priapism is a unique and unusual side effect of trazodone, and it has been reported in older individuals. Although this troublesome side effect is rare, some cases have resulted in permanent impotence. Concern over this problem has limited the use of trazodone.

INDICATIONS. Trazodone is indicated in the management of depression in patients who are expected to poorly tolerate the anticholinergic effects of TCAs.

Fluoxetine (Prozac)

Fluoxetine is a new antidepressant that has received a great deal of positive and negative publicity. Even more than trazodone, fluoxetine is a selective blocker of serotonin reuptake and has little or no effect on other neurotransmitter systems. It lacks anticholinergic activity and is much less sedating than trazodone.

The drug is well absorbed orally. One active metabolite has a half-life of more than 1 week. Pharmacokinetic study of this drug in the elderly is very limited.

Fluoxetine is highly protein-bound and has the potential of participating in additional drug interactions on this basis. Pharmacodynamic interactions have been reported with other psychotropic agents.

ADVERSE EFFECTS. Compared to TCAs, fluoxetine is associated with a higher incidence of **nausea, dyspepsia, loss of appetite, nervousness, agitation, insomnia,** and **headache.** These side effects appear to be particularly common in the elderly.

Fluoxetine may produce **modest weight loss** in patients being treated for depression, an effect that is perceived as desirable in the obese patient. The drug is less likely than TCAs to produce dry mouth, constipation, or sedation. It is less sedating than trazodone.

Fluoxetine slows the heart rate via a serotoninergic action at the level of the medulla. **Symptomatic bradycardia** as well as **orthostatic hypotension** have been reported rarely.

RECOMMENDATIONS. Fluoxetine shows promise in the treatment of depression in selected elderly patients because of its lack of sedative and anticholinergic effects. It is particularly suitable for the patient whose depression is complicated by fatigue but not for the patient with insomnia or agitation.

General recommendations regarding this agent in the elderly await further study. Presently, geropsychiatrists believe adverse effects can be minimized if initial doses are very small. As of the writing of this book, fluoxetine is only available as a 20-mg capsule and a liquid preparation. If the local pharmacy cannot prepare a small-dose capsule, the 20-mg dose can be given every other day if the capsule form is preferred.

Maprotiline (Ludiomil)

The structural configuration of maprotiline is that of a tricyclic antidepressant with a carbon bridge across its rings, and it is often referred to as a tetracyclic, but its properties are very similar to its tricyclic relatives. Limited study in elderly patients indicates that efficacy is comparable to that of other agents. Like the TCAs, it is lipophilic, highly protein-bound, and widely distributed. It is converted in the liver to pharmacologically active compounds. Maprotiline itself has a serum half-life averaging 2 days in young subjects; this is probably much longer in the elderly, making them subject to enhanced toxicity and great danger in case of overdose.

The potential side effects of maprotiline are roughly similar to those of other TCAs, owing to its pharmacologic profile. It has a somewhat higher tendency to cause **skin rash. Hallucinations** have been reported in elderly subjects taking ordinary doses.

The most highly publicized untoward effect of maprotiline has been its tendency to cause **seizures.** The incidence of seizures is low, and can be minimized if the daily dose does not exceed 200 mg; this dose cap probably should be lower in elderly patients, however. Maprotilene should not be given to patients with a history of seizures, nor should it be given in conjunction with agents known to lower the seizure threshold.

Because its ultralong half-life would lead to prolongation and possible enhancement of toxicity, maprotiline is not recommended as a first-line agent.

Amoxapine (Asendin)

Amoxapine is structurally related to loxapine, which is a potent antipsychotic agent, although it is considered a member of a separate subclass of TCAs, the dibenzoxazepines, and has predominantly antidepressant action. One of its active metabolites exerts antidopaminergic action and may be responsible for the fact that amoxapine has been reported to cause **parkinsonian symptoms,** including tardive dyskinesia, in elderly patients. Despite earlier claims that it has a lower risk of cardiotoxicity, it is not completely safe in this regard, but it is amoxapine's ability to produce parkinsonian side effects that has limited its use in this age group.

Bupropion (Wellbutrin)

Buproprion is unrelated to other available antidepressants and has a somewhat different pharmacologic profile. It has weak modulating effect on seritoninergic and dopaminergic systems but its exact mechanism of action is not known.

Bupriopion had been removed from the market in 1986 because it was found to have a higher likelihood than other antidepressants of producing **seizures.** This risk is dose-related but is greatest in people with a history of seizures, head trauma, or recent alcohol or benzodiazepine withdrawal. The seizure risk in the elderly is not known. After further study, the seizure risk was found to be rather low when dose precautions were followed, and the drug was reintroduced with stringent precautionary labeling.

Like fluoxetine, bupropion has a tendency to produce nervousness and agitation. Among the other reported side effects are nausea, constipation, weight loss, dry mouth, headache, insomnia, dizziness, and neuropsychiatric disturbances. Although this drug has not been extensively studied in geriatric patients, potential advantages over TCAs are that it does not possess significant anticholinergic effect, is less likely to produce orthostatic hypotension or sedation than TCAs, and does not produce cardiac conduction abnormalities. Whether it has advantages over fluoxetine remains to be seen.

IMPORTANT DRUG INTERACTIONS. Bupropion may be a hepatic enzyme inducer. For this reason, it is important to watch for reduced potency of concurrently administered drugs metabolized by that system. Likewise, other drugs that modulate bupropion's metabolic enzymes could alter its levels.

Monoamine Oxidase Inhibitors

Monoamine oxidase inhibitors (MAOIs) act by inhibiting monoamine oxidase, the nearly ubiquitous enzyme that degrades the biogenic amines. Antidepressant effect occurs in a delayed fashion as it does with other antidepressant agents. Monoamine oxidase levels may increase with age, making these agents theoretically applicable to the treatment of geriatric depression. Although MAOIs are effective antidepressant agents in the elderly, it has not been demonstrated that they are clearly superior to other agents.

Pharmacologic Considerations

The MAOIs are readily absorbed orally and are metabolized in the liver, peak levels occurring 2–4 hours after ingestion. Two MAOIs, phenelzine and isocarbamid, irreversibly deaminate monoamine oxidase; since new enzyme is not produced for up to 2 weeks, inhibition lasts for 2 weeks after the drug is out of the system. Thus, clinical effect outlasts the presence of the drug in plasma. A third member of this class of drugs, tranylcypromine, reversibly inhibits monoamine oxidase; it is structurally similar to amphetamine and exhibits a somewhat different clinical profile.

Adverse Effects

Like the TCAs, the MAOIs may cause **orthostatic hypotension.** This may occur as late as 4 weeks after initiation of therapy, necessitating continued blood pressure monitoring. The MAOIs are far more likely to cause **supine hypotension** than are the TCAs. Hypotension is believed to be due to inhibition of the normal breakdown of tyramine with enhanced production of a hydroxylated product that acts as a "false transmitter," impairing sympathetic outflow.

Although the MAOIs are said to lack anticholinergic activity, they have been reported to cause **confusion, dry mouth, constipation,** and **micturition difficulties** in some elderly patients. **Behavioral reactions** such as agitation and even psychotic symptoms have been reported in some patients being treated for depression. Tranylcypromine, which is structurally related to amphetamine, is more likely to produce agitative effects than the other MAOIs.

Some patients experience **drowsiness,** while others complain of **insomnia.** Altering timing of the dose may circumvent these problems, whether it is drug-related or due to the depression itself. Other adverse effects include **anorgasmia** or **impaired ejaculation.**

MAOIs do not impair cardiac conduction and can probably be used safely in patients with uncomplicated conduction system disease. Significant arrhythmogenicity and negative inotropy probably do not occur.

Important Drug and Food Interactions

Dietary tyramine can precipitate an adrenergic crisis in patients using MAOIs. A significant pressor response can occur if as little as 6 mg of tyramine is ingested, and 25 mg can result in hypertensive crisis. Severe headache, palpitations, stroke and even death are other potential consequences of this interaction. Tyramine is a precursor of the catecholamines, and dietary tyramine is normally degraded by monoamine oxidase in the liver and gastrointestinal tract. In the presence of MAOIs, tyramine levels are enhanced, and catecholamines can be displaced from presynaptic storage granules, enhancing their effect on alpha receptors.

A flurry of case reports in the early days of MAOI use prompted the imposition of severe dietary restrictions on patients taking these drugs. More experience has revealed that dietary restrictions can be limited to certain foods. However, the amounts of tyramine are highly variable, depending on processing and age of food, so that it is prudent to restrict entire categories of foods. Tyramine, which is produced by bacterial degradation of protein, is present to a greater or lesser extent in aged and fermented substances such as cheese, sausage meats, pickled herring, yogurt, alcoholic beverages, and any spoiled food. Cottage and cream cheese do not contain tyramine. Fava beans are restricted because the pods contain dopamine. Red wine, vermouth, beer, and ale often contain high levels of tyramine and must be avoided. Dietary restrictions must be observed for at

Table 8–3. Dietary Restrictions for MAOIs

Foods That Must Be Avoided
Cheese
Smoked or pickled fish
Chianti
Vermouth
Beer and ale
Banana peel
Fava beans
Sausage meats
Any meat that is not fresh
Brewer's yeast/yeast extracts
Meat extracts
Sauerkraut

Foods That Can Be Used Only in Limited Servings*
Other alcoholic beverages
Avocado
Raspberries
Soy sauce
Chocolate
Peanuts
Yogurt or sour cream if from unpasteurized sources

*Limited evidence that these pose a risk; standard precautions are that servings should not exceed ½ cup, 4 oz, or 120 ml.
Source: Adapted from McCabe.

least 1 day before, during, and for at least 2 weeks after taking MAOIs. A list of restricted foods is given in Table 8–3.

Concurrent use of the sympathomimetic agents such as amphetamine, methylphenidate, ephedrine, and phenylpropanolamine may result in hypertensive crisis or other symptoms as described above for the tyramine interaction. These sympathomimetic agents act by releasing neuronal stores of catecholamines and are more likely to adversely interact at that site with MAOIs than epinephrine itself, which is not fully dependent on monamine oxidase for its metabolic degradation. Many sympathomimetic agents are found in over-the-counter preparations, including cold medications, diet aids, nasal decongestants, bronchodilators, cough medicines, and eye drops, necessitating careful patient counseling. Sympathomimetic agents are often prescribed for urinary incontinence and respiratory disease and epinephrine eye drops are sometimes prescribed for glaucoma; the patient's other doctors must be informed of the drug regimen.

MAOIs may interact with sympatholytic antihypertensive agents, such as guanethidine, clonidine, methyldopa, and reserpine. Both hypotension and hypertension have occurred.

The combination of MAOIs with meperidine can cause a syndrome consisting of agitation, disorientation, alterations in blood pressure, tachycardia, hyperthermia, seizures, and muscle rigidity; it is believed to occur as the result of the combined seritoninergic effects of MAOIs and meperidine. This interaction does not seem to occur with other opioids with the possible exception of dextrome-thorphan, a mild antitussive with a similar seritoninergic action to meperidine. However, indirect evidence suggests that MAOIs may increase the potency of other narcotics.

MAOIs inhibit hepatic microsomal enzymes and may enhance the effect of drugs degraded by that system.

Contraindications

MAOIs are contraindicated in patients who are unwilling or unable to comply with a strict dietary-drug regimen.

Indications

MAOIs are indicated for the treatment of depression in patients who are unable to respond to or cannot tolerate TCAs or newer anti-depressants.

For a detailed discussion of the specialized use of MAOIs, the reader is referred to Arana & Hyman.

Is Alprazolam (Xanax) an Antidepressant?

Alprazolam is a benzodiazepine anxiolytic agent. It is structurally similar to the hypnotic agent triazolam but is less sedating. It has been claimed that alprazolam has intrinsic antidepressant activity independent of its ability to reduce anxiety. The mechanism of this putative antidepressant effect has been attributed to an increase in the sensitivity of postsynaptic serotonin receptors. However, most experts question these claims, pointing out that any benzodiazepine has the ability to provide initial symptomatic relief in depression.

The major drawbacks of alprazolam are those typical of the benzodiazepine class of drugs, namely the tendency to cause drows-iness, and the possibility of severe withdrawal syndromes after pro-longed use. Like other benzodiazepines, alprazolam lacks cardiac toxicity and anticholinergic activity. While alprazolam in particular has been used successfully in the management of classic panic disor-der, its use in the management of depression should be limited to adjunctive treatment, such as in the control of anxiety and insom-nia.

Benzodiazepines are discussed in Chaps. 6 and 7.

Psychostimulants (Amphetamine, Methylphenidate)

The psychostimulants were one of the earliest forms of pharmaco-therapy use for depression. Unfortunately, they have not been sub-jected to well-controlled studies. The use and study of these agents was all but abandoned with the advent of TCAs. Their reputation for efficacy in the treatment of depression comes from several flawed studies, and from widespread clinical use for a variety of psychiatric and behavioral disorders.

The agents in this group probably exert their effect by producing euphoria. They act by enhancing release and preventing reuptake of the catecholamines. It is doubtful that they are effective in depres-sion, but have been shown to increase attention, interest, and moti-vation in withdrawn, apathetic, and poorly motivated patients, par-ticularly those with dementia. The long-term efficacy in these settings has not been studied.

The psychostimulants are not approved for the treatment of de-pression by the FDA. However, they are often well tolerated by ger-iatric patients and have a different side-effect profile from other agents. They have been used occasionally in the treatment of refractory depression, and in patients whose underlying medical condition prohibits the use of other antidepressants.

Adverse Effects

The adverse effects of the psychostimulants are similar, differences being a matter of relative potency of the various agents. The most frequent adverse effects are **hypertension, headache, cardiac arrhythmia, nervousness, anorexia,** and **insomnia.** Psychostimulants can produce **psychotic symptoms** and **confusion,** and are more likely to do so in elderly patients. Excluding this type of confusional states, however, they are probably less likely than the TCAs to worsen dementia. Like other sympathomimetic agents, psychostimulants have the potential to precipitate **acute angle closure glaucoma.**

Drug interactions are similar to those that would be expected to occur with other adrenergic agents. Methylphenidate may participate in additional drug interactions, as discussed below.

Tolerance develops rapidly to certain effects, and the amphetamines and methylphenidate have significant abuse potential. They are best given in a controlled environment. Long-term use of the potent psychostimulants can result in a **withdrawal syndrome** consisting of depression, extreme fatigue, and increased appetite, so that these agents should be withdrawn gradually.

These drugs should not be used in patients with hypertension, ischemic heart disease, and tachyarrhythmias.

Specific Agents

D-AMPHETAMINE (DEXEDRINE, OTHERS). D-amphetamine is well absorbed, reaching peak plasma levels in 1–3 hours. It is metabolized in the liver, but a large portion is excreted unchanged in the kidney. The elimination half-life is 8–12 hours and is undoubtedly prolonged in elderly patients, although specific pharmacokinetic data are not available. Sustained-release preparations are available.

METHYLPHENIDATE (RITALIN). Methylphenidate is structurally related to amphetamine but is less potent. It is rapidly absorbed, reaching peak levels in 2 hours. It has an elimination half-life of approximately 2 hours in nonelderly adults but brain levels may persist a few hours longer.

Hepatic microsomal enzyme activity is inhibited by methylphenidate, so that it may enhance the action of drugs metabolized by that system.

The Place of Psychostimulants in Geriatrics

Psychostimulants are not ordinarily indicated in the management of depression. There may, however, be a place for these agents in the short-term management of apathetic or withdrawn patients, especially those with dementia, who are not candidates for conventional antidepressant treatment. Other antidepressants with stimulant activity, such as the MAOI tranylcypromine and the newer agent fluoxetine, would theoretically be useful in this setting, but there are no comparative studies.

There are no standard recommendations governing the use of psychostimulants in these situations. Doses used in studies of geriatric patients have ranged from 5–10 mg/day for d-amphetamine to 10–30 mg/day for methylphenidate.

BIBLIOGRAPHY

Arana, G.W., and Hyman, S.E. *Handbook of Psychiatric Drug Therapy.* (2nd ed.). Boston: Little, Brown, 1991.

Clark, A.N.G., and Manikikar, G.D. D-amphetamine in elderly patients refractory to rehabilitation procedures. *J. Amer. Geriatr. Soc.* 27:174–177, 1979.

Georgotas, A., McCue, R.E., Hapworth, W., et al. Comparative efficacy and safety of MAOIs versus TCAs in treating depression in the elderly. *Biol. Psychiatr.* 21:1155–1166, 1986.

Goldman, L.S., Alexander, R.C., and Luchins, D.J. Monoamine oxidase inhibitors and tricyclic antidepressants: comparison of their cardiovascular effects. *J. Clin. Psychiatr.* 47:225, 1986.

Kaplitz, S. Withdrawn, apathetic geriatric patients responsive to methylphenidate. J. Amer. Geriatr. Soc. 23:271–276, 1975.

McCabe, B.J. Dietary tyramine and other pressor amines in MAOI regimens: a review. *J. Amer. Diet. Assoc.* 86:1059–1064, 1986.

Rockwell, E., Lam, R.S., and Zisook, S. Antidepressant drug studies in the elderly. *Psychiatr. Clin. N. Amer.* 11:215, 1988.

Ruegg, R.G., Zisook, S., and Swerdlow, N.R. Depression in the aged: an overview. *Psychiatr. Clin. N. Amer.* 11:83, 1988.

Stauffer, J.D. Antidepressants and chronic pain. *J. Fam. Practice* 25:167–170, 1987.

Warner, M.D., Peabody, C.A., Whiteford, H.A., et. al. Alprazolam as an antidepressant. *J. Clin. Psychiatr.* 49:148–150, 1988.

Lithium

Mania is an uncommon cause of psychiatric illness among the elderly. However, whereas only a small proportion of individuals develop bipolar disorders in late life, others with earlier onset illness survive into late life and still others, who develop mania late in life, have had depressive episodes in the past. Recognition of these syndromes and their differentiation from other confusional disorders, including dementia, may pose diagnostic difficulties. These topics are discussed by Yassa et al. (see Bibliography).

Mania has been successfully treated in the elderly with lithium. Other agents, including neuroleptics and carbamazepine, are used adjunctively and are discussed elsewhere. This section is devoted specifically to the use of lithium (Eskalith, others).

PHARMACOLOGIC CONSIDERATIONS

Mechanism of Action

Lithium is a monovalent cation most often given as the carbonate compound. As demonstrated in human red blood cells, lithium is transported across cell membranes by several mechanisms. In one important system, it is transported into cells in exchange for sodium and is extruded from cells faster than sodium. In separate transport systems, lithium is exchanged for potassium or other intracellular cations. In the brain, lithium is believed to affect neurotransmitter systems through the "second messenger" phosphoinositide system. The fact that lithium has ameliorative effects on disparate behaviors, including mania, depression, and perhaps impulsivity, may be due to the fact that effects on the second messenger system lead to normalization of more than one neurotransmitter system.

Pharmacokinetics

Lithium is well absorbed from the upper small intestine. Absorption is delayed but not reduced by food intake. Lithium is almost entirely excreted via the kidney and is not bound to serum proteins. Approximately 80% is reabsorbed in the proximal convoluted tubule in competition with sodium; beyond the descending loop of Henle, the handling of lithium differs from that of sodium in that the former is excreted without undergoing further reabsorption.

Peak plasma levels are attained approximately 2–3 hours after ingestion of immediate-release forms of lithium carbonate. Lithium enters all body fluids and tissues, and equilibration with these compartments may occur slowly, so that excretion occurs slowly. Serum half-life varies proportionately with glomerular filtration rate; at initiation of treatment serum half-life is approximately 6–12 hours, but at steady state it is approximately 24 hours in nonelderly adults and reported to be 25%–50% longer in limited study of apparently healthy elderly. Half-life is further prolonged in the presence of frank renal insufficiency. Steady state is reached after 2–6 days when immediate-release lithium carbonate is given to patients with normal renal function, but may not be achieved for 7 days or more in elderly patients despite normal serum creatinine. The volume of distribution for lithium declines with age. All of these changes contribute to the fact that average steady-state serum lithium levels are higher at a given dose for elderly patients than for younger adults.

Lithium accumulates to varying degrees in many organs. Relative to its concentration in serum, concentration in thyroid gland may be 2 times, in bone up to 1½ times, and in salivary gland 6 times that in serum.

ADVERSE EFFECTS

Lithium frequently produces **thirst**. Although indirect evidence suggests that this could be partly a form of central **polydipsia** due to altered osmoreceptor sensitivity, lithium is known to produce a urinary concentrating defect and may produce **polyuria** with polydipsia on this basis. This is considered a functional defect of the distal tubule and is due to impaired renal response to vasopressin (nephrogenic diabetes insipidus), with polyuria generally subsiding when lithium is discontinued. This mechanism contrasts with alterations that occur early on in lithium therapy, when there is natriuresis and isotonic water loss; this resolves within days as compensatory mechanisms enhance renal sodium conservation. The status of sodium balance after long-term lithium therapy is uncertain.

Potentially serious consequences of the lithium-induced concentrating defect are **dehydration** and **hypernatremia**. Dehydration, in turn, can increase the risk of lithium toxicity. Normal elderly not taking lithium may have impaired thirst in response to dehydration, making it theoretically possible that those on lithium would be at increased risk of developing clinically significant dehydration. In those with central nervous system disease, the risk could be even greater.

Lithium enhances potassium excretion and may produce **hypokalemia**.

There is some evidence that long-term lithium use leads to irreversible renal problems, such as a progressive decline in glomerular filtration rate (GFR) or a permanent concentrating defect. Although specific histopathology has been described, the effect of long-term lithium use on renal function is controversial, and normal GFR after years of lithium ingestion has been documented. **Toxic overdose** has been reported to produce **acute renal failure** due to acute tubular necrosis. Other signs and symptoms of lithium toxicity are described below.

Diuretics such as thiazides and amiloride may ameliorate lithium-induced polyuria. The mechanism involves sodium diuresis, leading to decreased extracellular volume, reduction in GFR, decreased distal delivery of solute and water, with compensatory enhanced reabsorption of sodium and water proximally. Unfortunately, thiazides, but not amiloride, also enhance lithium reabsorption and lithium toxicity may result.

Lithium is associated with salivary gland atrophy. After several months of use, up to 70% of nonelderly patients complain of **dry mouth**. This problem may lead to an increase in dental caries and is potentially a more serious problem among the elderly. **Impaired taste acuity** has also been reported.

Nausea, vomiting, and diarrhea are dose-related side effects that may occur, especially at initiation of treatment.

Lithium inhibits the secretion of thyroid hormone from the thyroid gland and prolonged use has been associated with clinical **hypo-**

thyroidism. There is some evidence that the risk increases with age over 40 years and is highest in women. Since the incidence of primary hypothyroidism in general is highest in this group and increases further with advancing age, the risk of lithium-associated hypothyroidism may well increase in the later decades of life. Hypothyroidism seen after chronic lithium treatment is sometimes confused clinically with retarded depression, which must be distinguished from depression experienced by bipolar patients.

Chronic suppression of thyroid hormone secretion by lithium may lead to **euthyroid goiter.** This phenomenon has also been observed early in therapy and has later resolved. There is no evidence that lithium produces hyperthyroidism, and it could theoretically delay the onset of the disease in those who are predisposed.

Lithium reduces urinary calcium excretion and rarely has been associated with the development of **hyperparathyroidism** with **hypercalcemia.** Although the association with hyperparathyroidism cannot be discounted, a cause-and-effect relationship has not been firmly established, and the appearance of hypercalcemia could indicate an unmasking of preexisting disease by lithium. Hypercalcemia does not necessarily require the discontinuation of lithium, but if noted in the course of treatment it requires further investigation. Furthermore, hypercalcemia of any origin can produce a variety of cognitive and psychiatric disturbances and, in the setting of lithium therapy, these symptoms could be mistaken for a poor therapeutic response.

Some patients on lithium may experience **weight gain.** The reason for this is not known.

A variety of **skin rashes** have been reported, including exacerbation of psoriasis.

Lithium may affect cardiac conduction and is known to be associated with **electrocardiographic abnormalities,** most typically T-wave flattening similar to that seen in patients with hypokalemia. These abnormalities are felt to be related to intracellular flux of lithium and alteration in uptake of other ions by myocardial cells. Lithium has also been reported to produce **cardiac arrhythmias,** including sinus bradycardia, sinus arrest, and ventricular ectopy. Although these reports are rare, the problem has been largely described in older patients.

Lithium may produce **tremor,** which is clinically similar to benign essential tremor. This effect can be dose-related and appears to be more common in older individuals.

Lithium toxicity is generally manifested by **neurologic symptoms** such as ataxia, confusion, tremor, muscle twitching, seizures, stupor, and coma. **Confusional states, impaired memory,** and other neurologic or neuropsychiatric symptoms may occur at lower-than-expected serum levels, particularly in elderly patients.

As mentioned above, another serious consequence of overdose may be acute renal failure.

IMPORTANT DRUG AND NUTRIENT INTERACTIONS

Because lithium is handled by the kidney to a certain extent in a similar manner as sodium, drugs that alter sodium balance may alter lithium clearance. In general, drugs that produce natriuresis at the level of the distal nephron reduce lithium clearance and can increase lithium levels. A most important group, the thiazides, do this by interfering with distal tubular reabsorption of sodium, leading to a compensatory increase in proximal reabsorption of sodium, and along with it, lithium. These agents can reduce lithium excretion by 25%–50% in nonelderly adults and toxicity may occur if dose adjustments are not made. Drugs that exert a natriuretic effect elsewhere, such as furosemide, do not have this effect and are believed to produce no net change in serum lithium levels. The diuretic acetazolamide and presumably other carbonic anhydrase inhibitors, which are commonly prescribed for glaucoma, tend to increase lithium clearance and may decrease serum levels. Reports of interactions with other diuretics have been inconsistent; caution is advised when any diuretic is given in conjunction with lithium.

Nonsteroidal anti-inflammatory agents reduce renal lithium clearance, raising lithium levels. The effect seems to vary among various NSAIDs, being greatest with indomethacin and reportedly minimal with sulindac and aspirin; however, individuals vary in their response to this potential drug interaction, so that it is prudent to monitor lithium levels when any agent of this group is given. The mechanism has not been well defined but is felt to be related to impaired renal excretion of lithium.

Because lithium and sodium compete for proximal tubular reabsorption, a reduction in dietary sodium intake can increase the reabsorption of lithium and lead to increased lithium levels. Renal conservation of sodium may be impaired in late life, but the implications of this vis-à-vis lithium reabsorption are not known.

There is controversy surrounding whether there is a drug interaction between lithium and neuroleptics such as haloperidol and thioridazine, which are commonly used in combination with lithium in the management of mania. Extrapyramidal syndromes have been described in lithium-treated patients taking neuroleptics, but it is uncertain if these situations are due to the combination or the neuroleptic alone. It is prudent, nonetheless, to observe for neurotoxicity when the agents are used together.

There are scattered reports of interactions between lithium and calcium-channel blocking agents. Diverse reactions, including nausea, vomiting, and neurologic symptoms, as well as decreased lithium effect, have been reported to occur. The mechanism of this possible interaction is speculative and has been attributed to modulation of calcium in neuroregulatory processes.

Other potential interactions are summarized in Table 9–1.

PRECAUTIONS

Changes in sodium intake should prompt examination of serum lithium levels. The patient should be counseled to report any new dietary habits.

Thyroid function tests, including serum level of thyroid-stimulating hormone (TSH), should be performed at baseline and periodically.

Baseline EKG should be performed so that the use of lithium does not produce diagnostic difficulties in the elderly, in whom unrelated cardiac pathology is common.

Because of the risk of dehydration, lithium-treated patients require extra vigilance in certain situations. In the pre- and perioperative period, they should receive monitoring of electrolyte and fluid status; preoperative hydration may be required. Gastrointestinal

Table 9–1. Some Important Drug Interactions with Lithium

Agent	Effect
Thiazide diuretics	Increased lithium level
Furosemide	Inconsistent change in lithium level
Acetazolamide	Decreased lithium level
Phenytoin	Enhanced lithium effect
Nonsteroidal anti-inflammatory agents	Increased lithium levels (variable; see text)
Methyldopa	Enhanced lithium effect
Theophylline	Decreased lithium level
Iodine	Enhanced thyrotropic effect of lithium (may result in hypothyroidism)
Metronidazole	Increased lithium level
Tetracycline	Increased lithium level
Neuroleptics	Possible enhanced effect of lithium or neuroleptic
Tricyclic antidepressants	Increased mania, increased tremor
Carbamazepine	Increased neurotoxic symptoms
Calcium channel blockers	Scattered reports; see text

disturbances, fever, and exposure to high ambient temperatures also predispose to dehydration, altered sodium metabolism, and lithium toxicity. Renal function and serum electrolytes should be evaluated in these high-risk situations and periodically at other times.

INDICATIONS
The chief geriatric indications for lithium are acute mania and prophylaxis in recurrent bipolar disorders. Lithium is also used in certain subgroups of patients with unipolar depression.

LITHIUM LEVELS IN THE ELDERLY
The therapeutic range for maintenance lithium is the subject of debate. Standard recommendations are that the steady-state level should be maintained between 0.6 and 1.2 mEq/liter. However, some patients may be well controlled at lower levels, while others may develop toxicity when serum level is under 1.0 mEq/liter. It has been frequently recommended that the standard therapeutic range be adjusted downward for elderly patients, who are believed to exhibit heightened sensitivity to lithium, as manifested by a therapeutic or a toxic response at lower-than-expected serum levels. However, there is controversy over whether this phenomenon, when it occurs, is pharmacodynamic or due to age-dependent pharmacokinetic changes, and whether it is observed mainly in subgroups of frail elderly, specifically, those with dementia or other central neurological impairments.

As with all age groups, lithium levels should be interpreted with caution. In general, serum lithium should be maintained at the lowest possible level to prevent relapse, and in elderly patients serum levels above 0.8 mEq/liter should be avoided unless doses producing these concentrations are essential for symptom control.

If possible, serum lithium level should be measured at the trough, approximately 12 hours after the latest dose or immediately before the next dose. A morning fasting sample is often convenient for this purpose. The 12-hour serum lithium concentration is subject to the least amount of interpatient variability in all adults, including the elderly.

When initiating therapy or when changing dosage, it is important to keep in mind that since steady-state levels may not be achieved in older individuals for 7 days or longer, more frequent therapeutic monitoring at such times may be misleading.

DOSING

Initial dose: 150–300 mg bid.

Usual daily maintenance dose: 600–1200 mg in 2 or 3 divided doses, depending on serum lithium levels and clinical response. From a pharmacokinetic standpoint a bid schedule is generally sufficient. If gastric irritation occurs, a tid or qid schedule can be used.

Dose increments: Dose increases should generally not be made more frequently than once a week because of the tendency for steady state to be reached more slowly in aged patients. In frail patients or those with cardiovascular problems, dose increments should not exceed 150 mg.

Note: Dose should be further reduced in frank renal insufficiency. Sustained-release preparations are available; these are designed for bid administration and may be suitable for patients who cannot tolerate side effects related to rapid attainment of peak serum levels. Many elderly are adequately managed on bid dosing of immediate-release forms but sustained-release preparations could facilitate compliance in individual patients.

BIBLIOGRAPHY

Gelenberg, A.J., Carroll, J.A., Baudhuin, M.G., et al. The meaning of serum lithium levels in maintenance therapy of mood disorders: a review of the literature. *J. Clin. Psychiatr.* 50 (12, Suppl.): 17–22, 1989.

Himmelhoch, J.M., Neil, J.F., May, S.J., et al. Age, dementia, dyskinesias, and lithium. *Am. J. Psychiatr.* 137:941–945, 1980.

Rizos, A.L., Sargenti, C.J., and Jeste, D.V. Psychotropic drug interactions in the patient with late-onset depression or psychosis. Part 2. *Psychiatr. Clin. N. Amer.* 11:253–277, 1988.

Transbol, I., Christiansen, C., and Baastrup, P.C. Endocrine effects of lithium. I. Hypothyroidism, its prevalence in long-term treated patients. *Acta Endocrinol.* 87:759–767, 1978.

Yassa, R., Nair, N.P.V., and Iskandar, H. Late-onset bipolar disorder. *Psychiatr Clin N Amer.* 11:117–131,1988.

Antiparkinsonism Agents

Parkinson's disease is an idiopathic degenerative disease of the nigrostriatal system resulting in central dopamine deficiency, with decreases in norepinephrine, serotonin, and gamma amino butyric acid (GABA), and a functional increase in acetylcholine. Classic manifestations of Parkinson's disease are tremor, bradykinesia, and muscle rigidity. Other features include dysphagia with drooling, stooped posture, dysarthria, constipation, slowness of response, muscle aches from rigidity, micrographia, microphonia, progressive immobility, depression, and dementia. In general, treatment is palliative and does not slow the course of the disease, which eventually results in severe debility. New therapies, including tissue transplantation and recently released drugs, may be found to alter this poor prognosis, but more study is required.

Idiopathic Parkinson's disease is mostly a disease of the elderly, increasing greatly in incidence after age 55. Certain symptoms of classic Parkinson's disease are also seen in other disease states and are loosely referred to as *parkinsonism* or *Parkinson syndrome*. The most common cause of parkinsonism in the elderly is that due to drugs with dopamine antagonist activity, notably neuroleptic agents and metoclopramide. Less common causes include neurotoxic agents, head trauma (punch-drunk syndrome), Wilson's disease, and unusual neurodegenerative diseases that can mimic Parkinson's disease. Parkinsonism rarely occurs as a result of localized brain damage from atherosclerotic ischemia or tumor. Postencephalitic parkinsonism developed as a result of the great influenza pandemic of 1916, and is a unique example of an infectious agent causing Parkinson's disease. Only a few parkinsonian patients from this epidemic are living today.

DRUG TREATMENT

Medical treatment reduces symptoms of Parkinson's disease but, with the possible exception of selegiline (see below), has not been found to alter the inevitable neurologic outcome of the disease. In general, the agents in use do not prevent or reverse dementia and have little or no effect on depression, both of which may be endogenous features of the disease. Other symptoms, such as dysphagia, constipation, urinary disturbances, and confusion, are common in elderly parkinsonian patients and are often not improved and may be worsened or precipitated by medications used to treat the disease.

Drug therapy consists of correcting dopamine deficiency by replacing dopamine (levodopa, levodopa with carbidopa), stimulating postsynaptic dopamine receptors (bromocriptine, pergolide), augmenting endogenous levels of dopamine (amantadine, selegiline [deprenyl]), and reducing functional excess of acetylcholine (anticholinergic agents). Since the respective pharmacology of these agents differs, they are often used together for added benefit, but their toxicity may be additive as well. All agents have a high degree of central nervous system (CNS) toxicity, which is believed to be generally reversible. However, it is often hard to distinguish drug effect from disease, particularly when the symptom seems to persist after the drug is withdrawn.

Antiparkinsonian drugs should be instituted at low doses and increased gradually, with maintenance dose kept at the lowest effective level. This is particularly important for geriatric patients and for those being given other antiparkinsonian agents concurrently. All agents must be withdrawn gradually in order to avoid sudden exacerbation of parkinsonian symptoms.

SPECIFIC AGENTS

Levodopa; Carbidopa-levodopa Combination (Sinemet)

Pharmacologic Considerations

Levodopa (L-dihydroxyphenylalanine; L-Dopa) is a naturally occurring amino acid that itself has little or no pharmacologic effect but that exerts its action through its most important metabolite, dopamine. Levodopa is converted to dopamine by dopa decarboxylase (DDC), a pyridoxine-dependent enzyme that exists widely in the gastrointestinal tract, liver, and CNS. Levodopa enters the CNS only when present in the peripheral circulation at very high concentrations because it is rapidly converted in the periphery to dopamine, which does not cross the blood-brain barrier.

Peripheral conversion of levodopa to dopamine occurs primarily in the stomach. Unconverted levodopa is rapidly absorbed in the small intestine by an active transport system for the aromatic amino acids. There is wide interindividual variation in absorption, with peak plasma levels occurring between 30 minutes and 4 hours after oral administration. Levodopa undergoes saturable first-pass metabolism, so that it is possible to overwhelm the supply of peripheral DDC with large enough doses of levodopa. However, even at the highest tolerated doses, less than 5% of orally administered levodopa enters the brain.

Bioavailability of levodopa is decreased by concurrent ingestion of protein foods, delayed gastric emptying, and gastric hyperacidity. Absorption of levodopa is increased threefold in elderly subjects despite the fact that achlorhydria as well as delayed gastric emptying frequently exist. This enhanced absorption may be due to an age-related decrease in gastric DDC with the result that more unmetabolized levodopa is presented to the small intestine for absorption. Nonetheless, plasma half-life of levodopa, roughly 30–60 minutes, does not increase with age.

Bioavailability of levodopa is also diminished by vitamin preparations containing even small amounts of pyridoxine (B_6), but this effect does not occur when levodopa is given in combination with a DDC inhibitor as Sinemet (see below). Other bioavailability problems are modulated by this maneuver as well.

The doses required for therapeutic amounts of levodopa to enter the CNS produce high blood levels of dopamine and other levodopa metabolites, resulting in a high incidence of untoward dopamine-induced side effects. Thus, levodopa is almost always given with a peripheral DDC inhibitor, in this country as Sinemet. This combination therapy reduces the amount of levodopa required by 75% without sacrificing CNS penetration or central conversion to active dopamine.

Carbidopa does not cross the blood-brain barrier and exerts no pharmacologic effects when given alone. Toxicity has not been reported, so that there is currently no rationale for instituting levodopa alone except in patients known to be hypersensitive to carbidopa. Peripheral DDC tends to decrease with age, so elderly patients may do well on combinations containing low ratios of carbidopa to levodopa.

When to Begin Therapy

Controversy exists over whether treatment with levodopa should begin early or late in the course of the disease. Despite theoretical and laboratory evidence that chronic therapy with levodopa is self-limiting and possibly harmful, there is no direct evidence that it hastens clinical deterioration. In fact, chronic levodopa therapy could improve longevity by prolonging functional independence. There is no evidence that the effect of levodopa is finite; it may exert some effect even in the terminal stages of Parkinson's disease. For these reasons, many argue that levodopa should be started as early as needed.

In contrast, others argue that levodopa should be withheld early on. An early dramatic response will eventually give way to diminished response to therapy and troublesome side effects. Withholding therapy for a while might give the patient time to learn about the disease, and would give the physician time to learn about the effect of the disease on the patient's life-style.

In general, it is felt that therapy with levodopa should be started when the patient's symptoms interfere significantly with occupational or social functioning, or activities of daily living. Recent evidence indicates that early use of another drug, selegiline, may delay the need for levodopa (see below).

Adverse Effects

Side effects of levodopa are essentially those produced by dopamine. The incidence of peripheral side effects when levodopa is given in combination with carbidopa is strikingly lower than when levodopa is given alone. However, toxicity due to central dopamine effects is enhanced.

Levodopa may produce **gastrointestinal disturbances**. This may be due to a direct irritative effect on the gastrointestinal tract and gastritis can occur. More commonly, peripheral dopamine can induce nausea and vomiting by stimulating the chemoreceptor trigger zone in the area postrema, which lies outside the blood-brain barrier. Although these symptoms may limit therapy in some patients, they are diminished by reduction of dosage or by increasing the ratio of carbidopa to levodopa, and they often resolve over time.

Abnormal involuntary movements (dyskinesias) affect up to 80% of patients at some time during the course of treatment with levodopa. Dyskinesias are reversible, dose-related, and increasingly likely to occur with duration of therapy. Chorea and athetosis are the most common features; ballismus and myoclonus may also occur. Dyskinesias affect the head, trunk, lower face, neck, or extremities. Often such symptoms are more disturbing to family members or other observers than to patients themselves. Patients may actually feel quite well while experiencing dyskinesias, which tend to occur at the time of peak levodopa effect when disabling parkinsonian symptoms are minimal. However, movement disturbances may cause problems with the teeth, gums, and cervical spine. Respiratory and abdominal muscles may be affected and dyspnea and abdominal discomfort may result. Dystonia, an occasional form of dyskinesia, may cause pain or be in itself disabling.

Neuropsychiatric disturbances, including acute confusional states, toxic psychoses, hallucinations, drowsiness, nightmares, insomnia, delirium, delusions, or agitation, occur commonly. These symptoms are generally dose-related, and are of mild to moderate severity, but stupor and coma have been reported. These symptoms are to a large extent reversible, but occasionally appear to be irreversible. In such cases it is difficult to know how much is medication effect and how much is due to the disease itself. Cognitive disturbances are more common in the elderly, in patients with advanced Parkinson's disease, and in those with existing dementia.

Levodopa, but not dopamine, is a precursor in the synthesis of melanin and has occasionally been reported to **increase the growth of melanomas.** For this reason, the parkinsonian patient with melanoma should preferably be treated with agents other than levodopa.

Orthostatic hypotension is common but tolerance develops over time. Older patients often have underlying orthostatic hypotension due to venous insufficiency or impaired baroreceptor reflexes and are at higher risk. Symptomatic postural hypotension can be managed with patient education, by slowing dose increments, and with use of elastic stockings. In severe cases, low doses of fluorohydrocortisone have been given. The reason for orthostatic hypotension is unclear, but it may in some way be mediated through dopamine, which, at low concentrations, can produce vasodilation.

Although dopamine is a metabolic precursor to epinephrine and norepinephrine, and is itself a beta agonist, tachyarrhythmias occur only rarely in conjunction with levodopa administration. Even these cases are difficult to link directly to levodopa since many elderly have underlying cardiac disease, but vigilance is required.

Response Fluctuations

Although the dose-response of levodopa is generally satisfactory early in the disease, with symptomatic improvement lasting 12 hours or more after a small dose, favorable response wanes as the disease progresses. Although higher doses of levodopa have been instituted, response fluctuations occur and may become severe over time. These fluctuations take two forms. The "end-of-dose" or "wearing off" effect is a relatively predictable phenomenon characterized by the return of parkinsonian symptoms between doses, often worse the first thing in the morning. This is probably due to disease progression, resulting in the inability of the striatum to store exogenous dopamine. The end-of-dose effect can be managed by reducing the interval between doses, by giving the first dose of levodopa before arising, or by postponing the last evening dose, but without increasing the total daily dose.

The "on-off" phenomenon is characterized by rapid improvement shortly after the dose is given ("on") followed by the sudden resumption of symptoms at unpredictable intervals ("off"). This disabling phenomenon is less common than the end-of-dose effect and less well understood. It has been attributed to changes in levodopa kinetics coupled with entry of dopamine into the brain, which has lost its ability to store dopamine; alternatively, it may be caused by toxic metabolites of levodopa, which are preferentially produced in the deranged neuronal environment of advanced disease. The on-off phenomenon is managed by close observation of the patient to see if any pattern emerges, by reducing the interval between doses, and by administering levodopa at a fixed period in relation to meals. Adjustments in the medication regimen, such as cautious institution of bromocriptine or amantadine, may smooth out the dose-response curve.

Important Drug Interactions

Levodopa may worsen orthostatic hypotension produced by a variety of drugs, typically antihypertensive agents. Tricyclic antidepressants, which have a tendency to produce orthostatic hypotension, may actually lead to hypertension when given with levodopa.

Levodopa should not be given with monoamine oxidase inhibitors (MAOIs) because of the possibility of producing a hypertensive crisis. This interaction does not occur with ordinary doses of the selective MAOI selegiline, which is used for Parkinson's disease (see below).

Neuroleptic agents, which are potent dopamine antagonists, may counteract the efficacy of levodopa.

Contraindications and Precautions

Levodopa is contraindicated in patients with malignant melanoma or psychosis. It should be used cautiously in patients with unstable cardiac disease. Some experts caution that levodopa should not be used in patients with narrow angle glaucoma.

Dosing

Levodopa should be instituted as carbidopa-levodopa (Sinemet) unless the patient is known to be hypersensitive to carbidopa.

Carbidopa-levodopa is available in fixed ratios of 1:10 (Sinemet 10/100 or 25/250) and 1:4 (Sinemet 25/100). One tablet of Sinemet 10/100 is therapeutically equivalent to levodopa 400 mg given alone. **Initial dose:** Sinemet 10/100, ½ to 1 tablet bid. Dose increases should be made by increments of ½ to 1 tablet at 7–14 day intervals. The smallest effective dose should be given. Conservative dosing is appropriate in very elderly, debilitated, or demented patients because of the risk of neuropsychiatric and cardiovascular toxicity. **Maximum dose:** Sinemet 25/250 every 2 hours up to 8 tablets daily if tolerated. **Note:** Patients requiring treatment in the high dose range are generally receiving additional antiparkinsonian drugs. **These regimens are best prescribed in consultation with the neurologist.**

Additional carbidopa is occasionally needed as a noncombination preparation when individual dose titrations of levodopa and carbidopa are required. Peripheral DDC is saturated by carbidopa at total daily doses of 70–100 mg and there may be little gained by giving more. Daily doses of carbidopa over 200 mg should be avoided since the consequences of such dosing are not known.

Amantadine (Symmetrel)

Pharmacologic Considerations

MECHANISM OF ACTION. Amantadine is a stable hydrocarbon that was originally used as an antiviral agent and was found to have antiparkinsonian activity. It acts by releasing dopamine from intact central dopaminergic terminals and may delay reuptake of dopamine by neuronal cells. It also possesses anticholinergic action, which may contribute more to its toxicity than to its efficacy in

Parkinson's disease. In addition, amantadine has central noradrenergic actions and may produce mild amphetaminelike effects.

Amantadine is more effective than anticholinergic agents (see below), but less effective than levodopa. It is more effective in reducing bradykinesia and rigidity than tremor. It may act synergistically with levodopa and is often used with it.

PHARMACOKINETICS. Amantadine is rapidly absorbed from the gastrointestinal tract. Peak levels are attained within 2–4 hours, with maximum tissue levels occurring at around 48 hours. The average serum half-life is roughly 15 hours in the nonelderly, but the drug does not undergo significant metabolism and is excreted unchanged in the urine. Consequently, the serum half-life may be up to twice as long in geriatric patients.

Adverse Effects

Central nervous system effects are generally transient, reversible, and milder than with levodopa. Confusion, difficulty thinking, lightheadedness, hallucinations, anxiety, and insomnia are the most common of these side effects and are more likely to occur when the drug is given in conjunction with other antiparkinsonian agents. Amantadine has been reported to exacerbate seizure disorders but this is very unusual at ordinary doses.

Livedo reticularis and dependent edema may occur and are thought to be related to peripheral effects of released vasoactive neurotransmitters. Liver function abnormalities have also been reported with extended use of the drug. Owing to its anticholinergic effects, amantadine may produce urinary retention, constipation, and other atropinelike symptoms.

Cardiac arrhythmias have been reported rarely but should be considered as a potential risk in susceptible elderly.

As with other agents used for Parkinson's disease, side effects of the drug may be similar to symptoms of the disease itself and may appear to be irreversible when the drug is discontinued.

Important Drug Interactions

Amantadine may potentiate neuropsychiatric toxicity of other antiparkinsonian drugs and other centrally acting agents. It can potentiate the peripheral as well as central toxicity of anticholinergic agents. Caution should be observed when these agents are used together.

Amantadine has been reported to produce hypertension when used with MAOI antidepressant drugs.

Contraindications and Precautions

Amantadine should be used with extreme caution in patients with liver disease, or with a history of psychosis or urinary retention. Amantadine should not be given to patients with angle closure glaucoma.

Indications

Amantadine is indicated as adjunctive therapy in Parkinson's disease. It is frequently used in conjunction with levodopa to reduce the severity of symptoms during "off" periods. It is also useful as first-line monotherapy in selected patients with mild parkinsonism and is considered preferable to anticholinergic agents in this regard since it has a better therapeutic index. Unfortunately, certain patients treated with amantadine have an initial dramatic response that seems to wane after a few weeks to months, leaving them with only partial improvement. The reason for this is not known.

Amantadine has been used with varying success in the management of drug-induced parkinsonism. Its use in influenza is discussed in Chap. 32.

Dosing

Initial dose: 100 mg/day once or in 2 divided doses.
Note: Some patients may only tolerate smaller doses (i.e., 50 mg). A liquid preparation is available and can be used for this purpose.
Maximum dose: 100 mg bid. Some patients may benefit from higher doses.

Dose increments should be no greater than 50–100 mg total daily dose, and should be made after a minimum of 1 week.

Bromocriptine (Parlodel)

Pharmacologic Considerations

MECHANISM OF ACTION. Bromocriptine is a derivative of the ergot alkaloid lysergic acid, but is pharmacologically quite dissimilar. Bromocriptine is strongly dopaminergic. It acts by stimulating postsynaptic dopamine receptors in the corpus striatum, although some intact presynaptic substantia nigra neurones are probably required for its action.

PHARMACOKINETICS. Bromocriptine is rapidly absorbed from the gastrointestinal tract, reaching peak plasma concentrations within 1–3 hours. It is extensively metabolized in the liver, largely to inactive substances, with only small amounts excreted unchanged in the urine. Bromocriptine's duration of action (8–12 hours) outlasts its short plasma half-life of 3 hours, presumably because its effect is at the level of the dopamine receptor. The drug accumulates over time.

The average age of parkinsonian patients treated with bromocriptine is over 60 years, but the drug has not been specifically investigated in the very aged. At all ages, however, parkinsonian patients vary widely in the dose of drug required to elicit the same therapeutic response, regardless of the severity of the disease; this may partly reflect large variations in absorption and metabolism.

Adverse Effects

Lowering of systolic or diastolic pressure by 10 to 20 mm Hg occurs commonly with bromocriptine but small drops in blood pressure are generally asymptomatic. **Symptomatic orthostatic hypotension** may occur. Most striking is a **first-dose phenomenon** consisting of severe hypotension with syncope. This unusual effect is more common in elderly patients; it may be averted if initial doses are very small and given with the patient recumbent, ideally at bedtime. Hypotension occurs because bromocriptine inhibits the release of peripheral catecholamines. In general, tolerance to hypotensive effects develops within a few weeks.

Centrally mediated **nausea and vomiting** are less common than with levodopa preparations, but do occur. Tolerance generally develops to these effects within a few weeks.

Neuropsychiatric symptoms are more common with bromocriptine than with levodopa. These effects are dose-related but may not subside until several weeks after the drug is withdrawn. Confusion, paranoid delusions, vivid or frightening dreams, hallucinations, and psychosis may occur. Hallucinations are often vivid and colorful and may be mediated by a metabolite that is structurally similar to lysergic acid diethylamide (LSD). Bromocriptine has been reported to improve levodopa-induced depression, an effect that could in some way be due to the central serotoninergic properties of bromocriptine.

Dyskinesias caused by bromocriptine take the same forms as those caused by levodopa but are somewhat less common. They are dose-related and have not been reported in patients given low dose bromocriptine for hormonal disorders, adding support for the often forwarded argument that neuronal alterations in advanced Parkinson's disease are necessary for the induction of abnormal movements.

Like other antiparkinsonian agents that have peripheral dopaminergic activity, bromocriptine affects the vasculature and may cause **Raynaud's phenomenon, livedo reticularis,** and a tender, warm erythema and edema of the lower extremities (**erythromyalgia**).

Other side effects include allergic vasculitis, other dermatologic reactions, and hepatitis, but these are rarely seen at moderate doses recommended today. Headache and exacerbation of angina have been reported. Hypertension is rare.

Response oscillations (on-off and end-of-dose phenomena) are not a typical feature of bromocriptine, which has a longer duration of action than levodopa.

Important Drug Interactions

Bromocriptine may enhance not only the efficacy but also the toxicity of antiparkinsonian agents used concurrently. Dyskinesias and neuropsychiatric abnormalities are the most likely effects to occur with such combinations and dosage of one or the other agent may have to be lowered or the drug discontinued. Neuroleptic agents may counteract the therapeutic efficacy of bromocriptine.

Antihypertensive agents and bromocriptine may act in concert to lower blood pressure. Blood pressure should be monitored carefully, especially in the first few days of treatment, and dose adjustments made accordingly.

Contraindications and Precautions

Bromocriptine is contraindicated in psychosis. It should be used very cautiously in patients with unstable cardiac disease.

Indications

Bromocriptine is indicated as adjunctive therapy in Parkinson's disease. It is particularly suitable as an adjunct to levodopa in patients who develop response oscillations (on-off or end-of-dose phenomena) on the latter drug, in those in whom the efficacy of levodopa is waning, and in those who require lowering of the levodopa dose because of dyskinesias. If bromocriptine is added to a regimen containing levodopa, dosage of the latter generally needs to be lowered.

Because bromocriptine is less likely to produce gastrointestinal disturbances than levodopa, it may be used alone in patients unable to tolerate the latter. However, bromocriptine is rarely used alone as a first-line agent since it has a less favorable therapeutic index than levodopa-carbidopa and is very expensive. Moreover, the drug is usually not effective in patients who have failed to respond to levodopa ("primary levodopa failures").

Dosing

Initial dose: 1.25 mg once at bedtime. Dose increments of 1.25 to 2.5 mg are made at approximately 14-day intervals. It may take up to 3 months to achieve an adequate clinical response.

Note: Doses as high as 20–30 mg/day (in 2 or 3 divided doses) may be well tolerated. However, the exact dose should be determined by slow and careful titration with the goal of avoiding toxicity. If bromocriptine is being added to a regimen that includes levodopa, the dose of the latter is initially decreased to avoid additive toxicity.

Anticholinergic Agents

Pharmacologic Considerations

Anticholinergic (atropinelike) agents, once the mainstay of antiparkinsonian treatment, have taken a back seat to newer drugs. They are thought to act by reducing the functional excess of acetylcholine that is produced by dopamine deficiency in parkinsonism, thereby restoring normal cholinergic-dopaminergic balance in the central nervous system. Anticholinergic agents may also directly enhance dopamine by blocking its reuptake in synaptic sites. These agents exert well-known effects both centrally and peripherally, by blocking muscarinic receptors in many tissues.

The particular anticholinergic agents used in the treatment of parkinsonism are more active than natural belladonna alkaloids and synthetic derivatives that are used for their action on the bladder and gut, but have a relatively favorable therapeutic index for the elderly parkinsonian patient.

This category of drug also includes the antihistamines (histamine$_1$ blockers) that have sufficient central anticholinergic activity to be useful. Relatively speaking, antihistamines are only weakly anticholinergic.

Anticholinergic agents used for Parkinson's disease do not differ significantly in their effect from one another. However, individual patients may report that they respond to or tolerate one agent better than another. Specific agents are listed in Table 10-1.

Adverse Reactions

Anticholinergic agents in general are often poorly tolerated by elderly patients because of underlying disease in the affected organ system.

Although decreased salivation is often desirable in patients with Parkinson's disease, **dry mouth** in elderly patients may lead to periodontal disease, tooth loss, or intolerance of dentures.

Urinary retention is a potential side effect in elderly men with prostatic outlet obstruction and may even occur in previously asymptomatic or mildly symptomatic individuals. Elderly patients with other forms of bladder dysfunction are less likely to develop urinary retention, but anticholinergic agents should not be used in individuals with difficulty in bladder emptying. **Constipation** occurs frequently in elderly patients and more so in those with Parkinson's disease, and thus is a common side effect of agents with anticholinergic activity.

Anticholinergic agents cause **pupillary dilatation,** which may re-

Table 10-1. Some Anticholinergic Agents Used in Parkinsonism

Agent (Sample Brand)	Usual Dose
Trihexyphenidyl (Artane)	1-2 mg bid-tid
Benztropine (Cogentin)	0.5-1.0 mg bid
Antihistamine	
Diphenhydramine (Benadryl)	25-50 mg tid

sult in blurred vision and may precipitate acute angle closure glau-coma in susceptible individuals. These agents do not interfere with control of intraocular pressure in patients with chronic open angle glaucoma.

Central nervous system side effects occur commonly in elderly parkinsonian patients. The incidence of these effects is proportional to the dose of the anticholinergic agent and is highest among the very old and among those with dementia. Cholinergic deficits exist in the brains of many apparently normal elderly and are practically universal in parkinsonian patients with dementia. In such patients, anticholinergic agents occasionally precipitate frank dementia. Re-lated symptoms include milder memory impairments, mood change, somnolence, dizziness, delusions, and hallucinations. These effects are reversible with discontinuation of the drug or lowering of the dose. If they first manifest themselves when other antiparkinsonian agents are added to a regimen containing anticholinergic agents, it may be fruitful to first discontinue the anticholinergic agent rather than the more efficacious antiparkinsonian drug.

Abnormal involuntary movements are uncommon and dissimilar from those induced by levodopa and bromocriptine. They are usually of the buccolingual masticatory variety and rarely affect the limbs.

Tachycardia, a recognized effect of atropine, is less common in geriatric patients treated with anticholinergic agents, possibly be-cause underlying conduction system disease is frequently present.

Important Drug Interactions

Anticholinergic agents may potentiate atropinelike toxicity pro-duced by other agents with anticholinergic effect, such as tricyclic antidepressants, antispasmodics, and disopyramide. They may po-tentiate neuropsychiatric toxicity of other antiparkinsonian agents. By inhibiting gastric acid secretion, they may alter the absorption of drugs used concurrently.

Contraindications and Precautions

Anticholinergic agents are contraindicated in narrow angle glau-coma, urinary bladder outlet obstruction, and unstable cardiac dis-ease. They should be used with extreme caution in patients with de-mentia and organic psychosis.

Indications

Anticholinergic agents are indicated as adjunctive treatment in Parkinson's disease. However, they are sometimes useful in patients with minimal symptoms whose physician wishes to postpone treat-ment with levodopa. They are also occasionally used in patients unable to tolerate other agents. These drugs exert only a fraction of the antiparkinsonian effect of levodopa and, while they may help to ameliorate tremor and drooling, they are generally of limited efficacy in the management of disordered gait.

Anticholinergic agents are sometimes used to prevent or manage drug-induced parkinsonism, but their utility in that setting has been disputed.

Dosing

Usual dose ranges for these agents are summarized in Table 10-1.

New Drugs

Selegiline (deprenyl; Eldepryl)

Selegiline is a selective inhibitor of monoamine oxidase type B (MAO-B), the enzyme responsible for the degradation of dopamine. Unlike conventional monoamine oxidase inhibitors (MAOIs), which nonselectively inhibit MAO-A and MAO-B, selegiline prolongs the presence of dopamine in the central nervous system without participating in drug and nutrient interactions in the periphery at ordinary doses. Selegiline may also act synergistically with levodopa, allowing a reduction in the dosage of the latter. Recent evidence suggests that early use of selegiline may delay the need for levodopa by several months. These results and other evidence have been interpreted to mean that selegiline might be capable of delaying the progression of the disease itself, an effect not previously demonstrated by other drugs. It has been postulated that MAO inhibition counteracts progressive nigrostriatal degeneration, an "antioxidant" effect of the drug. Further study is required to clarify whether the drug affects pathophysiologic processes of the disease itself or, like other dopaminergic agents, is merely palliative.

Selegiline does not appear to improve the function of patients with moderate to advanced Parkinson's disease and presently should only be used in the early stages. Even in these cases, the benefits of selegiline may not be obvious for at least 6 months. High cost is presently an additional limitation of this drug.

Selegiline is metabolized to amphetamine and may produce **insomnia, cardiac arrhythmias,** and **alterations in blood pressure.** These metabolites may also account for antidepressant effect that has been observed in some patients. It may produce **adverse neuropsychiatric symptoms and dyskinesias** like other dopaminergic agents used in Parkinson's disease. At high doses (roughly 30 mg/day or more), selegiline loses its MAO-B selectivity and is capable of participating in the same drug and nutrient interactions as seen with conventional MAOIs (see Chap. 8). Such problems have not been encountered with antiparkinsonian doses currently recommended.

DOSING
Initial dose: 2.5–5.0 mg once daily.
Usual dose: 5 mg bid.

Pergolide (Permax)

Pergolide is a dopamine agonist related to but more potent than bromocriptine. It was recently approved for use as adjunctive treatment in Parkinson's disease and its current place in therapy is largely reserved for patients not tolerating bromocriptine. Elderly patients may be at higher risk than others for developing cardiac arrhythmias and hypotension from this agent, but may tolerate it better than bromocriptine.

DOSING
Initial dose: 0.05 mg.
Maximum dose: 1 mg tid.

NONPHARMACOLOGIC TREATMENT

Drugs that produce parkinsonian symptoms should be avoided if possible, since they are more likely to have these effects in elderly patients. The most common offenders include neuroleptic agents and metoclopramide. Methyldopa and reserpine have also rarely been reported to produce this problem.

Patients with Parkinson's disease should be encouraged to exercise. Active physical exercise may forestall the development of rigidity and passive range of motion exercise may prevent contractures. Secondary problems such as constipation, drooling, and depression should be managed aggressively in order to improve the quality of life. Toxicity from antiparkinsonian medications should be recognized early in order to prevent injury and medical complications. The home environment should be made safe and home care should be instituted when needed.

BIBLIOGRAPHY

Berg, M.J., Ebert, B., Willis, D.K., et al. Parkinsonism—drug treatment. *Drug Intell. Clin. Pharm.* 21:10, 1987.

Eisler, T., Teravainen, H. Nelson, R., et al. Deprenyl in Parkinson disease. *Neurology* 31:19–23, 1981.

Lieberman, A.N., and Goldstein, M. Bromocriptine in Parkinson disease. *Pharmacol. Rev.* 37:217, 1985.

Lieberman, A.N. Update in Parkinson disease, *N. Y. State J. Med.* 87:147–153, 1987.

Lees, A.J. L-dopa treatment and Parkinson's disease. *Q. J. Med.* 59:535, 1986.

Parkes, J.D. Adverse effects of antiparkinsonian drugs. *Drugs* 21:341, 1981.

The Parkinson Study Group. Effect of deprenyl in the progression of disability in early Parkinson's disease. *N. Engl. J. Med.* 321:1364–1371, 1989.

Wolters, E.C., and Calne, D.B. Recent advances in pharmacotherapy. Parkinson's disease. *Can. Med. Assoc. J.* 140:507–514, 1989.

Anticonvulsants

SEIZURES IN THE ELDERLY

Most seizure disorders in the geriatric age group are acquired, the most common antecedent pathology being stroke or head trauma. Less commonly, brain tumors are the cause. Seizures occur acutely, as in other age groups, from a variety of systemic derangements, drugs, drug withdrawal, or from acute intracranial disease. Hypoxic seizures are not uncommon and can be precipitated by choking episodes, transient heart block, or following cardiovascular surgery. The propensity for the geriatric patient to develop hypoxic seizures is probably due to the high prevalence of compromised cerebrovascular circulation.

In the vast majority of cases, the seizures are focal (simple partial), but they may become secondarily generalized in a significant number of these. The diagnosis is sometimes made in a workup for syncope. This does not mean that the seizure presented as simple loss of consciousness without motor symptoms, since syncope is commonly unwitnessed and the patient is often found on the floor, conscious but unable to get up.

In many cases, long-term use of anticonvulsants may be required in elderly patients, but there are instances when the drug can be permanently withdrawn. Because of the potential toxicity of anticonvulsants, it is important for reversible causes of seizures to be identified.

Poorly controlled seizures are commonly the result of noncompliance with the medical regimen. If the patient is functionally impaired or thought to be unreliable in any way, it is essential that the home situation be carefully evaluated and a means of supervision identified.

SPECIFIC AGENTS

Three drugs—phenytoin, phenobarbital, and carbamazepine—are almost always effective in controlling the types of seizures that afflict the elderly, namely, simple partial and generalized tonic-clonic seizures. For a complete discussion of these and other anticonvulsants the reader is referred to the readings in the Bibliography (see Eadie & Tyrer).

Phenytoin (Dilantin)

Pharmacologic Considerations

MECHANISM OF ACTION. Anticonvulsants in general bind to specific receptors in the brain and act on groups of neurons that are prone to develop bursts of electrical activity. These neurons may be so prone partly because of disinhibition due to abnormalities in neurons that normally act to inhibit them. In addition, there may be facilitation of transmission across synapses, leading to propagation of this abnormal activity. Phenytoin inhibits propagation of epileptogenic activity but is less effective in suppressing activity at the primary focus. However, phenytoin is very effective in controlling partial seizures and in preventing propagation and secondary generalization, and is thus highly effective in the management of the types of seizure disorders seen most commonly in the elderly.

The exact mechanism of action of phenytoin is not known, but it may act on chloride ion channels that control depolarization of the neuronal cell membrane, or it may act by altering excitatory or inhibitory neurotransmitters in the brain. Chronic use of phenytoin also causes folate depletion; low folate concentrations have been found to reduce epileptogenic activity under experimental conditions, but the contribution of this to the antiepileptogenic effect of phenytoin and other anticonvulsants is not known.

The anticonvulsant action of phenytoin occurs with a minimal amount of sedation at ordinary doses. However, geriatric patients tend to be more sensitive to the sedating effects of phenytoin than younger adults.

PHARMACOKINETICS. Phenytoin is well absorbed at the level of the proximal small intestine. Most available preparations have adequate bioavailability, but differences among brands do exist. Since phenytoin exhibits dose-related kinetics and has a narrow therapeutic ratio, small changes in bioavailability that could occur by a switch in brand could produce significant changes in serum drug levels and clinical effect.

Phenytoin has poor solubility properties, making intramuscular administration impractical. Because it tends to precipitate at physiologic pH and below, intravenous phenytoin requires specific preparation (see Dosing below).

Phenytoin is rapidly distributed to the site of action. It is approximately 90% bound to serum proteins, mostly albumin. Although the free or active fraction of drug tends to be higher in elderly patients, this is generally unimportant in chronic dosing because unbound drug is also more rapidly cleared. During illness, albumin levels may decline readily in geriatric patients, particularly those who are chronically debilitated. Although this could theoretically increase phenytoin sensitivity, the actual effect of serum protein fluctuations on phenytoin sensitivity is not known. A potentially important implication of phenytoin protein binding is that it may confound the interpretation of therapeutic drug levels (see below).

Phenytoin undergoes saturable metabolism by microsomal enzymes in the liver. Unlike most other drugs that are metabolized in this way, the enzyme system for phenytoin may be saturated at ordinary therapeutic doses. Plasma levels may increase rapidly as dose increments are made and toxicity may appear to occur abruptly. This phenomenon is particularly important in geriatric patients, in whom the early signs of phenytoin toxicity may be subtle. Another important implication of saturable kinetics is that the effects of drug interactions may be more pronounced when serum levels of phenytoin are at the high end of the therapeutic range.

Phenytoin metabolites are inactive. The major hydroxylated metabolite is primarily excreted in the bile or as glucuronide conjugates in the urine. Only a small portion of the drug is excreted unchanged by the kidney. Phenytoin is a potent stimulator of the hepatic microsomal enzyme system and there is some evidence that the drug induces its own metabolism. However, this results in only minor alterations in phenytoin levels and the clinical importance of this phenomenon is outweighed by the fact that the enzyme system becomes saturated as dose increases are made.

There is genetic variation in the ability to biotransform phenytoin, with unusually fast or unusually slow hydroxylators having been described. The half-life of phenytoin after oral administration ranges from 20 to 70 hours in most patients, but may be much longer in others. The half-life increases with increasing dose and at steady state it may be longer than 5 days. Half-life after intravenous administration is approximately 10–15 hours.

Metabolic clearance of phenytoin may decline in late life, as reflected by a 15%–20% reduction in the maximal rate of biotransformation (V_{max}). This could lead to more rapid saturation in the enzyme system, higher steady-state concentration, and earlier appearance of phenytoin toxicity at a given dose. However, the volume of distribution for phenytoin increases with age, which would balance the effect of increased V_{max}. Although there is controversy surrounding age-related pharmacokinetic changes for phenytoin in adults, the average therapeutic dose is believed to be somewhat lower in the elderly.

Use of Therapeutic Blood Monitoring

The accepted therapeutic range for phenytoin is 10–20 μg/ml. However, this range should be used as a guide and not a rule because many patients will remain seizure-free despite lower-than-expected levels and some will require higher levels to remain seizure free but will tolerate these high levels well. This variability depends presumably on the severity of epilepsy and the sensitivity to phenytoin. Many geriatric patients with epilepsy tolerate high levels poorly. This may be related to underlying central nervous system (CNS) disease and enhanced pharmacodynamic response. The ability of the patient to tolerate high levels is further dependent on his or her functional status, so that someone whose work required fine physical control or a high degree of intellectual output might notice subtle changes at low therapeutic levels while someone with fewer demands, such as a sedentary or functionally impaired patient, might not notice the negative motor or cognitive effects of the drug.

Cautious interpretation of drug levels in the elderly is important for other reasons. Age-related changes in protein binding may result in increased free or active fraction of the drug, but, since most laboratories measure total drug levels (bound plus unbound drug), the laboratory report may be misleadingly low. It has not been established that the determination of free drug levels contributes enough useful information to warrant routine use in preference to standard laboratory measures. However, the implications of drug binding should be kept in mind when interpreting results reported by the laboratory, particularly when a potentially competing protein-bound drug has recently been introduced. The pharmacodynamic response of the patient remains the most important consideration, so that if there are signs of toxicity in the therapeutic range, consideration should be given to reducing the dose. A few patients will paradoxically exhibit an increase in seizure frequency at toxic doses.

Adverse Effects

Dose-related side effects of phenytoin include **vertigo, ataxia, tremors, dysarthria, diplopia,** and **nystagmus.** Symptoms may be subtle in the elderly and are sometimes overlooked. Phenytoin is more likely to produce **sedation** or **confusion** in the elderly than in younger adults, effects that are probably also dose-related. Behavioral changes and other CNS symptoms may also occur, including **head-**

ache, delirium, intellectual deterioration, depression, psychosis, and involuntary movements. Electrophysiological signs of peripheral neuropathy have been described in patients on long-term phenytoin treatment, but this is generally asymptomatic.

Phenytoin very commonly produces rash and drug fever. Rash can be severe, with Stevens-Johnson syndrome being a rare but serious outcome.

Chronic use of phenytoin may produce osteomalacia. This has been attributed to the drug's enzyme-inducing effect, leading to accelerated vitamin D metabolism. Serum levels of 25-hydroxyvitamin D may decline, and hypocalcemia may occur. Reduced vitamin D levels imply preventable or reversible vitamin-D dependent bone disease. However, phenytoin also impairs vitamin K status by the same mechanism, reducing vitamin-K dependent protein (osteocalcin) in bone. Theoretically, both vitamins D and K would have to be given to prevent the bone disease, but there is conflicting information on the response of metabolic measurements of bone integrity and little information on whether nutrient supplements protect bone itself. The elderly are potentially at increased risk of phenytoin-induced osteomalacia because vitamin D status is frequently marginal and histologic evidence of osteomalacia is often present independent of anticonvulsant use. The tendency to produce osteomalacia is a property that may be shared by other anticonvulsants discussed in this chapter (see below).

Phenytoin may produce folate deficiency and, rarely, megaloblastic anemia. There is evidence that folate depletion actually reduces epileptogenic activity in the brain and folate repletion has been noted to restore the seizure diathesis. Phenytoin-induced folate depletion results in decreased metabolism of the anticonvulsant with consequent increases in phenytoin levels. When folate is given, phenytoin metabolism is again stimulated, reversing the increase in phenytoin levels. There is some controversy as to both the mechanism of folate depletion and whether the putative epileptogenic effect of this depletion is clinically important. Since megaloblastic anemia is a rare outcome, it is best to monitor hematologic parameters rather than to routinely give folate supplements. It is important to note that debilitated elderly are at baseline risk for folate depletion and that serum folate (unlike red-cell folate) measurements poorly reflect folate status.

Phenytoin has an inhibitory effect on pancreatic insulin secretion; although hyperglycemia may occur in some diabetics and can theoretically occur in individuals with impaired glucose tolerance, there is no evidence that phenytoin increases the risk of diabetes in the general population.

Phenytoin also induces lymphocytic proliferation and may produce lymphadenopathy. This "pseudolymphoma" can be mistaken for neoplastic disease but it is believed to be benign. Phenytoin has a variety of other effects on immune function and exhibits some immunosuppressant action. Severe hypersensitivity reactions of the bone marrow, liver, and other systems have been reported but are very unusual. Skin manifestations can range from simple rash to exfoliative dermatitis.

Hypotension or cardiac arrhythmia are largely effects of intravenous phenytoin and are more likely to occur in the elderly than in younger patients.

By stimulating the activity of delta aminolevulinic acid (delta-

ALA) synthetase, phenytoin can precipitate attacks of **acute porphyria.**

Phenytoin can **alter thyroid function tests.** Thyroxine may be displaced from serum-binding proteins, leading to decrease in total hormone level, but the euthyroid state is maintained.

Gingival hyperplasia, a common side effect in young patients, seems to be less of a problem as patients approach midlife and is relatively unusual in people over the age of 70 years. This may be because the mechanism involves uncontrolled growth of otherwise normal gingival cells, and may be confined to fibroblasts in young collagen. It does not occur in areas where there is no tooth.

Important Drug and Nutrient Interactions

Many drugs can interfere with the hepatic metabolism of phenytoin, increasing or decreasing its concentration. In addition, phenytoin can be displaced from protein binding sites by competing substances, thus increasing the free or active fraction of the anticonvulsant. Since this type of interaction also enables more drug to reach the site of metabolism, any clinical effect of the interaction should be transient. Nonetheless, drugs that interact at protein-binding sites should be administered cautiously.

As a potent hepatic enzyme inducer, phenytoin increases the metabolism of a number of drugs, reducing their effect. An important interaction occurs with corticosteroids, including dexamethasone, which is frequently administered to patients taking phenytoin. Phenytoin reduces the efficacy of corticosteroids but the latter reduce phenytoin levels, presumably by accelerating its metabolism. Clinical response to corticosteroids must be closely monitored and phenytoin levels should be followed. A phenytoin-warfarin interaction is complex. Increased warfarin sensitivity may be seen early on, followed by a decreased effect. Prothrombin time must be closely monitored throughout.

A summary of potential pharmacokinetic interactions is given in Table 11–1. The complex nature of phenytoin kinetics makes drug interactions unpredictable and difficult to prove. It is likely that published reports do not represent all the possibilities. Thus, it is prudent to be on the alert for interactions with any drug. Potentially interacting drugs are not contraindicated but must be given with caution and dose adjustments made when needed.

The impact of phenytoin on nutrients has been mentioned earlier. A poorly explained interaction with the drug has been described in patients who receive enteral feeding by tube. Although these reports are inconsistent, they suggest that enteral feeds impair the bioavailability of the drug more than would be expected with ordinary food. The problem does not seem to be due to an interaction with the feeding tube itself. A possible reason for the inconsistency in the reports may have to do with the complex kinetics of phenytoin rather than with any differences among the nutrient preparations, so that an "interaction" or lack of one could be related to whether the patient's phenytoin is at steady state when the drug levels are obtained. Nonetheless, in order to make absorption of this drug maximal and maximally predictable, tube-fed patients should receive the feed by the bolus method rather than continuously, if practical, so that the stomach remains empty for an adequate amount of time. Phenytoin should be given at least 2 hours away from the feed, after the tube has been flushed with water. Furthermore, the drug

Table 11-1. Some Drug and Nutrient Interactions with Phenytoin

May Decrease Phenytoin Levels	May Increase Phenytoin Levels
Enteral feeds	Cimetidine
Antacids	Isoniazid
Sucralfate	Omeprazole
Theophylline	
Folic acid	
Rifampin	
Dexamethasone	
Anticonvulsants*	

Phenytoin may reduce the effect or level of
Corticosteroids
Sex hormones
Digitoxin
Doxycycline
Folic acid
Haloperidol
Nortriptyline
Oxazepam
Meperidine
Theophylline
Warfarin

*Also known to increase or not change phenytoin levels. Phenytoin may also alter levels of other anticonvulsants.

should be administered at a constant interval with respect to feeding. Alternatively, drug levels should be carefully monitored and the dose adjusted as needed.

Contraindications
Phenytoin is contraindicated in patients with a history of hypersensitivity to the drug.

Precautions
Vitamin D status should be monitored by obtaining serum levels of 25-hydroxyvitamin D.

Because phenytoin does not completely dissolve, the oral liquid form is a suspension and it must be vigorously and adequately shaken before each administration.

Patients receiving intravenous phenytoin should have monitoring of vital signs during the infusion.

Indications
Phenytoin is a first-line drug in the management of seizure disorders in the elderly.

Other Uses
Phenytoin is used as adjunctive therapy in the management of neuropathic pain, such as trigeminal neuralgia and other neuropathic syndromes associated with paroxysmal or lancinating pain.

The drug has also been used for the management of cardiac arrhythmias, but is less commonly used today because other available drugs have a more favorable therapeutic-to-toxic ratio.

Dosing

Loading dose: 10–15 mg/kg. In urgent situations give in one dose; otherwise, in 3 divided doses over 6 hours. Intravenous and oral phenytoin are given at the same dose.

Note: When phenytoin is administered intravenously, it should be infused slowly, at a rate no greater than 50 mg/min. In order to avoid crystallization, the drug should be mixed in no more than 50 cc of saline and administered no more than 1 hour after preparation. Intravenous tubing should be flushed with saline or changed before administration.

Usual daily maintenance dose: 200–300 mg, depending on serum levels and clinical response.

Phenobarbital

Pharmacologic Considerations

MECHANISM OF ACTION. Phenobarbital inhibits propagation of epileptogenic activity, but may also suppress the primary focus. In addition to its anticonvulsant actions, it is a nonspecific central depressant and is more sedating than phenytoin. However, in contrast to shorter-acting barbiturates, phenobarbital exhibits its anticonvulsant action at doses lower than those that produce sleep.

PHARMACOKINETICS. Phenobarbital is slowly but well absorbed. It is extensively metabolized by the hepatic microsomal enzyme system. Like phenytoin, phenobarbital is a potent hepatic enzyme inducer, but it does not accelerate its own metabolism. Approximately 25%–50% of the drug is eliminated unchanged by the kidney.

The serum half-life of phenobarbital ranges from 2 to 6 days in nongeriatric adults. In the absence of a loading dose, steady state is not reached for approximately 20 days. The half-life is prolonged in liver disease. Study of phenobarbital kinetics in the elderly is limited; however, because a substantial minority of unchanged drug undergoes renal excretion, the half-life is likely to be prolonged with age.

Only approximately 50% of phenobarbital is bound to serum proteins.

Adverse Effects

The most common side effect of phenobarbital is **sedation.** Because tolerance to sedation commonly develops over time, the greatest importance of the sedative effect is during dose initiation when high loading doses may be given. High loading doses may produce profound somnolence or respiratory depression in aged individuals.

Phenobarbital can also produce **deterioration in gait, impairment of intellectual function, mood change,** and **other central nervous system effects** that are also seen with phenytoin, such as dysarthria, incoordination, and nystagmus. **Toxic overdose** can produce stupor, coma, and death.

Withdrawal symptoms may occur if the drug is discontinued abruptly; these consist of emotional lability, insomnia, tremor, diaphoresis, confusion, or prolonged seizures.

Osteomalacia has been described in patients who have been on phenobarbital for prolonged periods. As with phenytoin, the mechanism is believed to be at least partly related to accelerated vitamin D metabolism. **Hypocalcemia** may also occur. There is less information about phenobarbital's effect on other nutrients.

Other side effects of barbiturates are discussed in Chap. 7 in connection with the management of insomnia.

Important Drug and Nutrient Interactions

Phenobarbital participates in a very large number of drug interactions, mostly on the basis of its effect on hepatic enzymes. These interactions are summarized in Chap. 7. Because enzyme induction is probably a genetically variable process, the drug interaction is not predictable. A potential interaction should be anticipated when new drugs are started and the reversal of an interaction should be anticipated when phenobarbital is removed from the regimen. Since phenobarbital may stay in circulation for a prolonged period of time, one should watch for a change in the interaction for at least a month after the drug has been discontinued.

Interaction between phenobarbital and phenytoin has been reported but the effects described have been inconsistent, with levels of the latter decreasing, increasing, and staying the same.

Precautions

Like other barbiturates, phenobarbital must be tapered very slowly because severe withdrawal syndromes may occur if the drug is rapidly discontinued.

As with phenytoin, vitamin D status should be monitored in patients taking phenobarbital on the long term.

Indications

Phenobarbital is indicated for the management of epilepsy in the elderly if seizures cannot be controlled with phenytoin, and in patients who cannot take phenytoin or carbamazepine.

Dosing

Initial dose: 15 mg at bedtime. This is a test dose. Alternatively, give $\frac{1}{3}$ to $\frac{1}{2}$ of the anticipated daily maintenance dose. Increase by $\frac{1}{4}$ to $\frac{1}{3}$ of the daily maintenance dose every 7 days.
Note: Loading doses should be avoided.
Usual daily maintenance dose: 30 mg bid according to serum levels and clinical response.

Carbamazepine (Tegretol)

Pharmacologic Considerations

Carbamazepine is structurally related to the tricyclic antidepressants. However, it has wide-ranging anticonvulsant activity and is effective in controlling many types of seizures.

The mechanism of anticonvulsant action is in part similar to that of phenytoin, but the complex actions of carbamazepine are not well understood.

OTHER ACTIONS. An important action of carbamazepine is its ability to relieve the pain of trigeminal neuralgia. The drug is less effective in the management of other forms of neuropathic pain, such as diabetic neuropathy, and appears to be relatively ineffective in treating postherpetic neuralgia. There is conflicting evidence as to its efficacy in the management of phantom limb pain.

Carbamazepine stimulates the release of antidiuretic hormone and reduces free water clearance. This action has been harnessed in the treatment of central diabetes insipidus. However, a more important implication of this for the geriatric patient is the ability of the drug to produce symptomatic hyponatremia.

Carbamazepine has diverse effects on mood and has been used increasingly in recent years in the management of affective disorders (see Israel & Beaudry).

PHARMACOKINETICS. The rate at which carbamazepine is absorbed appears to be related to particle size and differs according to the preparation given. Food may increase absorption and sometimes patients experience dose-related side effects according to how the dose is timed with meals. Carbamazepine induces its own metabolism, so that while the serum half-life of the drug is greater than 36 hours after a single dose, it decreases to approximately 10–20 hours after chronic (1 month or more) administration. There is no information on carbamazepine kinetics in the elderly.

The major hepatic metabolite of carbamazepine is an active epoxide compound, which may be responsible to some extent for the drug's anticonvulsant and toxic effects. The proportion of circulating metabolite changes when the drug is given with agents that stimulate or inhibit hepatic enzymes, but the net effect on a clinical level is uncertain. Half-life of the epoxide is somewhat shorter than that of the parent drug. The active metabolite is transformed to inactive compounds that are excreted in the urine. Little active drug is excreted by the kidney. Parent drug is approximately 75% bound to serum proteins and active metabolite is less extensively bound.

Adverse Effects

Central nervous system side effects may occur in a dose-related fashion. These include ataxia, diplopia, dizziness, and lethargy. However, carbamazepine is less likely than phenobarbital to produce sedation and less likely than both phenobarbital or phenytoin to produce cognitive impairment. In fact, some patients experience improvements in behavior and mood, particularly when switched from other anticonvulsants. **Toxic doses** can produce worsening of seizures, respiratory depression, irritability, and coma.

Gastrointestinal disturbances, including nausea and vomiting, may occur, but tend to subside with time or reduction in dose.

Patients may experience dose-related side effects more acutely at different times of the day, relative to peaks in serum concentration. Timing of the dose may improve the patient's ability to tolerate the drug.

Like some of the TCAs, which are structural analogues, carbamazepine has been reported to produce the **syndrome of inappropriate antidiuretic hormone (SIADH)**. This side effect occurs most often among elderly patients. Signs of SIADH, such as confusion and restlessness, resemble those of carbamazepine toxicity; however, when hyponatremia is severe, seizures may be exacerbated.

Uncommonly, carbamazepine causes **disturbances in cardiac conduction**, including heart block and asystole. These problems have virtually always been reported in elderly patients who have been taking the drug for control of trigeminal neuralgia, for which relatively high doses are often required. These side effects are identical to those produced by TCAs, although they have been reported much less often with carbamazepine.

Also like the TCAs, carbamazepine has been reported to produce **acute urinary retention** with overflow incontinence.

As with the previously mentioned anticonvulsants, carbamazepine may produce **vitamin D depletion** and serum calcium levels may fall. Osteomalacia could theoretically occur with this drug, although the actual risk has not been determined.

Hypersensitivity reactions have been reported, including dermatitis, hepatitis, and pneumonitis. The most serious potential side effect is **aplastic anemia**, which can be fatal. However, this probably is much more rare than previously believed. **Leukopenia** occurs much more commonly, but this is almost always benign and can be transient. Because of fears that it can progress to a more serious form of **agranulocytosis,** if not generalized bone marrow suppression, hematologic parameters require periodic monitoring. **Thrombocytopenia** has also been reported.

Important Drug and Nutrient Interactions

Carbamazepine has been reported to reduce warfarin sensitivity, presumably by increasing the metabolism of the anticoagulant. Carbamazepine may also reduce the effect of theophylline preparations by a similar mechanism.

The effects of carbamazepine on concurrently administered anticonvulsants are inconsistent, but carbamazepine levels seem to be reduced by other anticonvulsants.

The toxicity of TCAs may be enhanced by carbamazepine; although an effect on their metabolism has been postulated, it is possible that carbamazepine enhances the pharmacodynamic action of TCAs. Carbamazepine has been reported to enhance CNS toxicity of lithium.

The effects of carbamazepine may be enhanced by concurrent administration of drugs that inhibit its metabolism, including cimetidine, erythromycin, and isoniazid.

As mentioned above, carbamazepine may produce vitamin D depletion. It has also been noted to produce a fall in serum folic acid levels, but these reports are inconsistent.

Because of its complex metabolism and its effect on liver enzymes, drug interactions should be anticipated even though they may not yet have been reported.

Pitfalls of Carbamazepine Serum Levels

Serum levels of carbamazepine do not correlate well with overall clinical effect. This is probably because it is somewhat difficult to time sample collection precisely. Peak and trough levels might be hard to predict because carbamazepine preparations tend to vary in their bioavailability. In addition, trough levels may change after the patient has been on the drug for several weeks. In the presence of other drugs that affect hepatic oxidative enzymes, the problem is further complicated because the ratio of active metabolite to parent drug varies according to whether the interacting drug is an enzyme inducer or inhibitor. In the case of enzyme inducers, including phenytoin and phenobarbital, the level of parent drug would be relatively decreased but anticonvulsant activity might be maintained because of an increase in the level of the active metabolite.

Serum levels of approximately 6–12 μg/ml are generally considered to be the therapeutic range, although this range may be somewhat dependent on the type of seizure being treated and whether hepatically active drugs (including other anticonvulsants) are being given concurrently.

Relatively high serum levels may be required for the control of trigeminal neuralgia. In this group of patients, side effects are common.

Contraindications

Carbamazepine is contraindicated in patients with known hypersensitivity reactions to the drug. It should generally be avoided in people with disease affecting the bone marrow.

Precautions

Complete blood count and serum sodium should be monitored periodically throughout the course of drug therapy. Because hyponatremia may both exacerbate seizures and produce symptoms identical to those of carbamazepine toxicity, serum sodium and drug levels should be measured when such symptoms occur.

Baseline EKG should be performed prior to institution of treatment. This is particularly important in patients who are about to undergo treatment for trigeminal neuralgia, for which relatively high doses may be attained.

Indications

Carbamazepine is less commonly used for seizure control in the elderly than other anticonvulsants, although it should be considered in patients whose cognitive capacities are unduly impaired by phenytoin or phenobarbital. A major application of this drug in the geriatric age group is in the management of chronic neuropathic pain syndromes. Although its efficacy in diabetic neuropathy and phantom limb pain is inconstant, carbamazepine is considered the drug of choice for trigeminal neuralgia.

Dosing

Starting dose: 100 mg at bedtime for 3–5 days. Increase daily dosage by 100–200 mg every 3–5 days until desired maintenance dose is achieved.
Usual daily maintenance dose: 200 mg bid–tid, according to serum levels and clinical response.
Note: The dose may need to be readjusted upward after several weeks because of changes that occur in clearance over time.
Dose in pain syndromes: The lowest effective dose should be given, but this varies over a wide range, depending on patient response. The average effective dose for pain control may be higher than the effective anticonvulsant dose. Although the patient may be very uncomfortable on account of pain, overly rapid dose increments may themselves be troublesome and should be avoided.

BIBLIOGRAPHY

Eadie, M.J., and Tyrer, J.H. *Anticonvulsant Therapy.* Edinburgh: Churchill Livingstone, 1989.

Haley, C.J. Phenytoin-enteral feeding interaction. *Drug Intell. Clin. Pharm.* 23:797–798, 1989.

Israel, M., and Beaudry, P. Carbamazepine in psychiatry: a review. *Can. J. Psychiatr.* 33:577–584, 1988.

Krall, R.L., and Resor, S.J. Drug treatment of epilepsy. *Semin. Neurol.* 7:128–138, 1987.

Mahler, M.E. Seizures: common causes and treatment in the elderly. *Geriatrics* 42(7):73–78, 1987.

Nation, R.L., Evans, A.M., and Milne, R.W. Pharmacokinetic drug interactions with phenytoin. *Clin. Pharmacokin.* 18:37–60, 131–150, 1990.

Antihypertensive Agents

HYPERTENSION IN THE ELDERLY

Any discussion of hypertension in the elderly must distinguish between hypertension and isolated systolic hypertension (ISH). Hypertension, regardless of etiology, is defined as systolic blood pressure greater than or equal to 160 mm Hg and diastolic pressure over 95. ISH is defined as systolic pressure over 160 and diastolic pressure less than or equal to 95 mm Hg. The incidence of hypertension increases with age until approximately the sixth decade and then levels off, but the incidence of ISH increases linearly with age. By age 75, between 27% and 43% of the American population, depending on race, sex, and criteria used, have ISH. The majority of elderly hypertensives have ISH while only a minority have diastolic hypertension.

There is ample evidence that correction of hypertension reduces cerebrovascular and cardiovascular morbidity and mortality, and that the benefits of treatment outweigh the risks. Although the group over age 60 has not been well studied, recent evidence from Europe indicates that treated elderly hypertensives, men more so than women, do benefit, but that those over the age of 80 (a group comprised mostly of women) do not achieve additional benefit. Since this group is predominantly female, it is possible that there are advantages to treating men over 80, but there is simply not enough data to clarify the risks and benefits of treating men of that age.

There is less information about the benefits of treating hypertension that is purely systolic. This form of blood pressure has been attributed to the increased stiffness and lack of distensibility of arteries known to occur with age, and it has been suggested that since this is essentially a normal age change, the resulting increases in blood pressure are normal as well. However, it has been repeatedly shown that systolic hypertension at any age is as great or greater a risk factor for stroke and ischemic heart disease than is diastolic hypertension.

The correlation of systolic hypertension and stroke risk does not mean that there is a cause-and-effect relationship. Although high systolic pressure results in high mean arterial pressure, which in itself could be harmful, the increased stroke risk could exist because intracranial arterial changes are simply part and parcel of the same arterial changes that produce hypertension. If the latter were true, correction of the blood pressure might not reduce the risk of stroke; in fact, aggressive treatment could reduce cerebral perfusion and perhaps increase the risk.

Results of the first randomized prospective trial examining this issue have been published very recently (see SHEP Cooperative Research Group). This trial showed that active treatment significantly reduced the risk of stroke and major cardiovascular events in a population with an average age of over 70 years, with a favorable trend for total mortality. Although only 14% of patients were 80 years of age or older, these individuals appeared to benefit as well. Since many patients were excluded for medical reasons, more study is required before the results of this study can be extrapolated to other members of the geriatric population, specifically to those who are very old and frail.

GUIDELINES TO TREATING HYPERTENSION IN THE ELDERLY

1. Blood pressure goals should be conservative. It is not necessary to lower blood pressure to youthful levels (e.g., 120/80) in elderly patients. In general, systolic pressure should not exceed but can be maintained at 160 mm Hg and diastolic pressure at 90–95. These goals should be further individualized, depending on the patient's overall function, ability to take and tolerate medications, and age. Overtreatment of hypertension may lead to hypoperfusion of vital organs and potentially serious symptoms. Aging is associated with impaired cerebroautoregulation so that drops in systemic arterial pressure may not be accompanied by immediate physiological shunting to underperfused areas of the brain. This pathophysiologic mechanism may be operating in other underperfused vital organs as well.

2. Very aged patients should be treated with particular caution. Toxicity may occur more readily, the risks of hypotension are greater, and the benefits of lowering blood pressure are probably limited. In such patients, the first goal should be the avoidance of side effects. The physician might elect not to treat the hypertension at all.

3. Many elderly patients currently being treated for hypertension do not actually require treatment. They may have at one time been treated for a level of blood pressure that is nowadays considered satisfactory in late life. If the patient's blood pressure history is undocumented or vague, cautious tapering of medication with periodic monitoring of blood pressure should be considered. This may be particularly important in patients with ISH, since systolic blood pressure tends to be more labile than diastolic pressure.

4. Older patients with ISH are more likely to suffer from a condition known as *pseudohypertension*, a situation in which arterial cuff pressure is significantly higher than intra-arterial pressure. Unfortunately, it is difficult to ascertain which patients have clinically important pseudohypertension. Unequal pulses, X-ray evidence of vascular calcification, and the subclavian steal syndrome are clues to the presence of severely calcified arteries. A bedside test known as *Osler's maneuver* has been suggested: While palpating the radial artery, the examiner inflates the blood pressure cuff above systolic pressure. If the radial artery is still palpable, the patient's cuff pressure is likely to be misleadingly high. Further study is required to determine the accuracy of this maneuver.

5. Initial doses should be low and dose increments should also be low and progress slowly. In general, the starting dose for an elderly patient should be no more than 25%–50% of the usual adult dose.

6. There is no "drug of choice" in treating the older age group. Treatment must be strictly individualized. An agent should be selected after careful consideration of the adverse effects that the patient is expected to develop and not on theoretical considerations based on general physiology of aging. Choice of agent can also be guided by the presence of other medical conditions that could be ameliorated by a particular agent (e.g., angina, arrhythmia, heart failure).

7. Antihypertensive agents produce a different spectrum of side

effects in the elderly, urinary dysfunction, constipation, edema, and confusion being typical examples. Orthostatic hypotension is more common and reflex tachycardia less common than in younger adults, presumably because of impaired baroreceptor mechanisms.

CHOICE OF AGENT

Certain physiologic observations have guided investigators to favor certain medications for older hypertensives. Renin levels and the renin response to diuretics decline with age, suggesting that diuretics would be a good choice. Beta receptor number or sensitivity may decline with age, suggesting that beta blockers might be less effective in older patients. However, it is more important to select an agent on the basis of its potential side effects than its mechanisms of action, for in fact, many agents may prove effective. Underlying disease makes the older patient susceptible to a wide range of side effects and, not uncommonly, the patient must make a long march through the pharmacopoeia before a tolerable agent is found.

DIURETICS

After years of popularity, diuretics have come under fire because of claims that they increase cardiovascular death by increasing the tendency to develop hypokalemia-associated arrhythmias and by producing hyperglycemia and hyperlipidemia. Although this has been disputed and is a subject of debate, careful monitoring and correction of hypokalemia can reduce the risk of arrhythmias, and monitoring of blood glucose is justified. The incidence and risks of diuretic-induced hyperlipidemia are not fully understood in any age group but this is a theoretical risk factor.

Diuretic therapy has been subjected to study in the geriatric population in long-term risk reduction trials (see Amery et al; SHEP Cooperative Research Group). **Judicious use of diuretics remains a safe, simple mode of therapy for treating most older patients** and thiazide diuretics may have an added benefit—that of maintaining bone integrity. The major drawback is that patients with urinary dysfunction may not tolerate diuretics and may fail to comply with treatment.

It is important to emphasize that most hypertensive patients experience a ceiling effect with diuretics, so that further hypotensive effect is generally not achieved beyond a given maximum dose. Increasing the dose further may, however, increase kaliuresis, hyperglycemia, and lipid levels. Because of altered pharmacokinetics, elderly patients most certainly achieve the ceiling effect with lower doses than do younger patients, a fact of great importance in dosing.

Thiazide and Thiazidelike Diuretics

The dozen or so members of the thiazide class of diuretics that are available in the United States are similar in pharmacological properties and differ mainly in their duration of action. Only the two most commonly used diuretics, hydrochlorothiazide and chlorthalidone, will be discussed in detail.

Hydrochlorothiazide (HydroDiuril, Esidrix, Others)

PHARMACOLOGIC CONSIDERATIONS
Mechanism of Action. Thiazide diuretics are sulfamoyl-containing benzoic acid derivatives. They produce volume depletion by enhanc-

ing sodium excretion in the proximal and distal tubules and collecting duct of the kidney. The major site of sodium loss is thought to be the distal segments because sodium that is filtered proximally may be absorbed in the loop of Henle. Acutely there is a compensatory increase in peripheral vascular resistance, but with chronic diuretic therapy vascular resistance decreases. The precise mechanism for reduction in vascular tone is not known.

Other Actions. Thiazides also enhance potassium excretion. Consequences of sodium and potassium loss include passive loss of chloride and metabolic alkalosis. In addition, thiazides also produce a net reduction in calcium excretion, either by stimulating parathyroid hormone release or by a direct effect on bone or gut. The anticalciuric effects of thiazides have been harnessed in the treatment of metabolic kidney stones, an infrequent problem in late life perhaps due to age-associated decline in dietary calcium absorption. A more important application of this effect may be the prevention of osteoporotic fractures (see Chap. 23).

Thiazides also produce magnesium wasting but this action is less well understood.

The ability of thiazides to raise uric acid levels is primarily a response to fluid depletion, which promotes tubular reabsorption of urate. This property is shared by other diuretics in use.

In renal insufficiency, the action of hydrochlorothiazide is blunted because inadequate amounts of the drug are delivered to the distal tubule, having been blocked by tubular organic acid en route.

Pharmacokinetics. Hydrochlorothiazide is well absorbed with peak plasma levels being attained at 1–4 hours and peak effect believed to occur shortly thereafter as active drug reaches the tubular lumen. Different preparations of this agent have not varied much in their absolute bioavailability. This fact may account for the popularity of hydrochlorothiazide, as inexpensive generic preparations are widely used. This does not necessarily apply to generic versions of the combination agent containing both hydrochlorothiazide and triamterene.

Hydrochlorothiazide is eliminated primarily by the kidney unchanged, but it is retained somewhat in erythrocytes. This latter property is probably responsible for its biphasic elimination half-life; the terminal half-life is 12–24 hours in nonelderly adults. Because of the renal route of elimination, the half-life is probably longer in late life, but this has not been well studied.

ADVERSE EFFECTS. Certain individuals may be particularly sensitive to the hypotensive effects of these agents and symptomatic **hypotension** may occur. This is most likely to occur in the very elderly or those with baseline diminished effective arterial volume.

By producing kaliuresis, thiazide diuretics frequently produce **hypokalemia**. The degree of potassium loss increases with increasing dose and may progress over time. Hypokalemia is not universal, however, and may actually be less common in geriatric patients than in younger adults. Therefore, potassium supplements should not be routinely added prior to measurement of serum potassium.

Hyponatremia may occur. It may be mild or profound, with serum sodium lower than 110 mEq/liter having been reported. It is unclear if this is due to enhanced release of antidiuretic hormone (ADH), enhanced renal response to ADH, or both. With aging, there is both an exaggerated hypothalamic ADH response to various provocative stimuli as well as an altered renal responsiveness to ADH. While the central and renal response to ADH may be further accentuated by thiazides, frank hyponatremia develops only in a small subgroup. It tends to develop early in the course of treatment unless additional factors are superimposed. Case reports of this phenomenon seem to be largely in elderly women.

Thiazides increase tubular reabsorption of calcium. There is increasing evidence that they have a beneficial effect on bone, making them particularly suitable for patients who also have osteoporosis. However, in certain patients, such as those with subclinical hyperparathyroidism, **hypercalcemia** may be precipitated.

Magnesium wasting may be produced by thiazide, but this is poorly reflected in serum magnesium levels. Although it is difficult to quantitate the clinical effects of tissue magnesium depletion, cardiac arrhythmias are generally considered the most important potential complication, particularly when digitalis preparations are being used.

Like other diuretics, thiazides may produce **prerenal azotemia.** This reversible problem is very common in older patients and is generally benign, but may be particularly marked in those with heart failure or other factors producing decreased effective arterial volume. Prerenal azotemia is to be distinguished from interstitial nephritis, which can lead to frank renal failure; this is an unusual hypersensitivity phenomenon that has been reported with thiazide and other diuretics.

Chloride loss results in increased serum concentrations of bicarbonate; **hypochloremic alkalosis** may be observed.

Thiazide diuretics may produce **hyperuricemia.** This property, shared by other diuretics in use, is ultimately related to volume depletion and increased urate reabsorption. Asymptomatic hyperuricemia requires no treatment. **Gout** may occur, in which case it is better to prescribe an agent other than a diuretic rather than to superimpose a hypouricemic agent.

Bladder disturbances are common among elderly patients treated with diuretics. Symptoms may consist of nocturia, urinary frequency, or frank incontinence. These "benign" symptoms may be debilitating to the patient, and may affect compliance.

The production of large volumes of urine may present as urinary retention in elderly men who have otherwise well compensated prostatic hyperplasia. This problem is actually more common with the use of powerful loop diuretics.

Thiazide diuretics produce small to moderate **increases in serum levels of low-density lipoprotein (LDL) cholesterol and triglyceride,** accompanied by increases or no change in high-density lipoprotein (HDL) cholesterol. These metabolic effects occur early on therapy and may not be maintained. Changes in serum lipid levels are thought to be mediated by a counterregulatory increase in the production of insulin and catecholamines, which, in turn, increase hepatic production of lipids. The clinical importance of these alterations is not known.

Thiazides may produce reversible **glucose intolerance** or **hyperglycemia** in susceptible individuals. Hyperosmolar coma has occasionally been reported. Impaired glucose tolerance has been attributed to potassium depletion, which is thought to reduce the sensitivity of the beta cell to glucose and the sensitivity of tissues to insulin. It is an effect that is common to all potassium-wasting diuretics.

Other side effects that have been reported with the use of thiazide diuretics include pancreatitis and blood dyscrasias. The importance and actual prevalence of these effects is not known. An association with acute cholecystitis has been reported and disputed.

Individuals who have demonstrated sensitivity to other compounds containing the sulfonamide moiety, notably the sulfonamide antibiotics, may exhibit cross-reactivity with thiazide diuretics.

IMPORTANT DRUG INTERACTIONS. Nonsteroidal anti-inflammatory agents (NSAIDs) may reduce the antihypertensive efficacy of diuretics, either by preventing diuretic-induced natriuresis or by some other effect on renal hemodynamics.

Thiazides may have some carbonic anhydrase inhibiting action, and when used in conjunction with carbonic anhydrase inhibitors such as acetazolamide (Diamox), severe hypokalemia may occur. Since systemic hypertension and ocular hypertension frequently coexist, these agents are often unwittingly prescribed together by separate physicians. The primary care physician should obtain a complete drug history from all glaucoma patients before prescribing diuretics.

Thiazides reduce renal lithium clearance; lithium toxicity may result. The complex interactions between diuretics and lithium are discussed in Chap. 9.

Thiazides and other potassium- and magnesium-wasting diuretics may increase the risk of digitalis-induced arrhythmias.

CONTRAINDICATIONS. Thiazide diuretics are contraindicated in patients with a history of significant hyponatremia. They should be used with extreme caution if at all in patients with untreated hyperparathyroidism and other hypercalcemic disorders.

PRECAUTIONS. Serum potassium, sodium, and calcium should be measured soon after a thiazide diuretic is instituted. Hypokalemia may develop over time, making periodic monitoring essential.

Digitalis-related cardiac arrhythmias may be provoked if serum potassium levels are low or even in the low normal range. This enhanced sensitivity to cardiac glucosides may also occur in the face of magnesium depletion or hypercalcemia. Patients who are also taking digitalis preparations should probably take potassium supplements routinely unless serum potassium level is clearly elevated. If digitoxic rhythm develops in the face of normal electrolyte and serum digoxin levels, magnesium depletion should be considered as a possible cause and appropriate action taken.

INDICATIONS. Hydrochlorothiazide and related thiazide diuretics are indicated for hypertension in elderly patients unless there is evidence of significant renal impairment. Patients with age-related decline in creatinine clearance masked by normal serum creatinine need not be excluded from thiazide treatment. Thiazides are also indicated in fluid-retaining and edematous states, including mild congestive heart failure or venous insufficiency.

OTHER USES. Thiazide diuretics are used in the management of metabolic renal stones composed of calcium oxalate, although this is a relatively uncommon problem in the geriatric age group.

There is a body of evidence that use of thiazide diuretics reduces the rate of osteoporotic fractures. Although not yet part of conventional treatment for osteoporosis, hypertensive patients with osteoporosis should be seriously considered for thiazide treatment. Glucocorticoid-induced osteoporosis may prove to be a specific application of thiazides, which reverse steroid-induced hypercalciuria and secondary hyperparathyroidism.

DOSING
Initial dose: 12.5 mg daily. Some patients may achieve adequate hypotensive or diuretic effect with even smaller or less frequent dosing, such as 6.25 mg daily or 12.5 mg 2–4 times per week. Such conservative dosing should be strongly considered for very old or frail patients.
Maximum dose: 25–50 mg daily.

Chlorthalidone (Hygroton)

Though structurally rather dissimilar from the thiazides, chlorthalidone possesses very similar pharmacologic properties. An important difference is that chlorthalidone has an extremely long duration of action. Although this prolonged duration of action makes chlorthalidone less desirable than other agents, it was the step 1 drug used in the SHEP study mentioned earlier.

PHARMACOKINETICS. Chlorthalidone is excreted primarily unchanged by the kidney. It also concentrates in erythrocytes and to a much greater degree than does hydrochlorothiazide. The elimination half-life varies from 24 to 72 hours in nonelderly adults, but may be doubled in older individuals. This is presumably because of age-related renal decline.

ADVERSE EFFECTS. The side effect profile is identical to that of hydrochlorothiazide. However, the prolonged half-life of chlorthalidone, accentuated in older patients, increases the likelihood and the degree of hypokalemia and perhaps other metabolic effects. Like hydrochlorothiazide, chlorthalidone possesses a sulfonamide moiety and may produce allergic reactions in patients sensitive to related drugs.

The anticalciuric action of chlorthalidone may reduce the formation of calcium oxalate stones, but its effect on bone has not been studied.

Contraindications and precautions addressed in the discussion of hydrochlorothiazide should be observed for chlorthalidone. Potential drug interactions are likewise similar.

INDICATIONS. Chlorthalidone is indicated in the treatment of hypertension when a diuretic is desired. However, its prolonged duration of action makes it theoretically less desirable than hydrochlorothiazide for elderly patients.

DOSING
Initial dose: 12.5 mg 3 to 4 times a week.
Maximum dose: 25 mg daily.

Indapamide (Lozol)

Indapamide is a nonthiazide diuretic, but shares the sulfamoyl moiety of that group of agents. It has been shown to lower blood pressure effectively in elderly patients, is less likely to produce hyponatremia, and retains its effect in renal insufficiency. Claims that it is less likely to produce hypokalemia have been disputed; potassium depletion may occur with chronic use. Indapamide may be less likely to increase serum uric acid levels than other diuretics, but this could be because it is a weaker diuretic. It appears to have less effect on serum lipid levels than thiazide diuretics and is sometimes promoted for this reason.

There is some evidence that indapamide is superior to hydrochlorothiazide in lowering systolic pressure, an observation that has not been fully explained.

Although other diuretics increase urinary phosphate excretion, indapamide has also been associated with decreased serum phosphate levels. It is not yet known if this feature has important clinical consequences.

Indapamide is extensively metabolized in the liver with little drug being excreted unchanged by the kidney. It is promoted as an agent with fewer adverse effects than thiazides but the importance of this is unclear. The thiazides have predictable and generally modifiable side effects and are presently much cheaper. Indapamide has no advantages in renal failure over older diuretics, such as furosemide.

Dosing
Usual dose: 2.5 mg/day.

Potassium-Sparing Diuretics

Triamterene (Dyrenium)

PHARMACOLOGIC CONSIDERATIONS
Mechanism of Action. Triamterene is believed to act by inhibiting sodium reabsorption in the distal tubule and collecting duct. At the same time, it inhibits the secretion of potassium into the tubular lumen. These actions occur independent of aldosterone.

Since the distal nephron normally handles only a small proportion of filtered sodium, the ability of triamterene to produce natriuresis and diuresis is modest, as is its antihypertensive action. Its chief applicability derives from its ability to spare potassium, as well as magnesium, so that it is generally used in combination with diuretics that waste these ions.

Triamterene has been used in combination in a major study of hypertension in the elderly (see Amery et al.), in which it appears to have been well tolerated.

Pharmacokinetics. Triamterene is extensively metabolized in the liver, with the production of an active, renally excreted metabolite. Diuretic action begins in about 2 hours when peak concentrations of the active metabolite are achieved. Elimination of triamterene and its metabolite is rapid with a half-life of 3–5 hours. Duration of action is probably somewhat prolonged with age since activity depends largely on the renally excreted metabolite. This is probably clinically unimportant when the drug is used once a day in combination with longer-acting hydrochlorothiazide (Dyazide, others).

ADVERSE EFFECTS. Triamterene may produce **hyperkalemia** in susceptible individuals. Those with renal insufficiency, even of a mild degree, are probably at greatest risk of this effect. Diabetes also is associated with an increased risk, but age alone is not. **Metabolic acidosis** may occur, as potassium reabsorption interferes with hydrogen secretion. Increased hydrogen concentration in plasma promotes efflux of intracellular potassium and promotes hyperkalemia further.

Although triamterene acutely increases urate excretion, chronic use can produce **hyperuricemia**, a property shared by other diuretics.

Triamterene may lead to the production of **renal stones** composed of triamterene or with triamterene as a nidus, but this is an uncommon complication. Many patients with this problem have had a prior history of renal stones. The relative risk to elderly patients is not known.

IMPORTANT DRUG INTERACTIONS. Triamterene is the diuretic most often implicated in renal insufficiency produced by concurrent use of NSAIDs and diuretics (see Chap. 2). The risk of this interaction may be increased in older patients.

Angiotensin converting enzyme (ACE) inhibitors may potentiate the potassium-sparing effect of triamterene; hyperkalemia can occur. Concurrent use of ACE inhibitors with potassium-sparing diuretics should be avoided.

Potassium supplements should be avoided except in the occasional patient in whom the combination of triamterene and a potassium-wasting diuretic does not correct hypokalemia. In such patients, serum potassium must be rigorously monitored.

CONTRAINDICATIONS. Triamterene is contraindicated in patients with hyperkalemia or renal failure. Although there is a disagreement over whether patients with a history of kidney stone are endangered by triamterene, it is best to select an alternative diuretic if possible.

INDICATIONS. Triamterene is indicated in patients requiring a diuretic who are unable to maintain normal serum potassium despite ordinary replacement doses of potassium, or in patients who cannot tolerate oral potassium supplements. It may be used in conjunction with a potassium-wasting diuretic in order to normalize serum potassium. Used alone, its antihypertensive action is less than the thiazide diuretics.

DOSING

Initial dose: 50 mg daily.

Maximum dose: 100 mg at once or in 2 divided doses.

Note: When given in combination with hydrochlorothiazide, the dose is intended to be given twice daily because of the short duration of action of triamterene. However, this is not always necessary to achieve the desired therapeutic effect.

Amiloride (Midamor)

PHARMACOLOGIC CONSIDERATIONS

Mechanism of Action. Amiloride is chemically related to triamterene and shares its mechanism of action. The two diuretics are roughly comparable in their potassium-sparing action. However, unlike triamterene, amiloride is water soluble and has not been reported to produce renal stones.

Pharmacokinetics. Amiloride begins to act within 2 hours. It is not metabolized but is excreted unchanged in the kidney. The duration of action in nonelderly adults is roughly 12–24 hours.

ADVERSE EFFECTS. Amiloride has not been reported to produce renal stones. Otherwise, amiloride has the same potential adverse effects as triamterene.

IMPORTANT DRUG INTERACTIONS. Hyperkalemia has been reported to occur when amiloride and indomethacin are used concurrently. It is probably prudent to avoid concurrent use of potassium-sparing agents and NSAIDs in general (see Triamterene above). Amiloride should not be given with ACE inhibitors.

Precautions regarding potassium supplements are those discussed in connection with triamterene.

CONTRAINDICATIONS. Amiloride is contraindicated in renal failure and hyperkalemia.

INDICATIONS. Amiloride is indicated as an alternative to triamterene. Claims have been made that its potassium-sparing effects are inconsistent, but this has not been verified. It is probably safe to use in patients with a history of kidney stones if renal function is normal.

OTHER USE. Amiloride may reduce lithium-induced polyuria. In contrast to thiazides, it has been reported to do this without increasing the risk of lithium toxicity.

DOSING

Usual dose: 5 mg daily, generally in combination with a thiazide diuretic.

Spironolactone (Aldactone)

PHARMACOLOGIC CONSIDERATIONS

Mechanism of Action. Spironolactone is structurally related to aldosterone and acts by inhibiting the action of aldosterone on the distal nephron. Sodium reabsorption is diminished and potassium reabsorption enhanced. Like other diuretics that act distally, spironolactone produces only modest natriuresis; however, its ability to lower blood pressure is probably as good as the thiazide diuretics. It is thought to be particularly suitable for the treatment of the edema of cirrhosis because of the high levels of aldosterone that tend to occur in that disease.

Pharmacokinetics. The onset of action of spironolactone is delayed by several days while the effects of aldosterone subside. The drug is extensively metabolized in the liver to metabolites with high and moderate activity. Spironolactone and its major active metabolite are extensively bound to serum proteins. The half-life of spironolactone is very short, while that of its metabolite has a biphasic elimination with a terminal half-life of up to 35 hours. The duration of action of spironolactone is approximately 48–72 hours. Some enterohepatic circulation occurs. Despite this and despite its extensive hepatic metabolism, it can be well tolerated in cirrhosis and in congestive heart failure.

Since spironolactone does not act independently of aldosterone, hyperkalemia and natriuretic response to spironolactone may vary from patient to patient, depending on individual physiologic status.

ADVERSE EFFECTS. Like other potassium-sparing diuretics, spironolactone may produce hyperkalemia. Metabolic acidosis may also occur.

Gynecomastia is a common side effect of spironolactone. This is due to the fact that spironolactone with its steroid nucleus is able to competitively inhibit androgen binding to tissue receptors. Impotence and reduced libido may occur as well. Although spironolactone may cause menstrual irregularities in younger adults, possibly by an antiestrogenic mechanism, the clinical effects on the postmenopausal woman are not well defined. Endocrinologic effects in general are most common at high doses and are reversible, but the risk of developing such problems at ordinary doses is theoretically higher in the geriatric patient because of age-related hormonal alterations. Because of this, it is important to distinguish drug-related symptoms from those that are due to physiologic or pathologic age-related problems.

IMPORTANT DRUG INTERACTIONS. Spironolactone decreases renal clearance of digoxin and may produce digoxin toxicity. However, serum levels of digitalis preparations must be interpreted with caution since they share structural similarity with spironolactone, and falsely elevated measurements on radioimmunoassay sometimes occurs.

As with other potassium-sparing diuretics, potassium supplement should be avoided (see Triamterene above).

INDICATIONS. The endocrinologic effects of spironolactone make it less desirable than other agents for elderly patients, who are theoretically at higher risk of these side effects. Its major indication is in the treatment of fluid retention in cirrhosis. It can also be used as an alternative to triamterene and amiloride in patients who cannot tolerate those agents.

Furosemide (Lasix)

Furosemide is a potent natriuretic agent and is highly effective in fluid-retaining states. Because of its short duration of action, acute salt-wasting is followed by compensatory sodium retention, and hypotensive effect is not maintained. Thus, it generally is not an ideal choice for the long-term management of hypertension in patients with normal renal function. For a full discussion of this drug, the reader is referred to Chap. 15.

CALCIUM CHANNEL BLOCKING AGENTS

Calcium channel blocking agents, as a group, are fairly well tolerated in the elderly, although important exceptions to this rule exist and will be noted below. These drugs are particularly useful in patients who also require treatment for angina and certain other cardiovascular disorders. Unlike the beta blockers, calcium channel antagonists do not possess adverse metabolic effects and do not produce bronchospasm.

Originally used to treat other cardiovascular disorders, they are frequently employed in the management of hypertension in older patients.

Pharmacologic Considerations

Mechanism of Action

These agents inhibit slow movement of calcium across cell membranes through "calcium channels," thereby reducing excitation of myocardial and vascular smooth muscle, and cardiac conducting tissue. Their antihypertensive action is thought to be related to vasodilation of vascular smooth muscle. However, they may prevent the compensatory increase in sympathetic activity that occurs as a result of vasodilation. In addition, some agents of this group possess weak natriuretic activity. It has been suggested that these actions help to sustain the antihypertensive effect and obviate the need for diuretic therapy that is often required with vasodilators such as hydralazine.

Selection of Agent

All calcium channel blockers are effective in reducing blood pressure. However, they differ from one another in specific actions, which can be harnessed in some circumstances but should be

Table 12-1. Properties of Commonly Used Calcium Channel Blocking Agents

Potential Side Effect in Elderly	Diltiazem	Nifedipine	Verapamil
Bradyarrhythmia	+	−	+ +
Heart failure	−	− ?	+
Flush	−	+ +	−
Edema	+	+ + +	+
Constipation	+ +	+	+ + +
Bladder disturbance	− to +	+	−

Potential of producing effect
− Little or none
+ Low
+ + Moderate
+ + + High

avoided in others. The properties of these agents are summarized in Table 12-1 and guidelines for selection are given in Table 12-2.

Diltiazem (Cardizem)

PHARMACOKINETICS. Diltiazem is rapidly absorbed and undergoes first-pass hepatic metabolism with peak serum levels occurring within 2-3 hours. Hepatic metabolism is saturable, so that the higher the dose and after continuous use the bioavailability increases and the elimination half-life lengthens. One major metabolite of diltiazem is partly active. Limited study indicates that the overall elimination half-life of 3-6 hours is prolonged with age. A long-acting preparation (Cardizem SR) maintains therapeutic blood levels for 12 hours in nonelderly adults. There is no information at present on its duration of action in older individuals.

Clearance of diltiazem is impaired in liver disease and heart failure. The drug is highly bound to serum proteins, specifically, alpha$_1$ acid glycoprotein.

Table 12-2. Guidelines on Selection of Calcium Channel Antagonist

To avoid:	Select:
Bradycardia	Nifedipine
Congestive heart failure	Nifedipine
Venous insufficiency	Diltiazem; verapamil
Constipation	Nifedipine; diltiazem
Asthma	All
Peripheral arterial disease	All (If edema develops, another selection from this group or another class of drugs should be made.)

Note: Selection of recommended agent is preferred over other calcium channel blockers in each case, but the expected protection is not guaranteed if the patient is highly susceptible. Nicardipine similar to Nifedipine in spectrum of effects.

ADVERSE EFFECTS. Diltiazem is generally better tolerated by older patients than other available calcium channel blockers, although exceptions to this rule certainly exist. **Dizziness** and **edema** occur uncommonly and **constipation** occasionally.

Diltiazem slows atrioventricular conduction; **bradyarrhythmias** may occur in susceptible patients but this is less common than with verapamil.

IMPORTANT DRUG INTERACTIONS. Diltiazem reduces renal clearance of digoxin and may potentiate digitalis-induced arrhythmias. Because diltiazem has an effect on atrioventricular conduction, the digoxin-diltiazem combination may lead to bradycardia on a pharmacodynamic basis as well. Concurrent use is not advised, but if necessary, digoxin dose should be reduced and the patient monitored closely. A pharmacokinetic interaction with digitoxin has also been described but the mechanism is unclear.

Concurrent use of diltiazem and beta adrenergic blocking agents may increase the likelihood of bradycardia.

Diltiazem may inhibit hepatic metabolism of theophylline but increases in serum theophylline levels are inconstant. Cimetidine may reduce diltiazem metabolism, increasing its effect.

CONTRAINDICATIONS. Diltiazem is contraindicated in patients with significant bradycardia or high degree of heart block.

INDICATIONS. Diltiazem is indicated for the treatment of hypertension and angina. It is highly suitable for elderly patients who require treatment for both conditions.

DOSING

Initial dose: 30 mg tid. Some patients may respond to 30 mg bid.
Maximum dose: 90 mg tid.
Note: Long-acting diltiazem (Carizem SR) is intended for bid dosing. The smallest available tablet is 60 mg.

Nifedipine (Procardia, Aldalat)

PHARMACOKINETICS. Nifedipine is well absorbed and is extensively metabolized in the liver. Half-life of the parent drug is only about 2 hours but a long acting form of nifedipine is now available. Its duration of action is more than 24 hours.

Nifedipine is extensively bound to plasma proteins.

ADVERSE EFFECTS. Nifedipine has the most potent vasodilating action of the available calcium channel antagonists. As a consequence, it is the most likely to produce **flushing, dizziness, headache,** and **edema.** These symptoms may be reduced in severity when the drug is taken in short dosage intervals. The newer long-acting form is said to reduce the incidence of these effects, with the exception of edema. Nifedipine appears to produce edema in elderly patients with a much greater frequency than in other age groups. This observation is probably related to the high incidence of underlying venous insufficiency or nonspecific hemodynamic changes that occur in this age group.

In contrast to diltiazem and verapamil, nifedipine often produces a **reflex increase in heart rate** and may produce tachycardia. This effect may not be as pronounced in elderly patients, because of blunted hemodynamic responses, and, in fact, the potential for increasing heart rate may make nifedipine suitable in patients with bradycardia.

Despite its propensity to produce edema, nifedipine has a mild natriuretic and diuretic effect. **Bladder disturbances** have been reported by older patients but these problems may be transitory. In fact, nifedipine may reduce the contractility of bladder smooth muscle and has been reported to increase urinary storage. Urine loss, nocturia, and urinary retention have all been reported.

Nifedipine may **worsen proteinuria and renal function** in hypertensive diabetics who have preexisting renal disease. This contrasts with the improvement that has been reported when such patients receive diltiazem or ACE inhibitors. This differential effect has not been fully explained but may have to do with internal renal hemodynamics.

Confusional states have occasionally been reported but are uncommon.

IMPORTANT DRUG INTERACTIONS. Decreased renal digoxin clearance has been reported to occur with nifedipine, but there is some controversy on this issue. If a patient on digoxin requires treatment with a calcium channel blocker, nifedipine is probably preferable to diltiazem or verapamil, since a pharmacodynamic interaction is less likely.

Although the pharmacodynamic effects of nifedipine are quite different from diltiazem, nifedipine has been reported to increase the negative inotropic and chronotropic effects of beta blockers. For a complete discussion of nifedipine interactions, the reader is referred to readings in the Bibliography (see Rizack & Hillman).

INDICATIONS. Nifedipine is indicated in the treatment of angina and is also suitable for the management of hypertension.

DOSING
Initial dose: 10 mg tid.
Maximum dose: 30 mg qid.
Note: A long-acting preparation of nifedepine (Procardia XL) is designed for once-daily administration

Verapamil (Calan, Isoptin)

This calcium channel blocking agent is used more frequently in the management of arrhythmias than hypertension. It has potent negative chronotropic and potential negative inotropic effects. In addition, it commonly produces constipation. For these reasons, verapamil should generally not be instituted primarily for the management of hypertension but should be reserved for hypertensive patients who also require management of atrial tachyarrhythmias.

Verapamil has been reported to relieve nocturnal leg cramps in elderly patients who did not respond to quinine. Paradoxically, nifedipine has been reported to worsen cramps.

Verapamil is discussed further in Chap. 15.

DOSE FOR HYPERTENSION
Initial dose: 40 mg bid-tid.
Maximum daily dose: 360 mg in divided doses. Some patients may tolerate total daily doses of 480 mg.
Note: Substantial-release verapamil (Calan SR, others) is designed for once-daily administration.

Newer Calcium Channel Blocking Agents

Nicardipine (Cardene) and israpidine (DynaCirc) are relative newcomers to this group of drugs. They are chemically related to nifedipine and thus similar to that drug in their hemodynamic effects. Nicardipine is known to be a potent cerebral vasodilator but there are no firm clinical applications of this action at this time. It is presently unclear if nicardipine and israpidine offer any new advantages over other calcium channel antagonists in the management of cardiovascular disease.

For nongeriatric adults, initial starting doses are 20 mg tid for nicardipine and 2.5 bid for israpidine. There is not yet enough experience with these agents on which to base specific recommendations for the elderly.

ANGIOTENSIN CONVERTING ENZYME (ACE) INHIBITORS

Pharmacologic Considerations

Mechanism of Action

Agents of this class act by binding to and inhibiting the action of angiotensin converting enzyme (ACE), which is responsible for the conversion of angiotensin I to active angiotensin II. Angiotensin II itself is a powerful vasoconstrictor, so that reductions in this substance lead to reduction in vascular resistance and lowering of blood pressure. Angiotensin II must also be viewed as a key segment of the renin-angiotensin-aldosterone cycle, which regulates functions such as fluid homeostasis, sodium metabolism, and renal perfusion. By interrupting this cycle, ACE inhibitors lower blood pressure by several mechanisms, and affect fluid homeostasis, renal autoregulation, and the handling of sodium and potassium. Age does not appear to alter the ability of these drugs to inhibit ACE.

The initial response to ACE inhibitors depends on certain physiologic factors present when therapy is instituted. Sodium depletion and hypovolemia activate the renin-angiotensin system and the response to ACE inhibition may be substantial. In fact, an initial exaggerated hypotensive response may be seen under these circumstances. However, low renin levels, as seen for example in elderly hypertensives, do not preclude an adequate response. Thus, despite evidence pointing to age-related impairment of the renin-angiotensin system, ACE inhibitors have been found to be effective antihypertensive agents in the elderly.

Other Actions

ACE is also responsible for the degradation of bradykinin, which has potent vasodilating properties, some of which are mediated by prostaglandin. The extent to which this system is responsible for antihypertensive effects of ACE inhibitors is not known, but it has been implicated in certain side effects.

Because ACE inhibition diminishes aldosterone secretion, ACE inhibitors promote sodium excretion and potassium retention. Use of ACE inhibitors in congestive heart failure is based on the increased peripheral resistance seen in that disease, and on their ability to blunt the compensatory increases in renin that occur when diuretics alone are used.

Several ACE inhibitors are now available. Clinical effects produced by these agents are similar, with variability due largely to pharmacokinetic differences.

Pharmacokinetics

The ACE inhibitors differ from one another in their duration of action. What these agents do have in common is that their elimination rate is proportional to renal function, so that all three tend to have prolonged serum half-lives in elderly patients.

Captopril (Capoten) achieves peak serum concentrations in about 1 hour, and has an acute onset of action within 30 minutes. Peak action occurs at 1–2 hours. It is extensively metabolized in the liver, but a significant proportion is excreted unchanged in the kidney. The serum half-life is relatively short at 3 hours or less, but the duration of action may be up to 12 hours. Elimination of captopril tends to be prolonged in older patients.

Enalapril (Vasotec) is a pro-drug that must first be converted in the liver to its active form, enalaprilat. Thus, its onset of action of 1–2 hours is later than that of captopril; this is further delayed in the presence of liver disease and severe congestive failure. Peak antihypertensive action may be delayed at 6–8 hours or more. Although this is not important in the usual long-term management of hypertension, it must be anticipated when treatment is first instituted in patients with congestive heart failure, who are at risk of an exaggerated hypotensive response. Enalaprilat is eliminated by the kidney, but much is retained in the serum bound to ACE, and its duration of action may be as long as 30 hours in some patients. Elimination half-life may be significantly prolonged with age.

Lisinopril (Prinivil), the newest agent of this group, is structurally related to enalaprilat and, unlike enalapril, its pharmacologic action does not depend on conversion to an active metabolite. However, its onset of action is at 1–2 hours and peak antihypertensive effect occurs at 5–6 hours or later. As with enalapril, this is not usually important in maintenance therapy of hypertension, but should be anticipated in patients at risk of an exaggerated hypotensive response. Like captopril, lisinopril does not undergo extensive hepatic metabolism and substantial amounts are excreted unchanged by the kidney. Its duration of action is approximately 24 hours in non-elderly adults. Even healthy elderly appear to eliminate lisinopril much more slowly than younger subjects, achieving higher concentrations at any given dose.

Adverse Effects

Serum potassium level tends to rise and **hyperkalemia** may occur with ACE inhibitors, due to inhibition of aldosterone secretion. However, this is unlikely to occur in the absence of renal insufficiency, potassium supplementation, severe sodium depletion, or the use of potassium-sparing diuretics or nonsteroidal anti-inflammatory drugs.

Dry cough is a common side effect observed with ACE inhibitors. It has been suggested that this symptom is somehow related to pulmonary accumulation of bradykinin, which is inactivated by angiotensin converting enzyme, but the exact mechanism is not known. ACE inhibitors have also rarely been reported to produce **angioedema**, another symptom that could be related to bradykinin accumulation.

Hypotension may occur with the first few doses of ACE inhibitors. This is more likely in patients with sodium depletion or volume contraction, presumably because of activation of the renin angiotensin system. Orthostatic hypotension is uncommon with ACE inhibitors, despite the absence of reflex tachycardia that would be expected with a vasodilator. The absence of orthostatic hypotension as well as reflex tachycardia has been ascribed to an effect on the parasympathetic nervous system, but the precise mechanism is not known.

Despite earlier reports, renal insufficiency now appears to be an unusual complication of ACE inhibitors. This is probably due to safer dosing and wider use in healthier individuals than in the past, when these drugs were reserved for very sick patients. In fact, recent evidence indicates that ACE inhibitors may retard the progression of renal disease in diabetics. **Renal failure** may, however, be produced **in patients with bilateral renal artery stenosis** because ACE inhibition impairs autoregulation of renal blood flow distal to the stenosis. Severe chronic heart failure is another condition associated with decreased renal perfusion pressure, and in this setting ACE inhibitors can produce **functional renal insufficiency** despite improvements in cardiac function.

Certain **other adverse effects** occur less commonly than previously thought. These include desquamative skin rash, skin ulcers, impaired taste, proteinuria, and neutropenia, effects that were associated with captopril, the earliest agent of this class in use. The reasons for earlier pessimistic reports may have been that captopril had been reserved for patients refractory to other cardiovascular agents. Now that captopril and other ACE inhibitors are in general use and at lower doses, fewer serious effects are reported.

Earlier in the evolution of ACE inhibitors, it was felt that hypersensitivity or allergic phenomena were due to the sulfhydryl group of captopril that is not contained in enalapril or lisinopril. However, these side effects may be common to all members of this class of drugs.

Elderly patients tend to tolerate ACE inhibitors very well. These drugs have no apparent effect on the metabolism of glucose or lipids, and they may attenuate the hyperuricemia produced by diuretics. They are less likely than many other antihypertensive agents to produce depression and decreased alertness. It is unclear whether this is related to the absence of central depressant effects, or to an enhancement of the feeling of well being.

Important Drug Interactions

ACE inhibitors should not be used concurrently with potassium-sparing diuretics or potassium supplements because of the danger of producing hyperkalemia. Concurrent use of nonsteroidal anti-inflammatory agents has been reported to reduce the antihypertensive action of ACE inhibitors, but this interaction probably occurs with other antihypertensive agents as well and is ultimately related to antinatriuresis.

Patients who have been taking other diuretics, such as furosemide or the thiazides, may develop an exaggerated hypotensive response to ACE inhibitors; initial doses should be cautious, especially in patients with hemodynamic compromise.

Contraindications and Precautions

Patients who have experienced a serious side effect from one member of the ACE inhibitor class should not use any ACE inhibitor.

Debilitated patients, who may be hypovolemic or otherwise unusually sensitive to the effects of these agents, should receive a test dose (no more than the equivalent of 6.25 mg of Captopril) and should be observed for the development of acute hypotension. Renal function and serum potassium should be followed in patients at risk for azotemia or hyperkalemia.

Selection of Agent

At present, there is no convincing evidence that any ACE inhibitor is safer or more effective than the others when used at appropriate doses. Selection should be made according to cost or desirability of the dose regimen. While the long duration of action of lisinopril makes it theoretically more useful when compliance is a problem, this could also be a disadvantage in elderly patients. It should be reserved for patients whose renal function permits adequate clearance.

Enalapril is often effective when given once a day, but many patients require twice daily dosing to achieve efficacy. This drug may also be ineffective in the presence of liver disease.

A twice-daily dose of captopril is effective in many patients. This is probably a reasonable starting regimen for hypertension in most elderly. If more frequent dosing is required, a longer acting agent is often preferable.

Indications

ACE inhibitors are indicated as first-line agents in the treatment of hypertension in elderly patients. They may be a particularly suitable alternative for patients who develop adverse metabolic effects on diuretics or beta blockers, those who cannot tolerate calcium channel antagonists, and those with depression or cognitive impairment. There is increasing evidence that ACE inhibitors may be helpful to diabetics who are showing signs of nephropathy manifested by proteinuria.

ACE inhibitors are also used as adjunctive treatment of congestive heart failure and are probably the most effective vasodilating agents available for this purpose.

Dosing in Hypertension

Initial dose: Captopril, 12.5 mg bid.
              Enalapril, 2.5 once daily to bid.
              Lisinopril, 5 mg once daily.

Some patients may achieve adequate initial pressure response from lower doses of these agents. Conservative dosing should be given to patients at risk of developing an exaggerated hypotensive response, namely those with volume contraction or sodium depletion.

Maximum daily dose: Captopril, 300 mg in 2 to 3 divided doses.
                     Enalapril, 40 mg in 2 divided doses.
                     Lisinopril, 40 mg once daily.

BETA ADRENERGIC BLOCKING AGENTS

Members of this large group of agents share one property—that of blocking beta adrenergic receptors in neural tissue and smooth muscle. Otherwise, these agents are pharmacologically rather different from one another. Their differences, which will be detailed below, should serve as a guide rather than a means of reliably predicting how the patient will respond. Guidelines for selecting beta blockers are described in Table 12–3.

Pharmacologic Considerations

Mechanism of Action

Beta blockers are structurally related to catecholamines and competitively inhibit their binding to beta adrenergic receptors in neural tissue and smooth muscle. There are two types of beta receptors: $beta_1$, which are found primarily in cardiac muscle and conducting tissue, and $beta_2$, which are found in smooth muscle of arterioles and bronchi. Beta receptor activity also mediates renin release in the kidney, urine storage in the body of the bladder, insulin release in the pancreas, and glycogenolysis in the liver. Blood pressure lowering is thought to be achieved at least in part by a reduction in cardiac output. It is not known to what extent other mechanisms are involved. Inhibition of renin release and central nervous system mechanisms probably play a lesser role.

Several types of beta blockers are available: nonselective agents, which block both $beta_1$ and $beta_2$ receptors; "cardioselective" agents, which have a greater affinity for $beta_1$ receptors; and agents that also possess some beta agonist properties ("intrinsic sympathomimetic activity"), which partly counteract the beta blockade. $Beta_1$ selective agents theoretically should avoid the side effect of bronchospasm in susceptible patients while retaining cardiac properties, but at the doses needed to achieve therapeutic effects selectivity is generally eradicated. Agents with intrinsic sympathomimetic properties are designed to counteract the production of bradycardia and perhaps claudication and hyperlipidemia, but once again, not all patients will be protected from these side effects.

One nonselective agent, labetalol, also possesses $alpha_1$ adrenergic blocking properties and partial $beta_2$ agonist properties. These characteristics prevent beta blockade from producing the vasoconstriction that occurs when alpha stimulation is unopposed, making labetalol theoretically more useful in patients with peripheral vascular disease.

Table 12–3. Guidelines on Selection of Beta Blockers (BB)

Condition	Recommendation
Bronchospasm	Avoid BB
Congestive heart failure	Avoid BB
Angina at rest	Avoid BB with ISA*
Depression or dementia	Atenolol, if tolerated
Diabetes mellitus (diet-controlled)	Selective BB: monitor glucose
Diabetes mellitus on medication	Avoid BB or consider pindolol
Hyperlipidemia	Avoid nonselective BB; monitor lipids
Bradycardia	Avoid BB; if necessary and if bradycardia asymptomatic, use BB with ISA
Peripheral vascular disease	Avoid BB; if necessary, use labetolol

*Intrinsic sympathomimetic activity

Beta blockers differ in their lipophilicity, with those most lipophilic being most capable of entering the central nervous system. It has been claimed that the less lipophilic are less likely to produce effects such as dementia and depression. While this is probably true, all beta blockers are capable of producing these symptoms in susceptible people.

Sensitivity to beta adrenergic stimulation and blockade appears to decline with age. This has been attributed to a decline in the number or the sensitivity of beta receptors, or both. Although it has not been shown that geriatric patients as a group fail to respond to beta blockers, some studies have demonstrated that a smaller proportion of older individuals achieve an adequate hypotensive effect with this class of agents than younger patients.

Pharmacokinetics

The pharmacokinetics of beta blockers such as propranolol are complex and vary widely from agent to agent. Clearance of these agents may be largely hepatic, largely renal, or mixed.

Hepatically cleared beta blockers such as propranolol are removed from circulation by extensive first-pass metabolism with production of some active metabolites. Age-related decline in hepatic blood flow is said to reduce the elimination half-life of these drugs, but there is controversy on this issue. As expected, most evidence indicates that beta blockers that are eliminated primarily by renal clearance are excreted more slowly with age. Importantly, pharmacodynamic response outlasts the presence of these drugs in serum, probably because of binding to beta receptors.

Most beta blockers are not highly bound to serum proteins. The binding of propranolol is complex, with a large portion being bound to alpha$_1$ acid glycoprotein, which tends to increase with age.

The properties of the various beta blockers are summarized in Table 12-4.

Do Older Patients Have Increased or Decreased Sensitivity to Beta Blockers?

Number or sensitivity of beta receptors tends to decline with age. While many older individuals do exhibit an adequate hypotensive response to beta blockers, several but by no means all studies have demonstrated that the proportion responding and the degree of response declines with age. This phenomenon occurs despite the fact that beta blockers tend to be eliminated from the body more slowly with advancing age. Although one could argue that this is the reason that many aged patients do respond to these drugs, it is also reasonable to attribute this variable response to physiologic variability of the geriatric patient and perhaps to chemical differences among the beta blockers studied in the various trials.

The clinical response to "intrinsic sympathomimetic activity" of certain beta blockers is not predictable in older patients. End-organ dysfunction, such as sinus node disease, may impair the response to adrenergic stimulation. Thus, normal mechanisms cannot be relied upon for the expression of partial agonist activity.

However, geriatric patients are far from being protected against side effects of beta blockers. Disorders that are more prevalent in late life, such as dementia, sick sinus syndrome, and congestive heart failure, increase the risk of specific side effects.

Table 12–4. Beta Blockers Commonly Used in Hypertension

Agent (Brand)	Elimination	Lipophilicity	Initial Dose (mg)
Nonselective			
Propranolol (Inderal)	H	High	20 bid
Nadolol (Corgard)	R	Low	20 once daily
Pindolol[a] (Visken)	H + R	Moderate	5 bid
Labetalol[b] (Normodyne; Trandate)		Moderate	100 bid
Cardioselective[c]			
Atenolol (Tenormin)	R	Very low	25 once daily[d]
Metoprolol (Lopressor)	H + R	Low–moderate	50 bid

H = Hepatic; R = Renal
[a]Has intrinsic sympathomimetic (partial beta agonist) activity (ISA).
[b]Has alpha$_1$ blocking activity and some ISA.
[c]See text.
[d]Further dose reductions may be required in renal insufficiency.

Adverse Effects

Beta$_1$ blockade may lead to **bradycardia, congestive heart failure, and cardiac conduction disturbances.** Beta$_2$ blockade may produce **bronchospasm** in susceptible individuals. All beta blockers, regardless of selectivity, are capable of producing these sides effects.

Beta blockade in the pancreas impairs insulin release and can **impair glucose tolerance.** In addition, by blunting tachycardia and sweating, beta blockade can **mask signs of hypoglycemia,** endangering the medically treated diabetic patient. Agents with intrinsic sympathomimetic activity are somewhat less likely to do this. However, it is important to point out that many aged diabetics tend to have impaired counterregulatory responses to hypoglycemia even if they are not taking beta blockers.

Blockade of beta$_2$ receptors in peripheral vessels leaves them vulnerable to unopposed alpha stimulation, so that vasoconstriction may result. This can lead to **Raynaud's phenomenon** or worsening of **arterial claudication.** Pindolol and labetalol may spare some patients these symptoms.

Central nervous system effects, such as **depression** and **dementia,** may be produced by beta blockers. Dementia may occur in a dose-related fashion, is reversible when the agent is withdrawn, and may not recur with substitution of a beta blocker with lower lipophilicity. **Drowsiness, lethargy,** and **sleep disturbances** may also occur. Beta blockers have rarely been reported to unmask or exacerbate **myasthenia gravis.** The mechanism is not fully understood, but it has been attributed to neuromuscular blockade, a phenomenon that has been demonstrated in vitro.

Orthostatic hypotension is uncommon, but may occur with labetolol, which blocks compensatory alpha$_1$ mediated vasoconstriction.

Bladder disturbances have been reported and are primarily seen in older patients. Although the urinary bladder is predominantly controlled by the parasympathetic system, adrenergic receptors are also found in the bladder body and outlet. Adrenergic stimulation tends to promote urine storage but the specific response of the bladder to blockade is unpredictable, owing to the variety of beta blockers in use and the complex innervation of the bladder. **Impotence** has also been reported.

Abrupt withdrawal of beta blockers may precipitate a **rebound** in ischemic symptoms or hypertension, which is thought to be due to beta receptor hypersensitivity. It is not known if age-related changes in beta receptors alter this phenomenon in any way. However, older patients may not manifest overt symptoms of rebound such as tachycardia or typical chest pain. The rebound effect is theoretically less likely with partial agonists, which are capable of activating the beta receptor to a limited extent.

Important Drug Interactions

Bradycardia may be potentiated by concurrent use of digoxin, diltiazem, verapamil, and other agents that suppress the conducting system. Heart failure may occur in susceptible patients taking other agents known to depress myocardial contractility, such as diisopyramide, verapamil, and, less often, diltiazem or quinidine.

By reducing hepatic blood flow and by binding to hepatic microsomal enzymes, cimetidine reduces the clearance of hepatically metabolized beta blockers. Other agents affecting hepatic enzymes may also increase or decrease levels of these beta blockers.

Beta blockers should not be used in conjunction with adrenergic agents that stimulate alpha receptors (epinephrine, phenylpropanolamine, ephedrine) because severe hypertension may occur as a result of unopposed alpha stimulation. The same mechanism occurs in pheochromocytoma.

When combined with central alpha$_2$ agonists, such as clonidine, beta blockers may produce paradoxical hypertension. This can occur during withdrawal of clonidine, presumably because beta blockade interferes with compensatory mechanisms that attenuate the clonidine withdrawal syndrome. This interaction does not occur with labetalol.

Contraindications and Precautions

Beta blockers are contraindicated in patients with congestive heart failure or significant bradycardia. Although partial agonists are tolerated by some patients with bradycardia, use of agents other than beta blockers should be considered first.

Patients being medically treated for diabetes should avoid beta blockers if possible because symptoms of hypoglycemia may be masked. Because of the possibility that glucose tolerance can be impaired by these agents, even untreated diabetics should receive additional blood glucose monitoring when beta blockers are instituted.

Beta blockers are contraindicated in patients with peripheral vascular disease who are exhibiting rest pain or more severe signs of ischemia. In patients with arterial claudication, labetalol or perhaps pindolol can sometimes be used without exacerbation of symptoms.

Beta blockers are contraindicated in known or suspected pheochromocytoma.

Dementia is not an absolute contraindication to the use of beta blockers, but agents from another class should be considered first in that setting.

Beta blockers should be withdrawn slowly in order to avoid rebound hypertension or exacerbation of ischemia.

Indications

Beta blockers are indicated in the treatment of hypertension, if there is no contraindication. Patients with diabetes, arterial claudication, dementia, and depression should use beta blockers only when they cannot tolerate other agents.

Beta blockers are indicated in the treatment of angina (see Chap. 13).

Other Uses

Beta blockers are used in the management of hypertrophic cardiomyopathy. Echocardiographic evidence of this entity exists in many elderly but its clinical significance requires further study.

Propranolol has been used with some success in the treatment of benign essential ("familial") tremor, a condition seen primarily in older patients. It is thought that this tremor is mediated by $beta_2$ receptors in peripheral muscle spindles, and that nonselective beta blockers, such as propranolol, are more likely to have a therapeutic effect. Agents with intrinsic sympathomimetic activity, such as pindolol, may actually increase tremor. Beta blockers may also be useful in the management of lithium-induced tremor.

Timolol, betaxolol, levobunolol, and metipranolol are beta blockers that are available as ophthalmic agents, which are used in the treatment of glaucoma. Ocular beta blockers are capable of producing the same spectrum of effects as oral beta blockers. This topic is discussed more fully in Chap. 34.

Beta blockers, notably propranolol, are used to suppress sympathomimetic symptoms of thyrotoxicosis while definitive treatment is readied or under way. This is considered very important in elderly patients with hyperthyroidism who readily develop cardiac complications. Propranolol is frequently continued for several weeks following radioactive iodine therapy because of the possibility of radiation thyroiditis and resultant thyrotoxicosis.

Use of beta blockers in the treatment of angina is discussed in Chap. 13.

Dosing

Pharmacokinetic and pharmacodynamic factors in older patients mitigate in favor of reducing doses, while decreased beta receptor sensitivity suggests that doses may need to be higher in older patients to achieve the same effect. Initial doses should be age-adjusted downward, to test whether the patient will suffer an adverse effect. If the initial dose is well tolerated, the dose can be titrated slowly upward. If ordinary (non-age-adjusted) dosages do not produce the desired effect, it is possible that the patient is not particularly sensitive to beta blockade and it may be preferable to switch to an agent other than a beta blocker rather than to continue raising the dose. Initial doses are given Table 12–4.

Selection of Agent

Selection of agent depends almost entirely on the patient's concurrent medical problems and proclivities. Guidelines are summarized in Table 12–3.

HYDRALAZINE (APRESOLINE, OTHERS)

Pharmacologic Considerations

Mechanism of Action

Hydralazine lowers blood pressure by producing arteriolar smooth muscle dilatation. This is believed to occur largely as a direct effect of the drug but other mechanisms could be involved. The effect of hydralazine is greatest in the precapillary bed. Because the drug lacks a direct effect on the autonomic nervous system, compensatory physiologic responses to its hypotensive effect are free to occur, the most important being reflex tachycardia and renin-induced sodium and fluid retention. These counterregulatory phenomena tend to reduce the drug's antihypertensive efficacy, unless concurrent therapy with diuretics or beta blockers is given.

Counterregulatory responses to hydralazine are less predictable in older patients. Reflex tachycardia is less likely to occur, because patients often have impaired sympathetic tone. Fluid retention also may be attenuated because of age changes in the renin-aldosterone system.

No compensatory mechanisms operate to reduce venous pooling produced by hydralazine. This feature is the basis for its use, though controversial, as a preload reducer in the treatment of congestive heart failure. Unfortunately, venous pooling has its drawbacks (see Adverse Effects below).

Pharmacokinetics

Hydralazine is well absorbed orally with peak plasma levels and antihypertensive action occurring within 1–2 hours. The drug is primarily metabolized by hepatic acetylation, a process with well-known genetic variability. "Slow acetylators" tend to have higher levels of hydralazine than "fast acetylators," particularly after oral use. This genetic factor seems to be a more important predictor of hydralazine disposition than age.

Although the average serum half-life is 4–6 hours, the antihypertensive action of hydralazine may last sufficiently longer so that blood pressure control can frequently be achieved with twice-daily dosing. This may be due to the fact that the drug binds to the vessel wall for a considerable period of time.

Adverse Effects

Hydralazine may produce **reflex tachycardia**, but this occurs less often in older patients because of impaired counterregulatory responses. While helpful in that situation, these blunted counterregulatory responses may also allow hydralazine to produce orthostatic hypotension, which is an unusual side effect in younger patients. Furthermore, some older individuals may develop reflex tachycardia. Caution is called for, particularly in patients with coronary artery disease.

Hydralazine has a tendency to produce fluid retention and **edema**, necessitating the addition of a diuretic.

Lupuslike reactions occur in 5%–15% of patients. As many as 50% of patients develop a positive antinuclear antibody reaction (ANA), but this is usually not a precursor to actual disease. Lupus reactions occur more commonly in "slow acetylators" and when high doses of the drug are used. The most common manifestations of this syndrome are joint pain, arthritis, rash, and pleuropericarditis. Renal and neurological symptoms have been reported but are rare. While older patients have a tendency to develop autoimmune phenomena in general, owing to age-related decrease in T cell function, they do *not* have a greater tendency to develop autoimmune *disease* and do not appear to be at excessive risk of developing hydralazine-related lupus.

Flushing and **headache** may occur but tend to subside with time. Nausea and vomiting have been reported fairly commonly in patients being treated for congestive heart failure, but this may be due to the high doses used.

Important Drug Interactions

The antihypertensive effect of hydralazine may be impaired by NSAIDs. This interaction with NSAIDs probably occurs with most other antihypertensive agents.

Contraindications

Hydralazine is contraindicated in patients with a history suggestive of systemic lupus erythematosus.

Precautions

A large proportion of older patients have low titers of autoantibodies in their serum, which can confound the diagnosis of drug-related lupus. Therefore, patients should be tested for the presence of antinuclear antibodies prior to starting hydralazine. A positive low-titer reaction in an elderly patient without lupuslike symptoms is not a contraindication to the use of hydralazine. However, in these situations, periodic determinations of ANA should be made, and a rising titer should prompt extra vigilance. This topic is discussed further in Chap. 14 in connection with procainamide.

Indications

Hydralazine is indicated for the treatment of hypertension in elderly patients who cannot take antihypertensive agents previously described in this chapter. It may be particularly suitable as an adjunct to beta blockers or diuretics in certain patients. Patients who have developed confusional states or lethargy on other antihypertensive agents may do quite well with hydralazine.

Hydralazine is also used as adjunctive treatment for congestive heart failure. However, despite the fact that it increases measures of cardiac output, hydralazine does not improve exercise tolerance beyond the beneficial effect conferred by digitalis and diuretics.

Dosing

Initial antihypertensive dose: 10 mg bid.
Maximum daily dose: 200 mg in 2 to 4 divided doses.

METHYLDOPA (ALDOMET, OTHERS)

Pharmacologic Considerations

Mechanism of Action

Methyldopa (dihydroxyphenylalanine) lowers blood pressure by a mechanism that is incompletely understood. The current view is that methyldopa enters the central nervous system where it is converted to alpha methylnorepinephrine, which can replace more potent norepinephrine as a neurotransmitter (the "false neurotransmitter" hypothesis). Methylnorepinephrine is an alpha$_2$ receptor agonist. Alpha$_2$ receptors are largely inhibitory so that the effect of methyldopa is to reduce sympathetic tone.

With chronic use, compensatory retention of sodium and water may occur. In general, this effect manifests as diminution of antihypertensive effect, which can be overcome with the addition of a diuretic.

Pharmacokinetics

Methyldopa is variably absorbed. The onset of action occurs at 2–3 hours. A portion is metabolized in the gut wall and a portion undergoes hepatic metabolism; several enzyme systems are involved, including widely distributed catechol-O-methyltransferase. Overall elimination half-life is variable at 2–7 hours. The duration and intensity of effect appear to be dependent on complex factors, including metabolic enzyme activity, which is subject to wide interindividual variation. Although there is little or no pharmacokinetic data available in older patients, the dose depends more on pharmacodynamic response. At all ages, duration of action outlasts the presence of the drug in plasma.

Adverse Effects

Geriatric patients are particularly susceptible to side effects such as **orthostatic hypotension** and **confusional states,** more so than are younger patients. Methyldopa may also produce **lethargy, depression, impotence, dry mouth,** and **nasal stuffiness. Bradycardia** occurs occasionally and probably represents an unmasking of sinus node dysfunction.

Methyldopa inhibits dopa decarboxylase, the enzyme responsible for the conversion of amino acids to dopamine. This effect may result in central depletion of dopamine and **parkinsonian symptoms** have been reported. This side effect is thought to be rare. In contrast to many other antihypertensive agents, methyldopa produces **diarrhea** more often than constipation. The mechanism is unknown.

Methyldopa is one of many agents capable of producing **autoimmune hemolytic anemia.** In the case of methyldopa, the mechanism involves the inhibition of suppressor T cells, which are responsible for regulating antibody production. Methyldopa-induced autoimmune hemolytic anemia may not occur until after several months of therapy, and the incidence increases with increasing dose and duration of therapy. Although 30% or more of methyldopa treated patients become Coombs positive, only a small proportion actually develop hemolytic anemia. This may be related to the fact that methyldopa tends to suppress macrophage activity as well. Suppressor T cell function, but not macrophage function, declines with age, making older patients theoretically more susceptible to immune reactions from methyldopa. Coombs positivity alone does not require that methyldopa be discontinued.

Hepatitis, a hypersensitivity reaction, has also been reported in about 5% of patients treated with methyldopa. That the number of cases is higher in older patients may merely reflect the increased incidence of hypertension with age. Other hypersensitivity reactions have been reported less commonly.

Important Drug Interactions

The antihypertensive action of methyldopa may be impaired by tricyclic antidepressants that possess central alpha$_2$ antagonist activity, but clinical effect is variable. Methyldopa may reduce the clinical efficacy of antiparkinsonian agents.

Methyldopa should not be used with beta blockers because paradoxical elevations in blood pressure may occur. The mechanism is unclear.

Confusional states may be precipitated when methyldopa is combined with haloperidol, monoamine oxidase inhibitors, and perhaps other centrally acting agents.

Methyldopa has been reported to produce bradycardia in patients taking digoxin; susceptible patients most likely have underlying carotid sinus hypersensitivity or sinus node dysfunction.

Contraindications

Methyldopa should generally be avoided in patients with a history of hepatic disease, depression, dementia, or hemolytic anemia.

Indications

Methyldopa is no longer considered a first-line agent in the treatment of hypertension in older patients, but it is indicated if other, better-tolerated agents cannot be used or are ineffective.

Dosing

Initial dose: 125 mg bid. Some patients may respond to lower doses. Such conservative dosing should be considered in very aged or frail patients.
Maximum dose: 500 mg qid.

CLONIDINE (CATAPRES, OTHERS)

Pharmacologic Considerations

Mechanism of Action

The mechanism of action of clonidine is similar to that of methyldopa in that it is a central alpha$_2$ receptor agonist. Stimulation of these receptors reduces sympathetic outflow to the periphery, diminishing sympathetic tone. Cardiac output is reduced, although this is not related to a direct effect on the myocardium, and resting heart rate is also reduced. Clonidine also has partial receptor antagonist activity. This is probably responsible for the fact that the drug exhibits a ceiling effect, with little further antihypertensive effect being achieved beyond a certain dose. High doses may, in fact, reverse the antihypertensive effect.

Unlike methyldopa and peripheral vasodilators, chronic administration of clonidine does not appear to be associated with significant sodium and fluid retention.

Pharmacokinetics

Clonidine is well absorbed orally with peak concentrations being achieved within 1–3 hours, and onset of action occurring as early as 1 hour. The drug is metabolized in the liver to largely inactive metabolites, but a significant portion is excreted unchanged by the kidney, and the clearance tends to be prolonged in older patients. A portion is excreted in the bile. The average serum half-life of the drug is 12 hours, but there is wide interindividual variability, with some non-elderly subjects demonstrating a half-life of up to 24 hours. The half-life may be trebled in patients with renal insufficiency. The duration of action correlates well with presence of the drug in plasma.

A transdermal preparation is available. It is designed to release a constant dose of the drug for a period of 7 days. This preparation unfortunately produces a high incidence of local skin reactions. Withdrawal syndromes may occur, as with oral clonidine.

Adverse Effects

Clonidine produces **dry mouth,** which can be particularly troublesome to patients who wear dentures, more so if they belong to the subgroup of older individuals that have diminished salivary gland function. **Dry eyes** and **dryness of the nasal mucosa** may also occur. Other effects include **drowsiness** and **lethargy.** Tolerance tends to develop to these effects after a few weeks. **Confusional states** have been reported, and are more likely to occur in older patients.

Like methyldopa, clonidine may unmask sinus node dysfunction, producing **bradycardia.** Although clonidine is less likely than many other antihypertensive agents to produce orthostatic hypotension, it may occur in susceptible patients.

If clonidine is abruptly withdrawn, certain patients may experience a **withdrawal syndrome** consisting of severe rebound hypertension, and other symptoms of sympathetic discharge such as tachyarrhythmia, nervousness, or agitation. Although this withdrawal phenomenon only occurs in some patients, it is prudent to taper clonidine slowly in all patients.

Important Drug Interactions

Clonidine and some, but not all, hypertensive agents may produce additive hypotensive effects. This is most likely to occur with diuretics, and is generally viewed as therapeutically desirable. It is less likely to occur with other sympatholytics.

As with methyldopa, concurrent use of tricyclic antidepressants may counteract the antihypertensive effect of clonidine. In addition, paradoxical hypertension with concurrent use of beta blockers has been described; this interaction may become manifest when clonidine is discontinued, presumably because beta blockade interferes with compensatory mechanisms that would attenuate the clonidine withdrawal syndrome. This apparently does not occur with labetalol, a beta blocker with $alpha_1$ antagonist effects; in fact, labetalol has been used to prevent this withdrawal phenomenon.

Contraindications

Clonidine should not be used in patients who are unable to comply with therapeutic regimens because of the danger that abrupt discontinuation might precipitate a withdrawal syndrome.

Precautions

Because of the risk of withdrawal syndromes, forgetful patients should only take clonidine if they live in a supervised environment.

Among antihypertensive agents, withdrawal syndromes are not unique to clonidine, although the phenomenon associated with clonidine seems to have received the most attention.

Indications

Clonidine is indicated in the treatment of hypertension. Although not a first-line agent, it is often well tolerated in the elderly. It is particularly suitable for patients who are unable to take regular oral medication, since a transdermal preparation is available.

Dosing

Initial dose: 0.05–0.1 mg by mouth once daily. Daily dose may be given at bedtime if desired.
Maximum daily dose: 0.6 mg in 2 to 3 divided doses.

GUANABENZ (WYTENSIN)

Guanabenz is closely related to clonidine in its mechanism of action, indications, and spectrum of adverse effects. There is little experience with this relatively new drug in geriatric patients. It does not appear to have any advantages over clonidine at this time.

PRAZOSIN (MINIPRESS)

Prazosin is uncommonly used in geriatric practice because of its purported tendency to produce dizziness and syncope during initiation of therapy. However, recent evidence that it may alleviate symptoms of benign prostatic hyperplasia (BPH) has renewed interest in the drug. The related drugs, terazosin and doxazosin, are discussed in the Bibliography readings (see Khoury and Kaplan).

Pharmacologic Considerations

Mechanism of Action

Prazosin acts by selectively blocking $alpha_1$ adrenergic receptors in the venous and arterial bed; arteriolar dilatation reduces systemic arterial pressure, while venous dilatation reduces central venous pressure. Selective blockade of $alpha_1$ receptors permits norepinephrine to bind to unblocked $alpha_2$ receptors, reducing the likelihood of reflex tachycardia. However, this selective action, along with venous pooling, can also impede compensatory mechanisms, so that orthostatic hypotension can be severe. This is a particularly important problem for many older patients, in whom impaired baroreceptor mechanisms are worsened by the presence of venous insufficiency.

The vasodilating effects of prazosin have been harnessed in the treatment of chronic congestive heart failure, where the drug is used as a preload and afterload reducer. Unfortunately, the development of tachyphylaxis limits its usefulness.

Prazosin also blocks $alpha_1$ receptors at the level of the bladder outlet, inhibiting smooth muscle contraction and reducing tone of the internal urethral sphincter. This action may prove beneficial to certain patients with BPH but may produce urinary incontinence in other groups of patients.

Pharmacokinetics

Prazosin is well absorbed, and undergoes extensive first-pass hepatic metabolism. The elimination half-life in nonelderly adults is roughly 3–4 hours, but the duration of antihypertensive action outlasts its presence in the blood. The volume of distribution is increased in older patients, and elimination may be somewhat prolonged. One of the tissues in which prazosin is avidly bound is the prostate gland.

Although prazosin is lipid-soluble, it does not appear to enter the brain significantly.

Adverse Effects

Symptomatic **orthostatic hypotension** may occur and is most often noted during initiation of therapy. This "first-dose phenomenon" usually subsides after the first few doses, but may recur each time the dose is increased. The risk of this effect most likely increases with age, but it can be minimized if precautions are taken (see below).

Prazosin may reduce the tone of the bladder outlet and produce **urinary incontinence.** This is most likely to occur in women with postmenopausal urethral incompetence.

Lethargy is uncommon and confusional states occur rarely if ever.

Important Drug Interactions

Nonsteroidal anti-inflammatory agents have been reported to reduce the antihypertensive effect of prazosin. This is a general property of NSAIDs that probably occurs with all antihypertensive agents.

Contraindications

Prazosin is contraindicated in patients with syptomatic orthostatic hypotension.

Precautions

Because of troublesome effects that can occur during initiation of therapy, treatment in certain elderly patients should be initiated at subtherapeutic doses. Those at highest risk are the very aged or debilitated, or those with a history of falling. The patient should be told of the possible effect, take the first doses while recumbent, and remain recumbent for 4–5 hours. This is most practical, of course, at bedtime. However, it should be emphasized that nocturnal dosing of troublesome medications can be hazardous in this age group. Drug-related falling episodes occur frequently at night, and would be a particular risk with a drug such as prazosin since orthostatic hypotension is more common after prolonged recumbency.

"First-dose" precautions should be taken for at least the first three doses, and again each time the dose is increased.

Indications

Prazosin is indicated as adjunctive treatment of hypertension in patients unable to take first-line agents. It may be particularly suitable in men with mild to moderate symptoms due to BPH, since a few patients have reported reduction in prostatic symptoms while on this drug (see Chap. 23).

Dosing

Initial dose: 0.5 mg.
Maximum daily dose: 15 mg in 2 to 3 divided doses.

RESERPINE

Reserpine, one of the first antihypertensive agents in wide use, is little used today because so many drugs are available that are purportedly better tolerated. It fell into disfavor among geriatricians because of its tendency to produce depression. In addition, reserpine stimulates gastric acid secretion and may exacerbate peptic ulcer disease. The degree of ulcerogenic risk posed by reserpine in humans is not precisely known, however, and the risks and benefits of this agent have not been carefully compared to those of more modern antihypertensive agents. Another worrisome side effect had been the development of extrapyramidal symptoms. This occurs after chronic use of high doses and is due to central depletion of dopamine. Doses currently in use are unlikely to produce this effect. Reserpine is an effective drug and may be less poorly tolerated than previously believed.

Reserpine lowers blood pressure by depleting catecholamines from storage vesicles in peripheral neural tissue and in the brain. Its antihypertensive action far outlasts its apparent short half-life in plasma, presumably because of tissue binding.

There is little published experience with reserpine in the current era of scientifically rigorous, controlled trials. Lower doses are now used than in the past. One recent retrospective study indicated that, with the exception of nasal congestion, reserpine was better tolerated in a group of elderly subjects than methyldopa (see Applegate et al.).

Reserpine is still used by some patients, particularly those for whom the drug was prescribed in the distant past. If the patient tolerates the drug, it need not necessarily be discontinued. Reserpine was selected as an alternate step 2 drug in the recently published SHEP study.

Another admonition regarding the use of this drug is that many new agents have been developed since the time that reserpine was in common use and as yet unknown drug interactions may exist.

Dosing
Usual dose range: 0.05–0.25 mg daily.

GUANETHIDINE (ISMELIN)
This drug acts by displacing norepinephrine from storage granules in peripheral neurons. Of all agents in use, it has the highest tendency to produce orthostatic hypotension, has a range of other troublesome effects, and participates in dangerous drug interactions. Because of its long duration of action, complications can be prolonged.

Guanethidine is useful in patients with hypertension refractory to other modalities, but it is poorly tolerated by elderly patients. Because there are now so many better-tolerated drugs from which to choose, there is little place for this agent in geriatric practice today.

NONPHARMACOLOGIC TREATMENT
The most important nonpharmacologic approach to treating older patients is to ensure that the diagnosis of hypertension is correct. As discussed above, the desirable level of blood pressure may be quite different for aged patients. Successful nonpharmacologic treatment not uncommonly consists of tapering and withdrawing the medication. In such patients, periodic monitoring of blood pressure is essential since it is not uncommon for blood pressure to rise subsequently.

Obese patients should exercise and attempt to lose weight. Unfortunately, weight control may be difficult in elderly patients, particularly if they are unable to engage in exercise. Dietary modifications should only be made if marginal nutrient deficiencies will not increase as a consequence. Modification of cardiovascular risk factors, such as cigarette smoking, hyperglycemia, or hyperlipidemia, may be easier to achieve in selected patients.

The efficacy of salt restriction in older patients is controversial. Age-related impairment of renal sodium conservation has been described, implying that sodium restriction might be unwise or ineffective. It is hard to imagine, however, that sodium restriction alone would produce consequences worse than those produced by diuretics. Clinical studies of the efficacy of sodium restriction in elderly hypertensives have shown conflicting results. If sodium restriction is recommended for the management of hypertension, it should be done only if it does not pose a significant burden on intake of other nutrients or on quality of life.

The possibility of reversible causes of hypertension should not be ignored in the geriatric patient. However, they are less likely to be found than in younger age groups. A possible exception to this is renal artery stenosis due to arteriosclerosis. Unfortunately, surgery for correction of arteriosclerotic renal artery stenosis is far less successful than for that due to fibromuscular dysplasia.

BIBLIOGRAPHY

Hypertension; Diuretics; Calcium Channel Blocking Agents

Amery, A., Brixko, R. Clement, D., et al. Efficacy of antihypertensive drug treatment according to age, sex, blood pressure, and previous cardiovascular disease in patients over the age of 60. *Lancet* 2:589–592, 1986.

Applegate, W.B. Hypertension in elderly patients. *Ann. Intern. Med.* 110:901–915,1989.

Ashouri, O.S. Severe diuretic-induced hyponatremia in the elderly. *Arch. Intern. Med.* 146:1355–1357, 1986.

Baltodano, N., Gallo, B.V., and Weidler, D.J. Verapamil vs quinine in recumbent nocturnal leg cramps in the elderly. *Arch. Intern. Med.* 148:1969–1970, 1988.

Freis, E.D. Critique of the clinical importance of diuretic-induced hypokalemia and elevated cholesterol level. *Arch. Intern. Med.* 149:2640–2648, 1989.

Gifford, R.W. Myths about hypertension in the elderly. *Med. Clin. North. Amer.* 71:1003–1011, 1987.

Khair, G.Z., and Kochar, M.S. Mild hypertension, diuretics, and cardiac arrhythmias: consensus amid controversy? *Am. Heart J.* 116:216–221, 1988.

LaCroix, A.Z., Wienpahl, J., White, L.R., et al. Thiazide diuretics and the incidence of hip fracture. *N. Engl. J. Med.* 322:786–790, 1990.

O'Malley, K., McCormack, P., and O'Brien, E.T. Isolated systolic hypertension: data from the European Working Party on High Blood Pressure in the Elderly. *J. Hypertens.* 6 (Suppl. 1):S105–S108, 1988.

Rizack, M.A., and Hillman, C.D.M. *The Medical Letter Handbook of Drug Interactions.* New Rochelle, N.Y.: *The Medical Letter,* 1989.

SHEP Cooperative Research Group. Prevention of stroke by antihypertensive drug treatment in older persons with isolated systolic hypertension. Final results of the Systolic Hypertension in the Elderly Program (SHEP). *J.A.M.A.* 265:3255–3264, 1991.

ACE Inhibitors; Beta Blockers; Others

Applegate, W.B., Carper, E.R., and Kahn, S.E. Comparison of the use of reserpine versus alpha-methyldopa for second step treatment of hypertension in the elderly. *J. Amer. Geriatr. Soc.* 33:109–115, 1985.

Croog, S.H., Levine, S., Testa, M.A., et al. The effects of antihypertensive therapy on the quality of life. *N. Eng. J. Med.* 314:1657–1664, 1986.

Findley, L.J., and Killer, W.C. Essential tremor: a review. *Neurology* 37:1194–1197, 1987.

Fitzgerald, J.D. Age-related effects of beta-blockers and hypertension. *J. Cardiovasc. Pharmacol.* 12 (Suppl. 8):S83–S92, 1988.

Frohlich, E.D. Methyldopa mechanisms and treatment 25 years later. *Arch. Intern. Med.* 140:954–959, 1980.

Khoury, A.F., and Kaplan, N.M. α-Blocker therapy for hypertension. *J.A.M.A.* 266:394–398, 1991.

Rotmensch, H.H., Vlasses, P.H., and Ferguson, R.K. Angiotensin-converting enzyme inhibitors. *Med. Clin. North Amer.* 72:399–425, 1988.

Williams, G.H. Converting-enzyme inhibitors in the treatment of hypertension. *N. Engl. J. Med.* 319:1512–1525, 1988.

Zubenko, G.S., and Nixon, R.A. Mood-elevating effect of captopril on depressed patients. *Am. J. Psychiatr.* 141:110–111, 1984.

Anti-Anginal Agents

ANGINA IN THE ELDERLY

The pharmacologic approach to treating angina in aged patients does not differ greatly from the approach in younger adults. However, the diagnosis is often more difficult, particularly in patients over the age of 80. Angina often presents atypically and ischemia may be silent or painless. In fact, typical angina, manifested as pressing substernal chest discomfort, is an unusual presentation of ischemic heart disease in the elderly. Thus, clinical end points cannot be easily determined and are often unreliable guides to prescribing.

Although cardiac pain is one manifestation of angina in the older age group, presentations commonly consist of dyspnea or fatigue on exertion, or sudden "unexplained" weakness with or without diaphoresis. Physiologically, this altered presentation is thought to be related to age-associated stiffness of the left ventricle. When myocardial ischemia occurs, the usual sequence of events is that left ventricular dysfunction occurs first and pain follows. In younger patients with a supple myocardium, the first manifestation in this series of events is pain. However, when ischemia is superimposed on an aged, stiff ventricle, impaired contractility is accentuated and symptoms of ventricular dysfunction tend to precede pain. Dyspnea or fatigue might cause the patient to rest, reducing ischemia and curbing pain. Some physiologists speculate that the absence of pain might be related to age-related impairment of pain perception or alterations in nervous transmission. Others suggest that the presence of noncardiac disease is what often confounds the diagnosis, or that physical limitations prevent the amounts of exertion that would cause real discomfort.

Like angina, acute myocardial infarction often presents atypically in late life. Since angina in some form is a common clinical predecessor of myocardial infarction, the physician must always be on the lookout for symptoms that could be attributed to cardiac ischemia.

NITRATES

Nitrates remain the mainstay of anti-angina therapy and are particularly suited to older patients because of their safety profile. They may be combined with calcium channel blockers or beta blockers when indicated.

Pharmacologic Considerations

Mechanism of Action

Nitroglycerin acts by improving the balance between myocardial oxygen supply and demand. The mechanism of action is based on the ability of nitroglycerin to directly produce smooth muscle relaxation in many peripheral vascular beds. At ordinary doses, nitrates dilate peripheral veins, reducing venous return to the heart (preload), and to a lesser extent they dilate peripheral arterioles, reducing the burden on the left ventricle (afterload), with the end result that myocardial work is diminished. If the coronary arteries are made to dilate, there is also an increase in nutrient oxygen supply to the heart. This mechanism may not contribute equally to the clinical effect in all patients.

The redistribution of blood volume to the periphery that occurs as a result of vasodilation tends to lower systemic blood pressure. While this has a therapeutic role in that it contributes to reduction in myocardial work, it occasionally leads to symptomatic hypotension and even syncope, a problem that may be more prevalent in aged and debilitated patients.

Forms of Nitroglycerin

There are various preparations of nitroglycerin available today. The bioavailability and onset and duration of action vary. Properties of nitroglycerin preparations are summarized in Table 13-1.

Sublingual nitroglycerin has a relatively rapid onset of action and is metabolized in the wall of the vessels themselves with small amounts being metabolized in the liver to relatively inactive substances. The onset of action depends to some extent on the rapidity with which the tablet dissolves but generally occurs within 1-2 minutes and subsides minutes later. Dissolution may be retarded when the oral mucosa is dry, a factor that could operate frequently in older patients.

Isosorbide dinitrate is a longer acting form which may be taken orally or sublingually. Oral drug undergoes extensive first-pass hepatic metabolism. Although this markedly reduces the bioavailability of native drug, long-acting active metabolites are formed in the process and contribute to clinical effect. However, reduced bioavailability of oral isosorbide necessitates higher doses than those needed for the sublingual form.

Pentaerythritol tetranitrate (Peritrate) and **erythrityl tetranitrate** (Cardilate) have not been widely studied but are available for oral use. They are intended to be used as intermediate-acting agents, comparable to isosorbide dinitrate.

Transdermal preparations are designed to deliver a constant dose of drug over a period of 24 hours. Like all transdermal drugs, the

Table 13-1. Commonly Used Nitrates

	Onset of Action	Duration	Usual Dose
Nitroglycerin Sublingual	1-3 min	20-30 min	$\frac{1}{200}$-$\frac{1}{150}$ gr
Isosorbide dinitrate Sublingual	2-5 min	1-4 hours	2.5-10.0 mg qid
Isosorbide dinitrate Oral	20-40 min	2-6 hours	5-40 mg tid-qid
Nitroglycerin Transdermal patch or disk	30-60 min	≤ 24 hours	5-20 mg for 12 hours only[a]
Nitroglycerin Ointment	30-60 min	2-8 hours	$\frac{1}{2}$-2 in; limit use to 12 hours[b]

[a]Efficacy of doses under 15 mg not known.
[b]One inch contains approximately 15 mg of nitroglycerin. One application lasts up to 8 hours depending on ambient skin conditions.

actual dose delivered may vary from patient to patient and throughout the day, depending primarily on local skin factors. Although the onset of action occurs at 30–60 minutes, the pattern and degree of response varies considerably among patients, and from brand to brand. This variability is probably less important than the fact that therapeutic blood levels are maintained for many hours, a property that would appear to be desirable for the purposes of angina prophylaxis, but which is probably responsible for the rapid development of tolerance that complicates the use of these preparations.

Intravenous nitroglycerin is used primarily in the acutely ill patient with crescendo angina and congestive heart failure. For a complete discussion of intravenous nitroglycerin the reader is referred to the Bibliography readings (see Sorkin et al.).

Tolerance

Tolerance (tachyphylaxis) to the therapeutic effects of nitroglycerin appears to be related to metabolic processes that occur within the vessel wall. This in-situ vascular metabolism may be required for pharmacodynamic action. When there is a constant source of nitroglycerin, as when long-acting preparations are used, the metabolic machinery becomes exhausted. Dosing that maintains a continuous therapeutic blood level may produce clinical tolerance within the first 24 hours of use, and efficacy seems to return after the patient experiences drug-free intervals. Tolerance is particularly swift with transdermal preparations and occurs somewhat less quickly with long-acting oral preparations. Tolerance is less common with the use of isosorbide dinitrate, since the dosing frequency required to achieve constant blood levels is probably not often achieved. Occasional "prn" use of sublingual nitroglycerin does not produce tolerance.

Various maneuvers have been recommended to minimize the development of tolerance. All of these maneuvers are designed to produce a significant drug-free interval. Tolerance to transdermal preparations may be reduced if the application period is not greater than a 12-hour period each day, or if the agents are used intermittently, restricted to vulnerable periods of the day. If angina occurs after the application period has ended, additional as-needed nitroglycerin may suffice. Otherwise, a beta blocker or calcium channel antagonist should be added.

Efficacy

The efficacy of transdermal preparations is an ongoing subject of controversy. The greatest efficacy appears to be attained with patches containing at least 10 mg, with the patch left on for no longer than 12 hours at a time. Efficacy has not been studied specifically in the elderly. In fact, conclusions about tolerance and minimum effective dose have been reached under experimental conditions that are largely irrelevant to geriatric patients. The subjects, rarely over 70 years of age, are exercising on a treadmill or bicycle, achieving workloads that are hardly ever achieved by older individuals in real life. In practice, efficacy is probably achieved at lower doses.

Adverse Effects

Nitroglycerin preparations are well tolerated by older patients. The most frequent side effect is **headache**, a problem that usually subsides even if cardiac tolerance does not occur. **Flushing and dizziness** may also occur as a result of cutaneous vasodilation. **Orthostatic hypotension** occurs more often in older patients than in younger ones, presumably because of venous insufficiency and impaired baroreceptor responses.

An occasional patient will experience acute **hypotension** and **syncope** from sublingual nitroglycerin. This is more likely to happen in patients who are very aged, debilitated, or hypovolemic, or in conjunction with acute ischemia. Hypotension may lead to **reflex tachycardia**. Rarely, **paradoxical bradycardia** may occur.

High doses of oral preparations may cause **gastrointestinal symptoms,** but this is unusual. Transdermal preparations may produce **contact dermatitis,** a problem that is sometimes overcome if the application site is rotated daily.

Important Drug Interactions

Other agents that lower blood pressure may increase the hypotensive response to nitroglycerin preparations. Headache and flushing can be exacerbated by potent vasodilators such as nifedipine. Medications that produce dry mouth can impair dissolution of sublingual nitroglycerin, impairing its action.

Contraindications

Nitrates should not be used in patients with obstructive hypertrophic cardiomyopathy, since outflow obstruction may be increased. Hypertrophic cardiomyopathy may occur more often in late life than previously believed.

Nitrate preparations should generally not be used in patients with a history of migraine headache.

Precautions

Patients should be told to sit or recline if possible, before taking sublingual nitroglycerin for the treatment of acute angina. This will reduce the likelihood of syncope should hypotension occur and is particularly important during the initiation of treatment when individual dose and response are not known. Once a patient's dose-response is determined, this precaution may no longer be required. Theoretically, nitroglycerin might be more effective when taken in the standing position because the drug and gravity act in concert to reduce venous return to the heart, lowering oxygen demand. However, this is not always practical or acceptable to the patient.

It has been suggested that abrupt withdrawal after prolonged therapy with high-dose nitrate therapy may produce rebound vasoconstriction with ischemic symptoms. Although this has been well documented in people with long-term industrial exposure to nitroglycerin, a rebound syndrome has not been particularly well documented with clinical use of the drug. Anecdotal observations of sudden death after sudden withdrawal of chronic therapy in heart failure patients have prompted some physicians to advise gradual tapering in these settings.

Special Considerations

Older individuals may have difficulty administering nitroglycerin preparations. Anxiety and tremor may make it difficult to retrieve and position a sublingual nitroglycerin tablet during an acute attack. Although this problem is far from universal, oral nitroglycerin spray has been suggested as an alternative. This preparation does not need to be inhaled and may be more rapidly absorbed than tablets in some patients. However, it is conceivable that not all patients would be able to use the dispenser correctly.

Transdermal patches and discs are practical and popular, but are difficult for many older patients to open. This may require changing to another brand. It may also be difficult for the patient to remove the patch from the skin, or to remember to remove the patch at the designated time.

Indications and Use

Sublingual nitroglycerin is indicated for the treatment of stable, acute angina, when attacks occur infrequently. When angina is predictable, for example, if it occurs when walking up an incline, patients frequently benefit by taking a nitroglycerin tablet just prior to the activity.

Transdermal nitroglycerin is indicated in patients with frequent angina episodes. In addition, these preparations are ideal for forgetful or dependent patients with limited home care. The preparation should be applied in the morning and remain on for no longer than 12 hours, in order to reduce the development of tolerance. Patients with nocturnal angina may use transdermal nitroglycerin at night as an adjunct to other treatment regimens. It is often practical to determine the patient's pattern of symptoms, using the patches specifically at critical periods of the day or less often.

Nitroglycerin ointment is less convenient. It is applied under a ruled paper patch that is nonadhesive. Dosing may be inexact, but this is probably less of a problem than compliance and inconvenience. The main advantage of ointment over transdermal patches is its lower cost. The paper can be taped to the skin or applied under a cloth wrist or ankle band if necessary.

Long-acting oral or sublingual pills may be a suitable alternative to transdermal preparations in many patients and may be clinically superior because tolerance develops less readily.

Dosing

The most commonly used dose of sublingual nitroglycerin is $\frac{1}{150}$ gr (0.4 mg). Although this standard dose is quite acceptable for most patients, smaller doses are sometimes required in patients exhibiting an unusually sensitive pressor response.

The efficacy of low-dose transdermal preparations has been questioned and some investigators claim that efficacy is not achieved unless dosages approaching 15 mg or more in 24 hours are used. However, in light of the absence of data on geriatric patients, it is sensible to begin with low initial doses.

Dose recommendations are summarized in Table 13–1.

CALCIUM CHANNEL BLOCKING AGENTS

Mechanism of Action

Calcium channel antagonists are thought to prevent angina by means of their arterial dilating properties, which reduce afterload and cardiac work. They dilate coronary arteries, although it is not known to what extent this action has clinical effect in all patients.

Agents of this class have varying degrees of direct myocardial depressant activity, but this may not be as important a factor in the suppression of angina than the drug's ability to reduce heart rate or blood pressure.

Drugs of this class are discussed in depth in Chap. 12 in connection with the management of hypertension. Verapamil is also discussed in Chap. 14.

Indications

Calcium channel antagonists are indicated in the management of angina in elderly patients. They are particularly suitable for those who also require management of hypertension and for those in whom nitrates produce insufficient relief of symptoms.

Selection of Agent

All calcium channel antagonists are effective anti-angina agents. Selection should be based on avoidance of adverse effects (see Chap. 12, Table 12–2).

BETA BLOCKERS

Pharmacologic Considerations

Mechanism of Action

Beta blockers inhibit the binding of endogenous catecholamines to beta adrenergic receptors. This results in decreased heart rate and myocardial contraction, particularly in response to exercise. This in turn lowers cardiac work and prevents exercise-induced tachycardia that could promote ischemia. Although blockade of arterial beta$_2$ receptors produces unopposed alpha stimulation and vasoconstriction, reduction in cardiac work is sufficient to reduce angina. This may not be the case in variant (Prinzmetal's) angina, in which coronary artery spasm is thought to be the principal pathophysiologic mechanism. The incidence of variant angina in the elderly is not known.

Agents such as pindolol have partial beta-agonist (intrinsic sympathomimetic) activity. Thus, when catecholamine levels are low, for example at rest, there is no competition for receptor sites and the beta blocker becomes a partial activator of the receptor, resulting in an increase in cardiac work and heart rate. While pindolol has been shown to adequately blunt exercise-induced tachycardia and relieve exercise-induced angina, it has the potential for being less effective, if not counterproductive, in the setting of rest angina or angina that occurs in patients who have low levels of exercise. Many geriatric patients fall into the latter category, and beta blockers with partial agonist action are not advised. A possible exception to this might be the occasional patient with significant bradycardia. However, in this situation, it is preferable to avoid beta blockers entirely; even partial agonists might be insufficient to raise the heart rate in the presence of sick sinus syndrome.

Labetolol, which has partial beta$_2$ agonist activity, is also a selective alpha$_1$ agonist; the latter property is felt to offset vasoconstriction that can be produced by beta blockers. There is disagreement as to whether labetolol is as effective as other agents in the treatment of angina, although it is a very satisfactory antihypertensive agent.

One potential problem with labetolol is its ability to produce postural hypotension.

Beta receptor sensitivity appears to decline with age, so that dose-response is less predictable for these agents than in younger age groups. In addition, many older patients have underlying cardiac conduction disturbances, notably sick sinus syndrome, which prevent normal cardioacceleration that occurs with exercise. These physiologic factors have led some to suggest that beta blockers might be less effective anti-angina agents in the elderly. However, there is no clinical evidence that aged patients fail to respond. In practice, use of beta blockers may be limited by side effects rather than lack of efficacy.

Beta blockers are discussed more fully in Chap. 12 in connection with the management of hypertension.

Selection of Beta Blocker

Selection of a particular agent depends on the accompanying vulnerabilities of the individual patient. Only propranolol, metoprolol, atenolol, and nadolol have received official FDA approval for use in angina. However, other beta blockers may be better tolerated by certain patients. In rest angina, beta blockers with intrinsic sympathomimetic activity (ISA) should generally be avoided.

Selection criteria are summarized in Table 12–3 in Chap. 12.

The Place of Beta Blockers in the Treatment of Angina

Beta blockers should be used for angina in late life when other agents are ineffective or not tolerated. Clinical end points may be very vague in the geriatric patient with ischemic heart disease because of the subtlety of symptoms. For this reason, the more predictable nature and narrower range of side effects accompanying nitrates and calcium channel antagonists generally make them preferable. However, beta blockers without ISA are highly suitable for the patient with ischemic heart disease following myocardial infarction. These drugs have been shown to reduce mortality and nonfatal ischemic events following myocardial infarction, an effect that has not been demonstrated with calcium channel antagonists or nitrates. The beneficial effect conferred by the beta blockers is felt to be related to protection against ventricular fibrillation and against ischemia, and possibly to other factors related to myocardial metabolism and platelet function. Despite theoretical considerations having to do with decreased beta receptor sensitivity, there is some evidence that the older patient achieves greater benefit from this intervention than younger adults.

In the treatment of angina, beta blockers may be used alone or in combination with nitrates. They are often well tolerated when combined with calcium channel antagonists but may increase the risk of bradycardia and left ventricular failure when used with verapamil or diltiazem in some patients.

Dosing

The initial dose of beta blocker should be lower than for younger adults. Once it has been established that the drug is tolerated, dose increases may be made. Many older patients may require doses at least as high as younger patients.

Dosages and selection criteria for commonly used beta blockers are summarized in Tables 12–3 and 12–4 in Chap. 12. The dosage in the treatment of angina should be determined according to the appropriate clinical end point.

NONPHARMACOLOGIC TREATMENT

Treatment consists of correcting modifiable risk factors, such as smoking, hyperlipidemia, hyperglycemia, and hypertension, and identifying medical problems such as anemia or thyroid disease. Occult blood loss and hyperthyroidism frequently manifest atypically in late life and may call attention to the heart rather than the underlying disease. Accompanying cardiac disease, such as aortic stenosis, may be at fault and should be sought. However, aortic murmurs are extremely common in geriatric patients and, as echocardiographic evaluation tends to demonstrate, these murmurs frequently do not represent significant pathology. Hypertension should be corrected carefully; overtreatment can be detrimental and the consequences of treating isolated systolic hypertension in the elderly are uncertain.

Modification of life-style may help the patient with angina, but restriction of physical exercise should only be imposed if symptoms are difficult to manage with medication. Patients with physical limitations may ambulate with lesser work loads if they use assistive devices maximally and correctly.

If pharmacologic treatment fails to control symptoms, selected patients, including those over the age of 80, may be treated successfully with cardiac surgery or angioplasty.

It has been said that angina treats itself. If a myocardial infarction occurs and involves an area that previously was the source of angina, the necrotic area may no longer produce noticeable symptoms. However, geriatric patients with exercise-induced angina may gradually have a reduction in symptoms if they become inactive because of skeletal limitations. In some cases, it may be possible to reduce or withdraw the medication. In all cases, the prescribing physician should keep in mind that the disappearance of classic symptoms does not mean that ischemic disease has resolved.

BIBLIOGRAPHY

Bayer, A.J., Chadha, J.S., Farag, R.R., and Pathy, M.S.J. Changing presentation of myocardial infarction with increasing old age. *J. Amer. Geriatr. Soc.* 34:263– 266, 1986.

Cohn, P.F. Silent myocardial ischemia. *Ann. Intern. Med.* 109:312–317, 1988.

Flugelman, M.Y., Halon, D.A., Shefer, A., Schneeweiss, A., Peer, M., Dagan, T., et al. Persistent painless ST-segment depression after exercise testing and the effect of age. *Clin. Cardiol.* 11:365–369, 1988.

Franciosa, J.A., Nordstrom, C.A., and Cohn, J.N. Nitrate therapy for congestive heart failure. *JAMA* 240:443–446, 1978.

Keram, S., and Williams, M.E. Quantifying the ease or difficulty older persons experience in opening medication containers. *J. Amer. Geriatr. Soc.* 36:198–201, 1988.

Nitroglycerin patches—do they work? *Med. Lett. Drugs Ther.* 31:65–66, 1989.

Olsson, G., Rehnqvist, N., Sjögren, A., et al. Long-term treatment with metoprolol after myocardial infarction: effect on 3 year mortality and morbidity. *J. Amer. Coll. Cardiol.* 5:1428–1437, 1985.

Sorkin, E.M., Brogden, R.N., and Romankiweicz, J.A. Intravenous glyceryl trinitrate (nitroglycerin). A review of its pharmacological and therapeutic efficacy. *Drugs* 27:45–80, 1984.

Other Important Cardiovascular Drugs

ARRHYTHMIAS IN THE ELDERLY

Cardiac arrhythmias are extremely common in late life but treatment is not always required. However, an essential component in evaluating the older individual with a new arrhythmia is to rule out secondary factors, such as drug treatment, thyroid disease, "silent" ischemia, and congestive heart failure. Both cardiac and thyroid disease may present atypically and may first manifest as an isolated arrhythmia. If no modifiable factors are present, the arrhythmia should only be treated with medications if the risks of treatment do not outweigh the benefits. A concerted effort should be made to suppress the arrhythmia when it produces untoward symptoms or places the patient at risk of ischemic events, cardiovascular decompensation, or sudden death.

Complex ventricular arrhythmias occur in 50% or more of older people without cardiac symptoms, as noted in studies of ambulatory (Holter) monitoring. There is no evidence that these arrhythmias untreated are associated with increased morbidity. Likewise, the coexistence of arrhythmias in persons with an episode of syncope may be circumstantial. Syncope is a common problem in the geriatric population and in most cases the precise cause of the event cannot be ascertained. Most "documented" causes of syncope are attributed to cardiac arrhythmias. However, it is important to realize that when a patient who reports a recent syncopal episode also demonstrates a cardiac arrhythmia, the two are not necessarily related.

The most commonly treated arrhythmia in the geriatric population is atrial fibrillation. This arrhythmia occurs in 5% or more of community-residing and approximately 20% of institutionalized elderly. It is associated with an increased risk of stroke, and when the ventricular rate is rapid, syncope and congestive heart failure may occur. In most elderly individuals, atrial fibrillation is a manifestation of nonlocalized conduction system disease, and the sinus node is frequently involved. The arrhythmia eventually becomes chronic, so that chemical or electrical cardioversion is generally unsuccessful in the long run. In fact, cardiologists point out that the association with sinus node dysfunction makes electrical cardioversion in these circumstances unwise because sinus arrest may occur. Treatment is directed at keeping the ventricular rate within the normal range. As conduction disease progresses, the atrioventricular (AV) node loses its ability to transmit electrical impulses, a process that is accentuated by aging. Thus, the patient should be followed periodically for the ultimate development of bradycardia, which will occur in a large proportion of patients. The use of warfarin in the long-term management of atrial fibrillation in the elderly is controversial (see Chap. 15).

Ventricular arrhythmias in the elderly are commonly seen in association with problems extrinsic to the conducting system or the heart. Important factors that can produce or potentiate ventricular arrhythmias include hypokalemia, hypoxemia, cardiac ischemia, hyperthyroidism, sympathomimetic drugs, digoxin, tricyclic antidepressants, and antiarrhythmic agents themselves ("proarrhythmic" effects). It is essential that these problems be attended to and cor-

193

rected if possible, before resorting to long-term antiarrhythmic therapy.

Antiarrhythmic agents must be used very cautiously in elderly patients because there is often a fine line between control of the arrhythmia and production of potentially disastrous conduction system deficits. Cautious dosing does not always protect the patient from cardiac toxicity, because the diseased, aged conducting system is exquisitely sensitive to low tissue concentrations of these drugs.

SPECIFIC AGENTS

In the elderly, atrial arrhythmias are usually treated with digoxin or verapamil, with quinidine and procainamide reserved for adjunctive treatment. Ventricular arrhythmias are generally treated with quinidine, procainamide being reserved for patients who cannot tolerate the former. Disopyramide tends to be poorly tolerated by elderly patients and is less frequently used. Newer agents are uncommonly used in geriatric practice and will be discussed only briefly.

CLASSIFICATION OF ANTIARRHYTHMIC DRUGS

Antiarrhythmic agents are traditionally classified according to their mechanism of antiarrhythmic action. The mechanisms described in this classification refer to therapeutic action; toxicity due to excessive doses or unduly sensitive conducting tissue may manifest in different ways. In addition, some overlap in mechanism of action occurs. The drugs are listed in Table 14-1.

Class I antiarrhythmic agents block the fast sodium channel, which is responsible for membrane depolarization of cardiac cells and the initiation of the action potential. Pure sodium channel blockers primarily affect ventricular conducting tissue and have little ef-

Table 14-1. Classification of Antiarrhythmic Drugs

Class	Agent
IA	Quinidine
	Procainamide
	Disopyramide
IB	Lidocaine
	Tocainide
	Mexiletine
IC	Flecainide
	Encainide
	Propafenone
II	Propranolol
	Metoprolol
III	Amiodarone
	Bretylium
IV	Verapamil
	Diltiazem
Cardiac glycosides	Digoxin
	Digitoxin

fect on the sinus node or the atrioventricular (AV) node. Subcategories have been delineated according to differential effects on various parts of the cardiac cycle. **Class IA** drugs decrease conduction velocity and increase the duration of the refractory period. They have a more pronounced effect on atrial conduction tissue than other class I drugs. **Class IB** drugs shorten the refractory period but have minimal effect on conduction velocity. **Class IC** drugs decrease conduction velocity but have no effect on the refractory period.

Class II drugs affect adrenergic receptors. This group consists primarily of beta adrenergic blocking agents. They act by suppressing automaticity and prolonging AV conduction, actions that are largely due to prevention of the dysrhythmic effects of catecholamines. For this reason, beta blockers that possess intrinsic sympathomimetic activity are not used to suppress arrhythmias. One beta blocker, sotalol, is considered a class III drug, and another antiarrhythmic agent, propafenone, possesses beta blocking action but is considered a Class I drug.

Class III drugs block potassium channels, slowing membrane repolarization. The refractory period is prolonged but there is minimal effect on conduction.

Class IV drugs block the slow calcium channel in sinus and AV nodal tissue. This slows conduction and increases the refractory period of the AV node, but ventricular tissue is not affected. Of the calcium channel blockers in use, only verapamil and diltiazem have this type of antiarrhythmic effect.

The **cardiac glycosides** are not generally included in the classification above, but they are important antiarrhythmic agents. They decrease conduction velocity of AV nodal tissue and may also affect the sinus node. Well-known digitalis-induced ventricular dysrhythmias are manifestations of toxicity, due either to excessive doses or ultrasensitive ventricular conducting tissue.

THE CARDIAC GLYCOSIDES—DIGOXIN AND DIGITOXIN

Structurally, the cardiac glycosides consist of an aglycone, which contains a steroid nucleus and is linked glycosidically to a sugar moiety. The aglycone is the cardiotonic portion. Digoxin and digitoxin differ only in one hydroxyl group on the steroid nucleus and are similar in potency but have vastly different pharmacokinetic properties.

Digoxin (Lanoxin, Others)

Pharmacologic Considerations

MECHANISM OF ACTION. Digoxin inhibits the action of sodium-potassium adenosine triphosphatase (NaK-ATPase), allowing more sodium to enter the cell, enhancing sodium-calcium exchange. More calcium is made available to contractile elements of the myocardium, resulting in greater force and velocity of myocardial contraction (positive inotropic effect). Analagous ionic events are thought to occur in conducting tissue with complex effects, the dominant one being increased vagal tone. Increased vagal tone slows conduction, prolongs the refractory period of the atrioventricular (AV) node, and slows the ventricular rate (negative chronotropic effect). There may be diminished NaK-ATPase activity in aged tissue, a factor that theoretically could increase sensitivity to digoxin, but on a clinical level enhanced sensitivity could well be due to pathologic factors, such as conduction system disease.

Hypokalemia, hypomagnesemia, and hypercalcemia enhance the sensitivity of the heart to the effects of the cardiac glycosides. Hypokalemia increases digitalis binding to NaK-ATPase; magnesium is required for activation of NaK-ATPase and its depletion potentiates intracellular loss of potassium and increases myocardial uptake of digoxin; calcium flux is ultimately responsible for the action of digoxin. Hypothyroidism and chronic lung disease also increase the sensitivity to digoxin, while fever, hyperthyroidism, and hyperkalemia reduce the sensitivity.

Digoxin also also causes peripheral venous and arterial constriction. It deposits widely in many organ systems, including neural tissue. The cardiac effects of digoxin may be partly mediated by neurotransmitter systems in the central nervous system.

PHARMACOKINETICS. Digoxin is primarily absorbed in the stomach and upper small intestine. The extent of absorption is variable, from as low as 60% to greater than 90%, depending on the product used, the dosage form, and the status of the gastrointestinal tract. Digoxin is not highly bound to serum proteins so that early peak plasma levels are followed by rapid disappearance from the serum and distribution to many body tissues. A lower serum level stabilizes at 4-6 hours. In nonelderly adults, steady-state concentrations are reached in 5-7 days if a loading dose is not given.

Digoxin is filtered by the glomeruli with some degree of tubular secretion and reabsorption. This process is decreased in low-flow states. Hepatic metabolism is minimal, and, in most patients, 70%-80% of ingested digoxin is excreted unchanged in the urine. Approximately 10%-15% is excreted in the bile and in a small number of patients significant amounts are converted to inactive metabolites by gut flora in the colon. Patients who metabolize the drug in this manner may have very high digoxin requirements.

The extent of absorption is not changed with age, but the rate of absorption may be delayed. However, because the concentration of the drug is much greater in the heart than in plasma, peak cardiac effect occurs later and correlates more closely with steady state rather than peak plasma concentration. These kinetics are important to keep in mind when monitoring serum digoxin levels (see below). Digoxin also deposits in skeletal muscle. Since muscle mass declines with age, digoxin has a lower volume of distribution in elderly patients.

Because the drug is primarily excreted in the kidney, average plasma clearance is about 50% lower, and steady-state plasma levels reached 2 or more days later in elderly than in young adults. The average half-life of digoxin at steady state is about 48 hours in older patients. However, because the extent of age-related decline in renal function is highly variable, digoxin pharmacokinetics are not always predictable in older individuals.

Adverse Effects

Digoxin may produce a wide variety of **cardiac arrhythmias** and **conduction system disturbances** ("digtoxic rhythms"). These generally occur when toxic levels of digoxin are achieved, but may also occur at subtoxic levels in a diseased myocardium that may be unduly sensitive to the effects of the drug. Cardiac toxicity is more likely to occur in patients with severe underlying conduction system disease, those with hypokalemia and certain other electrolyte disturbances, or patients taking other drugs that affect the heart. Typical digtoxic arrhythmias include premature ventricular depolarizations, often bigeminal or trigeminal, ventricular tachycardia or fibrillation, sinus bradycardia with junctional escape, accelerated junctional rhythm, atrial tachycardia with block, progressive degrees of atrioventricular block, premature atrial contractions, and occasionally, atrial fibrillation or flutter. Although some arrhythmias are considered typical digtoxic rhythms, their appearance in a person with a diseased heart may be coincidental. This diagnostic problem occurs commonly in geriatric patients.

The most common gastrointestinal side effect is **anorexia,** but **nausea** and **vomiting** may occur. These symptoms are mediated through the chemoreceptor trigger zone of the medulla. **Diarrhea** and **abdominal pain** occur less frequently. **Hemorrhagic necrosis** has been reported.

Digoxin also enters the brain and is capable of producing a wide variety of central nervous system symptoms, including **headache, delirium, confusion, hallucinations,** and **visual disturbances.** Visual disturbances include color distortion, blurring, and appearance of halos around objects. The elderly are particularly prone to digoxin-induced confusional states, which can occur in the presence of subtoxic digoxin levels and without other signs of toxicity. Because of the high incidence of dementia in the elderly, the cause may be missed. Other nonspecific symptoms such as **depression** and **lack of well being** may occur in geriatric patients and may also go unrecognized. **Neuritic pain** has been reported and has been attributed to a peripheral mechanism.

Gynecomastia has been reported in men, most of them elderly. The mechanism of this effect is not precisely known, but may be related to the fact that the structure of digoxin bears some resemblance to the sex hormones. Elderly men frequently have gynecomastia because of age-related hormonal alterations. Digoxin-induced gynecomastia is reversible on discontinuation of the drug. **Muscle weakness** and **fatigability,** which is related to deposition of digoxin in skeletal muscle, may be difficult to distinguish from the fatigue of cardiac disease. If caused by digoxin, these symptoms gradually disappear when the drug is withdrawn. **Urinary incontinence** has been reported but the mechanism is not known.

Important Drug Interactions

Cholesterol-lowering resins bind digoxin and reduce its absorption. Digoxin should be given 8 hours away from these agents. The absorption of digoxin can also be reduced by antidiarrheal agents containing pectin and kaolin (Kaopectate, others), antacids, and high fiber supplements. Absorption of the gelatin capsule form of digoxin does not seem to be much affected by these agents. Propantheline decreases gastrointestinal motility and increases absorption of digoxin, while metoclopramide increases gut motility and decreases absorption of digoxin.

Neomycin, PAS, and sulfonamides, which alter colonic flora, reduce bioavailability of digoxin for unknown reasons. This is in seeming conflict with the fact that antibiotics such as tetracycline and erythromycin increase bioavailability in the minority of patients whose gut flora is responsible for excessive metabolism of the drug to inactive metabolites, and whose digoxin levels increase after a course of these antibiotics. The patient should be observed for clinical change during and after a course of antibiotic treatment.

Quinidine may cause a 50% or greater increase in serum digoxin levels. The mechanism is thought to be related to displacement of digoxin from tissue binding sites and its release into plasma, and by a competition for renal sites of excretion. Enhanced cardiac effects and toxicity can result from this interaction and occur disproportionately in geriatric patients. For this reason, if quinidine is added to the regimen, the daily digoxin dose should be decreased by half. In the elderly, because of alterations in renal function, a new steady state may not be reached for at least 10 days and the patient should be observed for clinical change for up to 2 weeks after changes are made. Quinine and its derivative hydroxychloroquine participate in a similar interaction with digoxin and caution should be observed if these agents are given.

Digoxin levels may also increase significantly when verapamil is given concurrently. Although the effect is not as great as with quinidine, verapamil decreases the renal clearance of digoxin and toxicity may occur if the dose of digoxin is not decreased. In addition, the negative chronotropic effects of the two drugs may be additive. If verapamil is added to the regimen, it should be initiated at the smallest possible dose and the dose of digoxin should be decreased by 50%. Close monitoring should be done as with quinidine.

Diltiazem increases plasma digoxin concentration slightly and caution is required because the two drugs also interact pharmacodynamically. A pharmacologic interaction has been described with nifedipine but this may not be clinically significant.

Spironolactone, triamterene, and amiloride reduce clearance of digoxin by various mechanisms, necessitating close monitoring if these agents are added to the regimen. However, they can also induce hyperkalemia, which reduces the cardiac sensitivity to digoxin. Other diuretics, such as furosemide and the thiazides, may interact with digoxin in complex ways. Most important is their ability to waste potassium and magnesium, increasing sensitivity to digoxin. When diuretics are added to the regimen, electrolytes should be monitored closely and the patient watched for clinical change. Addition of diuretics to the regimen may allow discontinuation of digoxin in some circumstances.

These and other important interactions are summarized in Table 14-2.

Precautions

Electrolytes should be monitored periodically, particularly if patients are poorly nourished or are taking diuretics. In the presence of hypokalemia, hypomagnesemia, and hypercalcemia, digoxin-induced cardiotoxicity may occur even when drug levels are subtherapeutic. Alterations in sensitivity to digoxin may also occur in the presence of thyroid disease, fever, and chronic lung disease. Dose adjustments may have to be made in these situations and after recovery.

Most geriatric patients with chronic atrial fibrillation have diffuse, progressive conduction system disease. Although the patient may initially present with paroxysmal or sustained tachycardia, the risk of developing bradycardia increases as time goes on and digoxin may eventually have to be reduced in dose or discontinued.

The risk of digoxin toxicity is increased in the setting of acute myocardial infarction and its use in that setting is controversial. Caution is advised.

Table 14–2. Important Digoxin-Drug Interactions

Increased Digoxin Effect	Decreased Digoxin Effect
Qunidine	Antacides
Quinidinelike drugs	Bile acid resins
Verapamil	Corticosteroids
Diltiazem	Kaolin-pectin
Amiodarone	Antibiotics (see text)
Antibiotics (see text)	Metoclopramide
Flecainide	High-fiber supplements
Methyldopa	Sucralfate?
Anticholinergics	Phenytoin?
Potassium-wasting diuretics	
Nifedipine?	
Cimetidine?	
Oral hypoglycemic agents?	

Because of variations in bioavailability among brands and formulations of digoxin, clinical response should be monitored if changes are made.

Indications

Digoxin is indicated in the management of atrial flutter or fibrillation with a rapid ventricular response, and in supraventricular tachycardia. Although digoxin is frequently used to convert atrial fibrillation to normal sinus rhythm, in most geriatric patients atrial fibrillation is or will soon become chronic despite aggressive treatment. Therefore, in general the goal should be to normalize a rapid ventricular rate. If tolerated, verapamil may be preferable in patients with coexisting angina or hypertension, since these conditions can be ameliorated by verapamil. However, digoxin is clearly preferable to verapamil in patients with impaired left ventricular function.

Digoxin is useful in the management of congestive heart failure, although the benefits are modest in patients with normal sinus rhythm. In acute heart failure, digoxin is considered adjunctive treatment to diuretics, with or without vasodilators.

Digoxin may be used in the treatment of chronic congestive heart failure in patients with atrial fibrillation. If sinus rhythm is present, digoxin should be considered in patients whose heart failure is not controlled by sodium restriction, diuretics, or vasodilators. If the patient does not experience increased exercise tolerance or amelioration of other symptoms from digoxin, there is generally little reason to continue the drug.

Withdrawal of Digoxin

Some individuals, most of them elderly, have been taking digoxin for years without a clear indication. In other cases, the drug may have been prescribed for congestive failure, which could be adequately if not better and more safely controlled with diuretics. In as many as 70% or more of patients in these categories, digoxin has been withdrawn successfully. Many patients actually report an improvement in well being when the drug is discontinued.

Digoxin should not be blithely discontinued in all patients, however. A careful search should be undertaken to determine why digoxin was initiated. Even patients successfully withdrawn from this drug may have latent congestive failure. In such patients digoxin might prevent cardiac decomposition due to intercurrent insults such as respiratory infections, ischemic events, and dietary indiscretion. Although there is no physiologic reason to withdraw digoxin slowly rather than abruptly, gradual withdrawal gives the physician the opportunity to observe the patient closely for signs of increasing congestive failure or the appearance of arrhythmias. Once off digoxin, the patient should be closely followed.

Although it is impossible to predict with certainty which patient can discontinue the drug uneventfully, certain guidelines may be useful. In general, withdrawal should be attempted only in patients satisfying the following criteria:

1. No clear-cut indication for digoxin.
2. Faulty indication (anemia, sinus tachycardia, or peripheral edema without heart failure).
3. History of congestive failure with sinus rhythm, currently controlled.
4. No history of atrial tachyarrhythmia.
5. Absence of symptoms at subtherapeutic serum digoxin levels.
6. No audible third heart sound (S_3).
7. Easy access to physician or medical facility for close follow-up.

Formulations of Digoxin and Bioavailability

Digoxin is available in tablets, elixir, gelatin solution in capsules, and intravenous solution. Assuming 100% bioavailability for the intravenous form, absorption of tablets varies from 60% to 80%, the elixir 70% to 85%, and the gelatin capsule over 90%.

Although all available forms of digoxin satisfy current FDA requirements for bioavailability, absorption can be affected by factors such as particle size, which vary from one brand to another. Since digoxin has a narrow therapeutic index, variations in bioavailability can be important when brand or formulation is changed. There is no reason to switch from one brand to the other if the patient is doing well. In fact, the narrow therapeutic index of digoxin makes it prudent to treat certain patients with only one brand.

Dosing

Because of its narrow therapeutic index, it would be desirable to determine the dose of digoxin on the basis of objective calculations. Unfortunately, such precision depends on a number of factors, namely, exact bioavailability of the drug and patient peculiarities such as nonrenal metabolism, myocardial sensitivity, the presence of interacting drugs, lean (ideal) body weight, and creatinine clearance. These factors are all highly variable and physiologic variables are unpredictable in the elderly. Thus, it is practical to "digitalize" the patient using an empiric approach, which is time-tested and predictive of patient response. **Digitalization** signifies the saturation of body stores and achievement of steady-state plasma concentrations. Rapid digitalization consists of giving a loading dose and should be employed only when the clinical state demands that an effect be achieved rapidly. Slow digitalization is achieved over 10 or more days of a daily maintenance dose.

Even when dose is estimated, it is important to have as close an appraisal of the patient's renal function as possible. For rapid estimation of creatinine clearance, see Chap. 1.

In the geriatric patient, the average loading dose is approximately 75%, and average maintenance dose 50%, of the respective amounts recommended for younger adults. The lower loading dose is preferred because of the potentially greater cardiac sensitivity expected in an elderly patient. The lower maintenance dose is based primarily on the average 50% decline in renal clearance of the drug seen in elderly patients.

Intravenous digoxin is reserved for rapid digitalization, or when the patient is unable to take drugs orally. The intramuscular route is discouraged because it is very painful and may cause local muscle necrosis.

SLOW DIGITALIZATION

Initial oral dose:* 0.125 mg daily. Digitalization is achieved after approximately 10–12 days of daily maintenance dose depending on creatinine clearance.
Note: Patients with renal insufficiency should receive no more than 0.125 mg on alternate days as initial therapy.
Usual dose range: 0.125 to 0.25 mg daily. Dosage titrations in patients with arrhythmias should be further determined by clinical response.

RAPID DIGITALIZATION

Route	Initial Dose	Incremental Dose[†]	TLD[‡] (first 24 hr)
IV	TLD × 0.5	TLD × 0.25	0.5–0.75 mg
Oral	TLD × 0.5	TLD × 0.25	0.625–1.0 mg

*Based on tablet; for other formulations, see Table 14–3.
[†]At intervals of 4–8 hours after IV dose; at 6–8 hours after oral dose.
[‡]Total loading dose.

Serum Digoxin Levels

It has been suggested that currently used digoxin assays might lead to falsely high measurements in the elderly, but to date this question has not been resolved. More importantly, clinical response to a given dose, and in turn to a particular level of digoxin in the blood, tends to be less predictable in geriatric patients.

Blood should be drawn at least 5 to 6 hours after the oral dose of digoxin to give time for serum digoxin to equilibrate with digoxin in tissues. This is particularly important in the elderly in whom absorption and elimination may be delayed. Levels of 0.8 to 2.0 ng/ml of digoxin are considered to be in the "therapeutic range." Although lower levels are considered "subtherapeutic," symptoms and signs of toxicity can occur at normal or subtherapeutic levels because of electrolyte disorders, hypersensitivity of a diseased heart, or suscep-

Table 14–3. Digoxin Equivalents (mg)

Tablets or elixir	0.125	0.25	0.5
Gelatin capsule	0.1	0.2	0.5
Intravenous	0.1	0.2	0.5

tibility of other organs, such as the brain. Conversely, supratherapeutic levels may have to be attained before tachyarrhythmias are controlled in certain patients. Clinical improvement in heart failure may be achieved with very small doses of digoxin, and little additional improvement achieved when the dose is raised to achieve a "therapeutic level."

Digoxin levels should be used as an adjunct and not as a substitute for clinical judgment. Therapeutic monitoring may be particularly useful when clinical dilemmas exist, namely, if there is a need to clarify whether adverse symptoms are due to digoxin toxicity, whether a patient is complying with the regimen, or whether a patient who appears to require unusually large doses is malabsorbing or excessively degrading the drug. Routine monitoring is a waste of time and money, and may result in prescribing errors.

Digitoxin (Crystodigin, Purodigin)

Digitoxin is uncommonly instituted today, but is still being taken by some elderly patients who were first prescribed the drug years ago. For this reason, it is important for the physician to be aware that the pharmacokinetic properties of digitoxin are vastly different from the more familiar digoxin.

Pharmacokinetics

Like digoxin, digitoxin is absorbed in the stomach and smaller intestine, but, because of its greater lipophilicity, it is absorbed more extensively—nearly 100%—and with less variability. The plasma elimination half-life is 5–7 days and it takes 3–4 weeks before steady-state plasma levels are reached. Unlike digoxin, digitoxin is highly bound to serum proteins, so that higher total drug levels in the serum are attained than with digoxin; however, tissue binding is lower than with digoxin. The therapeutic range for serum digitoxin levels is approximately 15–25 ng/ml. Digitoxin is metabolized by hepatic microsomal enzymes to inactive metabolites, with only 15% being excreted unchanged in the urine. A small proportion (less than 10%) is metabolized to digoxin and excreted in the kidney and a small amount undergoes enterohepatic circulation. The liver has great reserve capacity for metabolism of this drug so that elimination half-time does not seem to be affected greatly by hepatic disease or by age, although it may be greatly affected by other drugs (see Important Drug Interactions below).

Intravenous digitoxin is available but is rarely used.

Adverse Effects

The potential adverse effects of digitoxin are identical to those of digoxin. These effects are not as readily reversed because the drug is eliminated very slowly.

Important Drug Interactions

Pharmacodynamic interactions occur as with digoxin. Otherwise, the spectrum of drug interactions is very different. Drugs that impair or stimulate hepatic enzymes can increase or reduce digitoxin levels and alter clinical effect. Although many such interactions were reported in the past, the uncommon use of this drug in recent years means that drug interactions with new drugs might not have been reported. Digoxinlike drug interactions occur with quinidine, verapamil, and diltiazem, but the mechanism has not been fully explained; the magnitude of these interactions is not as great as with digoxin.

Known interactions are summarized in Table 14-4.

Does Digitoxin Have a Place in Therapy?

There are few if any reasons to use digitoxin over digoxin today. Use of digitoxin waned when the better-absorbed, purified forms of digoxin became available. Despite the fact that age has little or no impact on digitoxin clearance, this drug is retained in the system for prolonged periods. Toxicity may occur as a result of drug interactions, electrolyte disorders, or end organ sensitivity. Recovery from digitoxin toxicity is inevitably a long process.

Dosing

Usual daily dose: 0.1 mg.

VERAPAMIL (CALAN, ISOPTIN)

Verapamil is a calcium channel blocking agent that has more potent effects on cardiac conduction than most other members of that class of drugs. Like other calcium channel antagonists, verapamil is effective in lowering blood pressure and in managing angina, but, because it is more likely to produce bradycardia, constipation, and a fixed cardiac output, in geriatric practice it is generally reserved for patients in whom arrhythmia management is also indicated. Other calcium channel blockers are discussed in Chaps. 12 and 13 in conjunction with hypertension and angina.

Pharmacologic Considerations

Mechanism of Action

Calcium channel blocking agents slow the movement of calcium across cell membranes through calcium channels, reducing excitation of myocardial and vascular smooth muscle and myocardial conduction tissue. Verapamil has the most potent effect of these agents on slowing atrioventricular nodal conduction and is useful in the management of atrial fibrillation and supraventricular tachycardia. Verapamil affects the sinus node less than the AV node and does not reduce heart rate if sinus node function is normal. However, the drug may unmask sinus node disease, producing bradycardia. Significant reductions in sinus rate have been observed in elderly patients with no history of overt sinus node disease.

Verapamil also has a more potent effect on cardiac and nonvascu-

Table 14-4. Known Digitoxin-Drug Interactions

Increased Digitoxin Effect	Decreased Digitoxin Effect
Quinidine	Barbiturates
Cimetidine	Rifampin
Ranitidine	Bile acid resins
Diltiazem	Alcohol?
Verapamil	
Potassium-wasting diuretics	

lar smooth muscle than other calcium channel blockers, which accounts for some of its adverse effects. Its negative inotropic effect has been harnessed in the management of hypertrophic cardiomyopathy, a clinical entity that may be more common in the geriatric population than previously believed.

Like other calcium channel blockers, verapamil is a peripheral vasodilator and is effective in reducing blood pressure in hypertensive individuals. It also enhances coronary blood flow and is useful in the management of angina.

Pharmacokinetics

Oral verapamil is well and rapidly absorbed from the gastrointestinal tract but undergoes extensive first-pass metabolism so that the oral dose is considerably higher than the intravenous dose. One metabolite has some pharmacologic activity. Only small amounts of the parent compound remain unmetabolized and available for renal excretion. The serum half-life of oral verapamil is roughly 4–6 hours in nonelderly adults, but hepatic metabolism is saturable so that after continuous use less ingested drug is metabolized and the half-life can be much longer, ranging from 5 to 12 hours. Half-life tends to be further prolonged with age and in liver disease.

Verapamil is highly bound to serum proteins, including alpha$_1$ acid glycoprotein. This protein has been noted to increase in concentration with age, leading to a decrease in the free or active fraction of certain drugs, but the clinical importance of this effect has not been well delineated.

Adverse Effects

Because of its potent effect on atrioventricular conduction, verapamil may produce **bradyarrhythmias,** including **atrioventricular (AV) block.** This occurs more frequently with verapamil than with other calcium channel blockers. The risk of bradycardia is enhanced when the drug is used in conjunction with digoxin or beta blockers, which also slow AV conduction. Its effect on the sinus node is less potent and patients with truly normal sinus node function do not develop bradycardia on this account. However, occult sinus node dysfunction is common in elderly cardiac patients so that caution should be observed. More serious arrhythmias have been more commonly described in patients with accessory conduction pathways and are not commonly encountered in geriatric practice when ordinary doses are used.

Verapamil's effect on the sinus node is also great enough to prevent a compensatory increase in heart rate when its vasodilatory effects lead to lowering of blood pressure. The resulting fixed cardiac output may be clinically important in patients with impaired myocardial contractility, since verapamil has a potent negative inotropic effect; **congestive heart failure** occurs occasionally. This is not a common side effect because vasodilation produces decreased afterload, which tends to compensate for the negative inotropic effect. In patients with chronic congestive heart failure, however, reduced afterload is insufficient to make up for the negative inotropic effect and heart failure may worsen.

Another potential cardiovascular effect of verapamil is **hypotension.**

Constipation is a very frequent side effect experienced by elderly patients taking verapamil and may limit compliance with the medication.

Other side effects include **dizziness, flushing,** and **leg edema.** Mental confusion has been reported but is thought to be extremely rare.

Important Drug Interactions

Verapamil reduces the clearance of digoxin and may increase serum digoxin levels as much as 70% in patients being treated for atrial fibrillation. Although digoxin-induced arrhythmias may result, the two drugs can be given together safely if digoxin dosage is adjusted early, according to clinical criteria or digoxin blood levels. Since verapamil and digoxin share the property of slowing AV nodal conduction, they may also potentiate each other's effect on a pharmacodynamic basis. This may have therapeutic benefit, but if care is not exercised, high-degree AV block can result. A similar action has been described with digitoxin but the effect is of a smaller magnitude. A verapamil-quinidine interaction has been less well defined.

Concurrent use of beta blockers may result in bradyarrhythmias as well as potentiation of negative inotropic effect. The combination of verapamil and disopyramide may result in congestive heart failure in susceptible patients. Verapamil may potentiate the hypotensive effect of other antihypertensive agents.

It is claimed that verapamil participates in interactions with drugs that are cleared by or that influence the hepatic microsomal enzyme system, such as rifampin (reduced verapamil effect), cimetidine (increased verapamil effect), and theophylline (possible increased theophylline toxicity). Although clinical interactions of this nature have not consistently occurred, caution is advised.

Although verapamil is highly protein-bound, no displacement interactions have thus far been reported on this basis.

Contraindications and Precautions

Verapamil is contraindicated in patients with symptomatic bradycardia or hypotension, and should be avoided if possible in patients with congestive heart failure. The drug should be instituted very cautiously in patients with constipation; laxatives may be required.

Verapamil is contraindicated in ventricular tachycardia (VT). Narrow complex VT may be almost indistinguishable from paroxysmal atrial tachycardia, for which intravenous verapamil is commonly given. A patient with evidence of new myocardial ischemia and no prior history of supraventricular arrhythmias may well have VT, in which case another agent should be selected.

Verapamil or Digoxin for Rapid Atrial Fibrillation?

As compared to digoxin, verapamil has a more rapid onset of action in the acute situation. In the chronic situation, it is more effective in controlling tachycardia exacerbated by exercise and adrenergic stimuli and provides additional therapeutic benefit in the patient with hypertension or angina. It is less likely to produce confusional states than digoxin and has a more favorable therapeutic-to-toxic ratio, all other factors being equal.

As a practical matter, however, digoxin is probably used more often. It is a more logical choice in the setting of congestive heart failure. It is well accepted by geriatric patients because it does not produce constipation and need be taken only once a day. Digoxin's less favorable therapeutic index does require caution, however, in patients who are unreliable or on complicated medication regimens.

Indications

Verapamil is indicated in the treatment of supraventricular tachycardia and rapid atrial fibrillation. Intravenous verapamil is used when rapid correction of the tachyarrhythmia is needed.

This drug is an effective antihypertensive and anti-angina agent. However, patients with angina or hypertension who do not require drug therapy for an atrial arrhythmia may tolerate other calcium channel antagonists better than verapamil (see Chaps. 12 and 13).

Verapamil is indicated in the management of hypertrophic cardiomyopathy. It has also been reported to relieve nocturnal leg cramps in elderly patients who did not respond to quinine.

Dosing

Oral

Initial dose: 40 mg tid.
Usual daily dose range: 160–360 mg in 2 to 3 divided doses.
Note: Slow-release preparations of oral verapamil (Calan SR, others) are available.

Intravenous (For Acute Conversion of Tachyarrhythmias)

1.0–2.5 mg over 60 seconds. If hemodynamically stable, repeat bolus at 5–10 minute intervals. In paroxysmal atrial tachycardia, a bolus of 5–10 mg may be required.

BETA BLOCKERS

The chief geriatric application of beta blockers in the management of cardiac arrhythmias is as adjunctive treatment of rapid supraventricular arrhythmias. When added to other negative chronotropic agents the dose must be given cautiously because bradycardia may occur unexpectedly.

Beta blockers may also be given to patients with recent myocardial infarction. There is evidence that these drugs prolong survival in such patients, although it is not known if this is due to an antiarrhythmic effect or some other mechanism. Drugs that possess intrinsic sympathomimetic activity should not be used for this purpose.

Beta blockers are discussed more fully in Chap. 12.

QUINIDINE

Pharmacologic Considerations

Mechanism of Action

Quinidine acts by decreasing conduction velocity and decreasing excitability of specialized conducting tissue of the atrium and ventricle. It depresses myocardial contraction in the ventricle, but this exerts little or no clinical effect at ordinary doses. As a class IA antiarrhythmic drug it resembles procainamide and disopyramide in its mechanism of action. Quinidine is chemically related to the antimalarial agent quinine, however, and shares some of its properties and toxicities as well.

Quinidine also has vagolytic and alpha-adrenergic blocking properties, actions that together can increase the heart rate and enhance atrioventricular conduction. The alpha blocking effect leads to afterload reduction, which may compensate for the small negative inotropic effect of the drug.

Pharmacokinetics

Quinidine is well absorbed by the gastrointestinal tract as both the sulfate (various brands) and the gluconate (Quinaglute, others), although the latter is somewhat more slowly absorbed than the former. Onset of action may occur as early as 30 minutes. The drug is metabolized in the liver to active and inactive metabolites that are excreted in the kidney. Approximately 20% of the drug is excreted unchanged by the kidney. The average serum half-life is about 4 hours, but the range is very wide. Elimination is prolonged in the presence of congestive heart failure and appears to be prolonged with age.

Adverse Effects

At the high dosage end, quinidine may excessively prolong conduction, leading to widened QRS complex. In severe cases, **heart block** or **asystole** may occur. The QT interval may become prolonged, increasing the risk of **ventricular arrhythmias,** including ventricular tachycardia and fibrillation. QT prolongation is generally, though not always, dose-related. Rapid supraventricular arrhythmias may also rarely occur.

Quinidine may produce **syncope.** This has been attributed to a proarrhythmic action but it could also be a direct result of vasodilation mediated by alpha blockade. Hypotension per se is unusual at ordinary doses.

Gastrointestinal symptoms are common, particularly diarrhea and dyspepsia. It has been reported that quinidine gluconate is better tolerated in this regard, perhaps because of its slower absorption rate, but this has been disputed. Older patients occasionally perceive the diarrheal effect as a beneficial decrease in constipation. Gastrointestinal symptoms are sometimes seen in conjunction with tinnitus, flushing, disturbed vision, and altered mental status. This complex of adverse symptoms, **cinchonism,** is not seen with other antiarrhythmic agents, but is a toxicity peculiar to quinidine and other drugs derived from cinchona.

Rash and **hypersensitivity reactions** may occur. **Autoimmune hemolytic anemia** and **thrombocytopenia,** though relatively uncommon, may affect the elderly disproportionately. These hematologic reactions tend to present suddenly after several weeks of therapy.

Lupuslike reactions have rarely been reported and are far less likely to occur than with procainamide (see below).

Important Drug Interactions

Many drugs that affect cardiac conduction may produce additive effects with quinidine. In addition to antiarrhythmic drugs, tricyclic antidepressants and phenothiazines promote quinidine cardiac toxicity.

Quinidine increases the serum level of digoxin. A quinidine-digitoxin interaction also occurs but to a lesser degree. The digoxin interaction is mediated in part by competition between the two drugs for renal elimination. In contrast to nonelderly adults, patients over the age of 70 experience toxicity from the combination of digoxin and quinidine at a much higher rate than would be expected from the sum of reactions produced by either agent alone. Thus, elderly patients tend to have additive toxicity from this interaction. If quinidine is added to a digoxin regimen, the dose of the latter should, on the average, be reduced by half.

Quinidine levels may be increased by coadministration of drugs that impair hepatic metabolic enzymes, such as cimetidine. Likewise, quinidine efficacy may be impaired by enzyme inducers such as rifampin, barbiturates, and phenytoin. Verapamil may also increase quinidine levels.

Quinidine can inhibit synthesis of vitamin-K-dependent clotting factors, increasing sensitivity to warfarin.

Other drugs with alpha-adrenergic blocking action, such as prazosin, may precipitate syncope when used in conjunction with quinidine.

Contraindications

Quinidine is contraindicated in patients with known allergic history to quinidine or related compounds, such as quinine sulfate. It is also contraindicated in patients with untreated bradyarrhythmias or heart block.

Indications

Quinidine is indicated in the treatment of symptomatic or unstable ventricular arrhythmias. It is also indicated as adjunctive treatment in supraventricular tachycardia and rapid atrial fibrillation that fail to respond to other agents. In atrial arrhythmias, quinidine should not be used without digoxin or verapamil, which stabilize the AV node and prevent the vagolytic action of quinidine from worsening tachycardia.

Dosing

Initial dose: 200 mg tid-qid as quinidine sulfate. This is not a loading dose. Complete antiarrhythmic effect may not occur for several days.
Usual dose range: 200–300 mg tid-qid.
Note: Quinidine gluconate (Quinaglute) 325 mg is equivalent to 200 mg of quinidine sulfate. An extended-dose form of quinidine sulfate (Quinidex) is available.
Intravenous route: This route should generally be avoided in elderly patients because of the risk of hypotension.

PROCAINAMIDE

Pharmacologic Considerations

Mechanism of Action

Procainamide is similar to quinidine in its antiarrhythmic mechanism of action. However, it does not have significant vagolytic or alpha blocking action.

Pharmacokinetics

Procainamide is well absorbed and acetylated in the liver to an active metabolite, N-acetylprocainamide (NAPA), which has some of the antiarrhythmic actions but less immunogenic effect than the parent compound. The rate at which this step occurs is genetically determined, with individuals being classified as *fast* and *slow* *acetylators*. Slow acetylation prolongs the duration of action of procainamide and increases the proportion of parent drug to NAPA in the system. Speed of acetylation is probably not changed with age. However, both NAPA and at least 50% of parent drug are excreted by the kidney, which results in prolongation of antiarrhythmic action with age. Unless dose adjustments are made, this may reduce the safety margin for certain patients.

The half-life of procainamide is only 3–4 hours, but that of NAPA is more than twice as long. While both are further prolonged somewhat in older patients, a potentially favorable consequence of this is that efficacy can be easier to achieve than in younger adults, who require inconveniently frequent dosing. Sustained-release procainamide has a half-life of 5–7 hours in nonelderly adults and produces more predictable serum levels.

Significant protein binding of procainamide does not occur.

Adverse Effects

Like quinidine, procainamide may produce high degrees of **heart block, bradycardia,** and **ventricular arrhythmias.** Prolongation of the QT interval or the QRS complex may be present before the production of ventricular arrhythmias.

An important adverse effect of procainamide in the elderly is its ability to produce a **lupuslike syndrome.** In contrast to hydralazine-related lupus, the risk may increase with age, in part because procainamide is eliminated more slowly and in part because of age-associated suppressor T-cell dysfunction. Procainamide is probably one of the most common causes of this syndrome and produces antinuclear antibody (ANA) in as many as 80% of cases, although only a small proportion of these patients develop symptoms. The syndrome occurs after several months of treatment but its appearance may be delayed by two years or more in fast acetylators. It is generally manifested as arthralgia, arthritis, pleural effusion, or pericarditis; anemia and other hematologic involvement is uncommon, dermatologic involvement rare; neurologic symptoms rarely if ever occur and renal disease has not been reported. Procainamide-induced lupus usually resolves when the drug is discontinued but in some cases months may elapse before resolution. It is important and often difficult to distinguish an actual lupuslike reaction from other pathology. Many elderly patients taking no medications may have low titers of autoantibodies in their serum, including ANA, and coincidental joint pathology is extremely common.

Other hypersensitivity reactions are unusual. **Neutropenia** occurs rarely and is not thought to be immune-mediated. Central nervous system toxicity is likewise rare. **Gastrointestinal disturbances** may occur but are much less common than with quinidine.

Important Drug Interactions

As with quinidine, drugs that affect cardiac conduction can produce additive cardiotoxicity.

Elimination of procainamide may be reduced by concurrent administration of histamine$_2$ blockers, including cimetidine and ranitidine. This interaction is thought to be mediated by competition for renal elimination rather than impaired hepatic metabolism.

Pharmacokinetic interaction with digoxin has not been described. However, concurrent use of digoxin may increase the cardiac effects of procainamide on a pharmacodynamic basis.

Contraindications

Procainamide is contraindicated in patients with untreated high-grade heart block. It should not be used in patients who have a history of drug-related lupus.

Precautions

All elderly patients about to embark on therapy with procainamide should have baseline determination of ANA because many will have low titers of spontaneously occurring autoantibodies. A careful rheumatologic history and physical evaluation should be done as well. These precautions are advised for diagnostic purposes only, since neither the presence of spontaneous autoantibodies nor a history of osteoarthritis is a contraindication to the use of procainamide. If baseline ANA has not been done, and if the patient's new symptoms are confined to the joints, serum should be tested for the presence of IgG antibodies to single-stranded DNA, which are present in high titers in this syndrome as well as in systemic lupus erythematosus (SLE) but should be absent in normal elderly. This diagnostic strategy differs in the younger patient in whom SLE is more often part of the differential diagnosis. In patients with SLE, regardless of age, positive titers of antibody against native, double-stranded DNA will be found, but should be absent in drug-induced lupus. If a diagnostic dilemma cannot be resolved, the drug should be discontinued.

ANA should be monitored during therapy. If levels rise progressively, the drug should generally be discontinued, even though lupuslike symptoms have not become manifest. This precaution is particularly important in elderly patients in whom symptoms may be subtle or not voiced.

Indications

Procainamide is indicated in the same circumstances as quinidine. However, because of the potential for producing lupuslike reactions, it should only be used in patients unable to tolerate quinidine.

Intravenous procainamide can be substituted for lidocaine if that drug is contraindicated.

Serum Levels

When monitoring serum levels, it is important to measure both parent drug and NAPA because of the antiarrhythmic activity of both substances. NAPA levels may exceed those of the parent drug in many patients, especially elderly ones.

Serum levels of drug do not substitute for serologic testing if lupuslike reaction is suspected.

Dosing

Initial oral dose: 250 mg tid-qid as procainamide.
Note: Although this is not a loading dose, complete antiarrhythmic

effect may be established within 24 hours because of the drug's short half-life. However, the half-life of NAPA tends to be prolonged with age, so that pharmacologic effects may not be maximal for up to 48 hours.

Usual dose range: 250–750 mg every 4–6 hours as procainamide. Sustained-release forms of procainamide (Procan SR, others) can be given 2 to 3 times a day.

Intravenous dose: 12 mg/kg over 30 minutes followed by continuous infusion of 2 mg/min. Some patients may require higher doses to suppress arrhythmias.

Note: Intravenous procainamide should be reserved for emergencies. While younger adults may tolerate doses up to 6 mg/min, this is likely to be excessive for geriatric patients because excretion of the active substances tends to be prolonged.

DISOPYRAMIDE (NORPACE)

Pharmacologic Considerations

Mechanism of Action

Disopyramide exerts its antiarrhythmic effect by the same mechanisms as quinidine and procainamide. Disopyramide has potent negative inotropic action but, unlike verapamil and quinidine, does not reduce afterload that would compensate for reduced left ventricular function. This factor often limits the usefulness of disopyramide in patients with cardiac disease beyond the conducting system. In addition, disopyramide has potent anticholinergic action. This probably contributes less to its electrophysiologic effects than to unwanted side effects.

Pharmacokinetics

Disopyramide is well absorbed. Its hepatic metabolism includes one active, renally excreted metabolite with less than half of the antiarrhythmic action of the parent drug but with far greater anticholinergic effect. A substantial portion of disopyramide is excreted unchanged in the kidney. The average duration of action of disopyramide is 7 hours in healthy nonelderly, but tends to be significantly prolonged in some older individuals.

Adverse Effects

Disopyramide produces a high incidence of **atropinelike** side effects, including dry mouth, blurred vision, constipation, confusional states, and urinary retention. Urinary retention, hesitancy, and frequency are very common in elderly men treated with disopyramide and generally require that the drug be discontinued. It may also precipitate acute angle closure glaucoma.

Because of its potent negative inotropic effects, disopyramide may produce **congestive heart failure** in patients with underlying myocardial impairment. Congestive heart failure is a reported side effect in as many as 50% of patients with a prior history of cardiac decompensation, but in only a small proportion of those with no history of overt myocardial disease. **Exacerbation of ventricular arrhythmia** may also occur.

An uncommon side effect of disopyramide is **hypoglycemia**. As with most cases of drug-induced hypoglycemia, this has been most often reported in elderly patients. This phenomenon may be related to insulin resistance but the precise mechanism is not known.

Important Drug Interactions

Cardiac conduction disturbances may be potentiated by concurrent use of antiarrhythmic and related drugs. These interactions are discussed in connection with quinidine (see above). In addition, agents that affect myocardial contractility, such as beta blockers or verapamil, may potentiate the negative inotropic effects of disopyramide, leading to heart failure.

Agents that stimulate the hepatic microsomal enzymes system, such as phenytoin and rifampin, may accelerate the metabolism of disopyramide, reducing its effect. Likewise, enzyme inhibitors have the potential of increasing the effect of disopyramide, although to date such interactions have not been reported.

Contraindications

Disopyramide is contraindicated in congestive heart failure, states of urinary retention, and in patients with a history of acute angle closure glaucoma.

Indications

Disopyramide is indicated in patients who require control of ventricular arrhythmias but who cannot tolerate quinidine or procainamide.

Dosing

Initial dose: 100 mg bid-tid.
Usual daily dose range: 300–500 mg in 3 or 4 divided doses. Long-acting forms of disopyramide (Norpace CR, others) are available.

LIDOCAINE

Pharmacologic Considerations

Mechanism of Action

Like other class I antiarrhythmic drugs, lidocaine acts to suppress ventricular arrhythmias by stabilizing myocardial cell membranes. It is effective in suppressing ventricular arrhythmias but has little effect on atrial tachyarrhythmias. It does not suppress the sinus node and may increase heart rate directly or by producing reflex tachycardia in response to its peripheral vasodilating action.

The effect on ventricular conduction seems to be greatest in the diseased myocardium. For this reason, it may be more effective in patients being treated for arrhythmias in conjunction with myocardial ischemia than in those without additional evidence of organic heart disease. Likewise, cardiac toxicity is enhanced.

Pharmacokinetics

Lidocaine cannot be given orally because extensive first-pass hepatic metabolism limits its bioavailability. After an intravenous bolus, antiarrhythmic effect occurs within 90 seconds. The drug distributes widely, and shortly after administration plasma levels decline rapidly with a half-life of 10–20 minutes. After the rapid distribution period, there is a slower decline in levels with a half-life of 2 hours. The second phase is dependent on hepatic metabolism and hepatic blood flow. The drug is metabolized by oxidative processes with the production of some pharmacologically active substances. The distribution phase occurs readily in geriatric patients, but overall elimination tends to be slowed and half-life of parent drug and renally excreted active metabolites is prolonged. Like other drugs that are eliminated by hepatic extraction, lidocaine is eliminated more slowly when there is reduced hepatic blood flow, as in congestive heart failure, liver disease, and probably advanced age. However, the prolonged half-life of lidocaine seen in elderly individuals without heart failure may be related to an increased volume of distribution rather than impaired hepatic clearance. Moreover, the elimination half-life is not prolonged in all elderly patients.

Lidocaine is about 70% bound to alpha$_1$ acid glycoprotein, a serum protein that is an acute phase reactant and that increases on the average with age. The implications of this to lidocaine pharmacokinetics are not known.

In congestive heart failure there is increased peripheral vascular resistance. This leads to a shunting of blood away from skeletal sites to the brain and heart, allowing the drug to distribute with greater rapidity to those organs. Cardiac and central nervous system toxicity can be enhanced in this setting.

Adverse Effects

Adverse effects are more frequent in geriatric patients than in younger adults. This is due not only to altered pharmacokinetics, but to the increased susceptibility at the tissue level to the effects of lidocaine. In elderly individuals, toxic side effects tend to occur at lower blood levels of this drug than expected.

Central nervous system (CNS) toxicity is common in the older age group, and is dose-related. Lidocaine is best known for its propensity to produce seizures as a manifestation of this toxicity. However, geriatric patients are also particularly prone to other side effects, such as confusion, delirium, and lethargy. Neurological impairment increases the risk of CNS side effects. Related toxicity includes visual disturbances, paresthesias, dysarthria, dizziness, tremor, and muscle twitching.

Cardiac toxicity is also dose-related, although individuals with myocardial or conducting system vulnerabilities may be exquisitely sensitive to smaller than expected levels of the drug. Serious toxicity may occur if dosing is not age-adjusted and sometimes occurs even at very low doses in sensitive individuals. Lidocaine can suppress escape rhythms, slowing the ventricular response in atrioventricular block. Patients with sinus node disease may develop sinoatrial conduction disturbances or sinus arrest.

Lidocaine is excreted in the saliva and may produce a **metallic taste** and **anesthesia of the tongue.**

Topical lidocaine used for local anesthesia is capable of producing systemic effects in susceptible individuals.

Important Drug Interactions

By reducing hepatic blood flow, agents such as propranolol and cimetidine may reduce the elimination time of lidocaine, enhancing its action. Hepatic metabolism of lidocaine can be reduced by drugs that inhibit microsomal enzymes, such as cimetidine.

Contraindications

Lidocaine is contraindicated in patients with a history of hypersensitivity reactions to local anaesthetics. It should not be used in patients with untreated high-degree heart block.

Precautions

Patients with acute myocardial infarction and other disease states may have resistant arrhythmias. Increasing dosage may not suppress these arrhythmias but may lead to lidocaine toxicity.

Dosing

Initial dose: 1 mg/kg given as intravenous bolus; this may be repeated once if necessary after 20–30 minutes.
Maintenance dose: 1–2 mg/min (20–40 μg/kg/min) as continuous infusion, begun after the initial dose.
Note: Dosing must be individualized according to the clinical situation. Some patients may require higher doses to suppress arrhythmias.

NEWER ANTIARRHYTHMIC DRUGS

A number of other antiarrhythmic agents are now available but their use in geriatric practice is limited. Although, in the long run, some of these agents may prove to be safer than older drugs, there is less experience with them at this time. Thus, they should be prescribed to geriatric patients only after cardiology consultation, using electrophysiologic testing when appropriate. Even in younger patients, these drugs are generally reserved for specialized use. For a complete discussion of these and other antiarrhythmic agents, the reader is referred to Purdy and Boucek (see Bibliography.)

Flecainide (Tambocor) and encainide (Enkaid) are highly effective in suppressing ventricular ectopic beats, even when other agents have failed to do so, and have also been used in the management of supraventricular arrhythmias. They were selected for study in the postinfarction Cardiac Arrhythmia Suppression Trial (CAST), because their favorable side-effect profile and intermediate duration of antiarrhythmic action made them suitable for long-term study. However, both drugs were found to increase mortality rather than improve survival as compared to placebo and were withdrawn from the trial. Although age was not found to be a factor, only 5% of subjects were over the age of 75. Cardiac as well as total mortality was increased, with cardiac mortality attributed to proarrhythmic events. Despite this, it is presently unclear whether the proarrhythmic effect attributed to these two agents is greater than that produced by other antiarrhythmic agents, because comparative studies have been very limited in scope. The risk of proarrhythmia is greater in patients with structural heart disease, those with a history of ventricular tachycardia, and those taking other cardiotropic medications, but it has not been possible to accurately identify all patients at risk. Since most geriatric patients with arrhythmias also have some cardiac structural abnormalities and since blood levels would likely be higher than average for a given dose, it is theoretically possible that they would be at increased risk. Indirect evidence of an age-associated risk comes from the fact that a pilot study that preceded CAST, but showed the drugs to be safe, excluded patients over the age of 75.

Flecainide has negative inotropic effect, though probably no greater than Quinidine and possibly less than disopyramide. In addition, it has some anticholinergic activity and has been rarely reported to produce urinary retention. Encainide is a less potent negative inotrope than flecainide. Its pharmacokinetics are complex and subject to genetic variability, but the duration of antiarrhythmic action is relatively consistent, and the drug can be given as infrequently as twice a day. Elimination of both drugs, particularly encainide, is prolonged in renal failure and, to a certain extent, with age. Although generally well tolerated, both flecainide and encainide can produce dizziness and visual disturbances in a significant minority of patients.

Results of the CAST study led to highly restrictive labeling of flecainide and encainide, and for the moment they should be reserved for the treatment of refractory symptomatic arrhythmias or for patients who cannot tolerate other agents. In the future, if comparative studies show these drugs to be as safe as older agents, they might be particularly applicable to the elderly because they may actually be better tolerated in the long run. If they are given to geriatric patients, downward dose adjustments should be considered. Dose increments of encainide should be made less often than for younger adults.

Propafenone (Rhythmol) is a complex drug that was recently released. It is classified as a IC antiarrhythmic agent, sharing some features with encainide and flecainide. Because of this similarity, propafenone has been released with the same restrictive labeling as the other two agents. Propafenone also has mild beta adrenergic blocking activity and may produce typical side effects associated with those agents. It participates in a number of pharmacokinetic drug interactions.

Tocainide (Tonocard) is a lidocaine analogue that is similar in its mechanism of action, but is less extensively metabolized and can be given orally. This drug has few advantages over quinidine and can produce a large number of annoying side effects, most common among them being gastrointestinal and central nervous system disturbances. Most of these side effects are not serious but they tend to be poorly tolerated by elderly patients. Agranulocytosis has been reported.

Mexiletine (Mexitil) has effects similar to tocainide both in spectrum of action and the high incidence of side effects. In addition, mexiletine participates in a number of pharmacokinetic drug interactions.

Amiodarone (Cordarone) has an extremely long half-life and its strong protein- and tissue-binding properties cause it to accumulate in many organs. It is associated with an unusual range of toxicity, including pulmonary infiltrates, thyroid disease, skin changes, visual changes, central nervous system aberrations, and hepatitis, which may not subside readily because of the drug's slow elimination. Although it is said to have a low likelihood of worsening ventricular arrhythmias and does not impair myocardial function, it should be used only when other agents have failed. It is rarely if ever used in geriatric practice.

MANAGEMENT OF CONGESTIVE HEART FAILURE

As compared to younger adults, congestive heart failure in the elderly is more often associated with reversible factors, including anemia, acute blood loss, hyperthyroidism, and medications that depress myocardial function. The physician should identify these factors before embarking on long-term drug treatment for heart failure. Unfortunately, underlying heart disease is commonly present in these cases as well.

The symptoms of heart failure in the aged may be subtle, presenting as weakness and decreased exercise tolerance rather than dyspnea, orthopnea, or gross pulmonary edema. Heart failure is frequently the only presenting symptom of acute myocardial infarction, which is frequently "painless" in the elderly.

Physical findings may also be misleading. Crepitations in the lung bases may be chronic and may be due to old scarring or, in sedentary or nonambulatory patients, to basilar atelectasis. Peripheral edema is frequently due to venous insufficiency. Venous insufficiency is often asymmetric and edema may be asymmetric even when heart failure is present. Jugular venous distension may be unrelated to cardiac function but due to compression by branches of the aged, ectatic aorta. This finding is confined to the left jugular vein and does not subside when the patient is erect.

Selection of drugs should be guided by the patient's ability to tolerate them. Diuretic therapy is essential but may be poorly tolerated as older cardiac patients are particularly susceptible to symptomatic dehydration, orthostatic hypotension, and prerenal azotemia. In addition, bladder dysfunction may prevent the patient from complying with a full diuretic regimen.

Digoxin should be given if necessary and should be part of the regimen in patients who also have rapid atrial fibrillation. The vasodilators of choice are the angiotensin converting enzyme (ACE) inhibitors. These agents dilate both the venous and arterial bed, thereby reducing preload and afterload. To date, they seem to be quite well tolerated by older patients. Nitrates act primarily on the venous bed and reduce preload; they are very well tolerated by elderly patients and may increase exercise capacity, but tachyphylaxis can occcur. Hydralazine acts primarily on the arterial bed, and although it may increase indices of cardiac output, it does not actually increase exercise tolerance further when added to a regimen that contains diuretics and digoxin. Multiple drug regimens reduce patient compliance, may contribute little to clinical outcome, and should be discouraged in most patients.

The most widely used diuretic in congestive heart failure is furosemide, which will be discussed here. Also discussed is metolazone, which is reserved for special circumstances. Other diuretics, digoxin, and drugs used as vasodilators are discussed in other sections and the Bibliography (see Malloy & Lopez).

Furosemide

Pharmacologic Considerations

MECHANISM OF ACTION. Furosemide inhibits sodium and chloride reabsorption in the ascending loop of Henle. This portion of the nephron is responsible for reabsorbing up to 30% of the filtered sodium load, so that interference at this location results in marked diuresis. Acutely, loss of volume also reduces blood pressure. However, due to the short duration of action, compensatory mechanisms soon halt this action. Patients with normal renal function are unlikely to experience sustained lowering of blood pressure with furosemide. A possible exception to this rule could theoretically be the many older individuals with occult impairments in creatinine clearance, but this has not been well established.

Furosemide may produce loss of a number of other ions, including magnesium and calcium. Depletion of these ions is not associated with its action on volume or blood pressure. There is interindividual variation in response to furosemide with some patients achieving diuresis at lower doses than others.

PHARMACOKINETICS. Furosemide is rapidly absorbed. Rate and extent of absorption do not appear to be diminished by gut edema of congestive heart failure. The extent to which furosemide undergoes hepatic metabolism is not known, but it appears that a substantial amount of its elimination occurs via the kidney. The duration of action in nonelderly adults is 4–6 hours, but this may be significantly prolonged in older individuals, to the extent that many are troubled by the need to urinate throughout the day and even night.

Adverse Effects

Furosemide may produce important **disturbances in electrolyte balance,** notably hypokalemia, hyponatremia, and magnesium depletion. Hypercalciuria may occur, but the clinical implications of this have not been fully explored. Rapid volume depletion may produce symptomatic **hypotension,** particularly if the intravenous route is used.

Like all diuretics, furosemide may produce **bladder disturbances.** The rapid production of large volumes of urine may overwhelm the capacity of the bladder to store urine and patients with marginal bladder control may develop frank **incontinence.** Because its duration of action is prolonged in older patients, even morning doses may produce **nocturia.** These problems frequently interfere with patient compliance. Patients should be instructed to take furosemide at the time of day or night that is the most convenient for them.

Men with prostatic hyperplasia may develop acute **urinary retention** from the sudden delivery of large volumes of urine to the bladder. This commonly occurs in the elderly male who is admitted to the hospital, becomes bedridden and constipated, and is instructed to use a urinal in bed rather than stand. Urinary retention may develop in anyone with potential outlet obstruction.

Large doses of furosemide may produce **tinnitus** or **deafness.** This is most likely to occur in patients with renal failure and those receiving large intravenous boluses of the drug. A potential additive risk may exist when other ototoxic drugs are being administered concurrently. Acute ototoxicity is unlikely to occur with ordinary oral doses used for hypertension and congestive heart failure, but chronic hearing loss has been reported in older patients receiving moderate doses of oral drug. The frequency of this problem is not known but is believed to be low.

Important Drug Interactions

Ototoxic drugs, such as the aminoglycosides, can theoretically potentiate the ototoxic effect of furosemide. This is most likely to occur in patients with renal insufficiency who receive large doses of the latter.

Furosemide combined with other potassium-wasting diuretics may produce severe hypokalemia or azotemia.

Digitalis preparations and furosemide are a useful combination, but in the face of potassium or magnesium depletion, digitalis toxicity may occur.

Precautions

Monitoring of serum electrolytes is essential, especially when digitalis preparations are being given concurrently. Blood urea nitrogen (BUN) should also be checked periodically. In patients who develop severe prerenal azotemia from furosemide but whose heart failure or edema remain uncontrolled, it is often best to give adjunctive treatment rather than increase the dose of furosemide further. Elastic stockings or compression bandages may be helpful in controlling leg edema if further salt restriction is impractical or ill-advised.

Indications

Furosemide is a first-line agent in the treatment of moderate to severe congestive heart failure and may be used in other fluid-retaining states when thiazides or thiazidelike diuretics are ineffective or contraindicated.

When a diuretic is desired, furosemide is indicated for the treatment of hypertension or other fluid-retaining states in patients with renal insufficiency. It is less likely than the thiazides to produce sustained hypotensive effect in patients with normal renal function.

Furosemide is also used in the treatment of hypercalcemia. In this setting, sodium intake must be increased to enhance hypocalcemic effect.

Dosing

Initial dose: 10–20 mg. If diuresis is not achieved, the dose should be increased by 50%–100% and all drug given in one dose. This is more likely to produce diuresis than if the new dose is divided. Once the appropriate dose is realized and if further diuresis is required, additional doses can be given at 4–12 hour intervals.

Usual daily dose range: 20–80 mg. Higher doses are often required in renal insufficiency.

Metolazone (Zaroxolyn, Others)

Metolazone is a thiazidelike diuretic that is particularly useful in patients with fluid-retaining states refractory to furosemide. Unlike thiazides, metolazone has important action in the proximal as well as distal tubule, and does not lose its effect in renal insufficiency. In fact, it may be particularly useful in that setting. It is sometimes used in conjunction with furosemide to enhance the diuretic action of the latter. It is thought to enhance the effect of furosemide by proximally blocking sodium reabsorption, thereby increasing delivery of sodium to the loop of Henle where furosemide exerts its action. Thiazide diuretics are also able to act in a synergistic fashion with furosemide but only if renal function is relatively normal.

Metolazone is an extremely potent diuretic and kaliuretic agent, particularly when used in conjunction with furosemide. Elderly patients in general are more prone to the development of diuretic-related azotemia than younger patients, and metolazone may greatly increase the risk; profound prerenal azotemia can occur.

Precautions

Because of the possibility of azotemia and severe hypokalemia, especially when metolazone is used in combination with loop diuretics, electrolytes, BUN, and creatinine should be measured very shortly after therapy is instituted and at frequent intervals thereafter. If metolazone is given to a patient taking a loop diuretic, the dose of the latter should be reduced.

Indications

In geriatric patients, metolazone should be reserved for refractory fluid-retaining states, in which it may be used cautiously in combination with a loop diuretic.

Dosing

Downward dose adjustments are recommended in geriatric patients with congestive heart failure because the potency of this agent may lead to severe azotemia, especially when given with furosemide.

Initial dose: 1.0–2.5 mg 3 times per week. Certain patients may require less frequent dosing. Dose increases should not be made more frequently than once every 2–3 weeks. Higher doses are generally required in renal insufficiency.

Other Diuretics

Commonly used diuretics are discussed in Chap. 12 in conjunction with the treatment of hypertension. These drugs are suitable for the management of fluid-retaining states and mild congestive heart failure in patients with normal renal function.

BIBLIOGRAPHY

Abernethy, D. R., Schwartz, J. B., Todd, E. L., et al. Verapamil pharmacodynamics and disposition in young and elderly hypertensive patients. Altered electrocardiographic and hypotensive responses. *Ann. Intern. Med.* 105:329–336, 1986.

Cush, J. J., and Goldings, E.A. Southwestern internal medicine conference: drug induced lupus: clinical spectrum and pathogenesis. *S. Med. J.* 290:36, 1985.

Doherty, J. E. Clinical use of digitalis glycosides. *Cardiology* 72:225–254, 1985.

Fisch, C. (Ed.). William Withering: an account of the foxglove 1785–1985. *J. Amer. Coll. Cardiol.* 5 (5 Supp A):3A–123A.

Gallagher, K. L., and Jones, J. K. Furosemide-induced ototoxicity. *Ann. Intern. Med.* 91:744–745, 1979.

Klein, H. O., and Kaplinsky, E. Digitalis and verapamil in atrial fibrillation and flutter. Is verapamil now the preferred agent? *Drugs* 31:185–197, 1986.

Kreeger, R. W., and Hammill, S. C. New antiarrhythmic drugs: tocainide, mexiletine, flecainide, encainide, and amiodarone. *Mayo Clin. Proc.* 62:1033–1050, 1987.

Malloy, M. J., and Lopez, L. M. Management of congestive heart failure in the elderly. *Drug Intell. Clin. Pharm.* 22:788–792, 1988.

Mooradian, A. D., Grieff, V. L., Bressler, R., Reed, R. L., and Marcus, F. I. Digitalis in the elderly. *J. Amer. Geriatr. Soc.* 37:873–882, 1989.

Podrid, P. J., Schoeneberger, A., and Lown, B. Congestive heart failure caused by oral disopyramide. *N. Engl. J. Med.* 302:614–616, 1980.

Purdy, T. E., and Boucek, R. J. *Handbook of cardiac drugs.* Boston: Little, Brown, 1988.

Rodin, S. M., and Johnson, B. F. Pharmacokinetic interactions with digoxin. *Clin. Pharmacokin.* 15:227–244, 1988.

The Cardiac Arrhythmia Suppression Trial (CAST) investigators. Preliminary report: Effect of encainide and flecainide on mortality in a randomized trial of arrhythmia suppression after myocardial infarction. *N. Engl. J. Med.* 321:406–412, 1989.

Walker, A. M., Cody, R. J., Greenblatt, D. J., et al. Drug toxicity in patients receiving digoxin and quinidine. *Am. Heart J.* 105:1025–1028, 1983.

Antithrombotic Agents

Two broad categories of agents are used to prevent intravascular coagulation leading to clinical thromboembolic disease—anticoagulants and antiplatelet agents. These agents also prevent further propagation of preformed thrombus. Members of a third group, fibrinolytic agents, act to directly lyse preformed thrombus, and are used in settings of acute thrombus formation, such as acute myocardial infarction. A discussion of the fibrinolytic agents streptokinase and tissue plasminogen activator, which are subject to highly specialized use, is beyond the scope of this book. Readers interested in this topic are referred to the Bibliography readings (see Wittry et al.; Cairns et al.).

Anticoagulants alter the manufacture or metabolism of proteins involved in the coagulation cascade. The coagulation cascade is a series of enzymatic reactions that culminates in the production of fibrin and intravascular trapping of blood cells, a process that tends to occur in areas of low flow, such as the venous bed or a dysfunctional cardiac atrium. For this reason, anticoagulants are used in conditions such as deep vein thrombosis, pulmonary embolus, and cardiogenic thromboembolic disease. The most frequently used anticoagulants in the United States are warfarin and heparin.

Antiplatelet agents alter the production or aggregative adhesive properties of platelets, decreasing the tendency to form fibrin-containing microemboli. Arterial endothelial damage stimulates platelet aggregation and ultimately leads to the formation of microthrombus. The high flow of blood in the arterial bed favors this process by facilitating contact of the platelet with the arterial wall and by increasing local turbulence and endothelial injury. Thrombus forms as a result of disturbance of arterial circulation, usually in the setting of arteriosclerosis. This is the basis on which antiplatelet agents have been utilized for the prevention of stroke, transient ischemic attack (TIA), and myocardial infarction. Because platelet activation can ultimately result in stimulation of the coagulation cascade, anticoagulants can theoretically be useful in these situations as well. The preferred antiplatelet agent now in use is aspirin.

Although the choice of antithrombotic agent has traditionally rested on pathophysiologic factors leading to clot formation, there are certain situations in which it is unclear which approach—anticoagulation or antiplatelet therapy—is superior, and there are several situations in which the efficacy of either type of agent is unclear. Helpful guidelines have been published by the American College of Chest Physicians regarding the use of antithrombotic agents (see Bibliography). The recommendations put forth by that group are based on a wide range of studies of varying scientific weight. In general, these recommendations can serve as a guide for geriatric patients. However, it is important to emphasize that no studies on which the published recommendations are based have focused specifically on elderly subjects. For this reason, important controversies should be evaluated specifically with the geriatric patient in mind.

THE ATRIAL FIBRILLATION CONTROVERSY

At least 5% of community-residing and up to 20% of nursing-home elderly have chronic atrial fibrillation, making the geriatric population an important target group for preventive treatment. Patients with chronic atrial fibrillation have a fivefold or greater risk of stroke than those with sinus rhythm, the risk being further increased with age and in the presence of additional cardiac pathology, in particular rheumatic mitral valve disease, dilated cardiomyopathy, and congestive failure. In contrast, the risk of stroke is relatively low when atrial fibrillation is present without evidence of any other heart disease (*lone atrial fibrillation*). Lone atrial fibrillation is probably rare in elderly individuals.

The risk of stroke in the setting of transient episodes of the arrhythmia (*paroxysmal atrial fibrillation*) is substantially lower than in chronic atrial fibrillation, even in elderly patients. This observation is seemingly inconsistent with the belief that the greatest risk of stroke exists at the onset of the arrhythmia. However, this risk is probably also dependent on the duration of the paroxysmal rhythm and is probably higher for episodes that persist for days to weeks than for truly transient episodes lasting seconds to minutes.

The risk of systemic embolization increases when cardioversion is given to patients who have had atrial fibrillation for longer than 3 days, leading experts to recommend prophylactic anticoagulation for patients about to undergo elective cardioversion. There is no reason to suggest that geriatric patients have a different risk of systemic embolization in this setting. However, cardioversion itself should be applied sparingly in the elderly, especially if the duration of atrial fibrillation is not known; sinus rhythm is seldom maintained in this patient population because conduction system disease tends to be widespread, and the frequent involvement of the sinus node increases the risk of sinus arrest when cardioversion is employed.

The risk of recurrent stroke in patients with atrial fibrillation is only slightly higher (25%) than in those without atrial fibrillation (20%). There is no reliable clinical or neuroimaging method of distinguishing between carotid artery embolic, cardioembolic, and thrombotic stroke and, even in patients with a history of stroke, one cannot rely on the mere presence of atrial fibrillation to establish an association. In fact, it has been argued that atrial fibrillation can predispose to stroke by leading to diminished and inconsistent cardiac output, leading to ischemic stroke in susceptible individuals, most of whom would be elderly.

Alternatively, chronic atrial fibrillation is believed to increase the risk of stroke by predisposing to the formation and propagation of atrial thrombi. However, indirect evidence indicates that 25%–35% of strokes experienced by patients with atrial fibrillation are not cardiogenic but are due to other lesions. Thus, if the goal is to prevent the propagation of thromboemboli, anticoagulation may fail to reduce the stroke risk for a significant number of elderly.

Recent primary prevention studies suggest that antithrombotic therapy reduces the risk of stroke in patients with atrial fibrillation (see Bibliography). However, as of the writing of this book, available evidence indicates that aspirin is ineffective in patients over the age of 75. Low-dose warfarin may prove to be the treatment of choice, but data on its efficacy is somewhat limited for the geriatric age group. Age-adjusted analysis is crucial because the risk-benefit ratio of anticoagulation could be greater for the elderly.

Recommendations

Because the risks of anticoagulation may outweigh the benefits in certain individuals, prophylactic anticoagulation should only be given to patients at high risk of thromboemboli and at low risk of complications. Thus, anticoagulation for primary prevention in elderly patients with atrial fibrillation should be strongly considered if there are additional risk factors for cardiogenic embolism, including rheumatic valvular heart disease, mechanical heart valve, dilated cardiomyopathy, or congestive heart failure, or if additional risk factors for thrombotic disease are superimposed, such as prolonged bedrest, abdominal or orthopedic surgery, or hip fracture. In those with no additional risk factors for embolism, anticoagulation with low-dose warfarin should be considered in robust patients who are highly motivated and reliable. Such patients are arguably similar to the "young-old" for whom efficacy data is available. Further recommendations await the outcome of prospective studies geared at those over the age of 75 years.

Patients should receive anticoagulation only if they are highly reliable and do not have risk factors for complications, such as a tendency to fall, a history of bleeding, or a complicated medication regimen.

In patients with chronic atrial fibrillation and a history of thromboembolic episodes, anticoagulation should be strongly considered. However, in the case of stroke, because the risk of recurrence is not much greater for the patient with atrial fibrillation than for the patient without atrial fibrillation, anticoagulation should only be considered for patients who are clearly at low risk of developing complications.

Routine anticoagulation is not recommended for patients with transient episodes of atrial fibrillation when there are no signs of systemic embolization.

Anticoagulation is recommended for 3 weeks prior to and 2–4 weeks after elective cardioversion in patients who have had atrial fibrillation for longer than 3 days, if there is no contraindication. However, only highly selected patients in the geriatric age group who have established atrial fibrillation should be selected to undergo this procedure.

THE STROKE CONTROVERSY

The incidence of stroke increases dramatically with age, and with age a greater proportion of strokes are due to thrombotic or thromboembolic events and a smaller proportion to intracranial hemorrhage. Thus, even in the absence of atrial fibrillation, older patients would be expected to derive at least as great a benefit from antithrombotic therapy as younger patients. Unfortunately, clinical trials may exclude aged patients, include small numbers, or fail to analyze the data by age.

Overall, aspirin reduces the risk of stroke and TIA in patients with **prior evidence** of thromboembolic cerebrovascular disease (*secondary prevention*). There is no evidence that antithrombotic therapy prevents noncardioembolic stroke in previously unaffected people (*primary prevention*). Since antithrombotic agents can increase the risk of hemorrhagic stroke in susceptible individuals, and since it is not possible to accurately predict who is susceptible, patients without a prior history of stroke or TIA may not only fail to benefit from aspirin or other antithrombotic treatment, but may develop an increased risk of stroke. This has in fact been demonstrated in studies of patients receiving various antithrombotic agents for the primary or secondary prevention of myocardial infarction but who had no symptoms of cerebrovascular disease (see The Aspirin-Myocardial Infarction Controversy, below).

Although there is some evidence that aspirin does not reduce the risk of recurrent TIA or stroke in women, this finding has not been universal.

Geriatric patients have not been well studied as a specific group. The failure of aspirin to benefit people over age 75 in the Stroke Prevention in Atrial Fibrillation study (see Bibliography) underscores the fact that the elderly must be studied as a separate group before non-age-adjusted data can be applied to them. In that study, the failure of only the elderly to benefit once again reminds us that geriatric patients often have multiple risk factors for stroke.

Little is known about the effects of antithrombotic therapy in multi-infarct dementia. Multi-infarct dementia is a poorly defined syndrome traditionally believed to result from lacunar infarcts in small arteries that penetrate deep structures of the brain. This syndrome accounts for at least 30% of dementia cases in the geriatric population. The term "vascular dementia" has also been applied to dementia related to cerebrovascular disease, since patients with classic stroke can develop dementia; these patients are probably often classified as having multi-infarct dementia and some of them would be expected to have lower rate of stroke recurrence on aspirin. However, claims that aspirin is useful in the prevention and management of this syndrome require further study.

While antiplatelet therapy remains the hallmark of stroke prevention, there are many who advocate the use of anticoagulants in the management of acute thrombotic stroke-in-evolution, but this indication requires further study. Likewise, there are those who advocate the use of anticoagulants in patients who have "breakthrough" TIAs despite antiplatelet therapy. This is one logical option, but it is also important to rule out cardiogenic emboli and temporal ("giant cell") arteritis in such situations.

Recommendations

Although geriatric patients have not been well studied, low-dose aspirin should be given to those who have a history of TIA or non-hemorrhagic stroke. Aspirin should be considered over warfarin in geriatric patients with a history of classic TIA even in the setting of atrial fibrillation, because there may be a lower risk of bleeding complications and because it is likely that arteriosclerotic disease exists in the carotid system and elsewhere. This recommendation is based on the known benefit of aspirin in classic TIA and not on recent evidence from primary prevention studies of atrial fibrillation that warfarin is superior to aspirin.

Although the benefits to women are unclear, the risks of antithrombotic doses of aspirin are very low in patients without a bleeding diathesis or peptic ulcer. Thus, consideration should presently be given to treating female patients as well as male patients.

Antithrombotic therapy should not be given for primary prevention of stroke because it is not possible to accurately identify all patients at increased risk of hemorrhagic stroke.

THE ASPIRIN-MYOCARDIAL INFARCTION CONTROVERSY

There is evidence that aspirin reduces the risk of recurrent myocardial infarction, although this question has not been well studied in the elderly. There is also evidence that aspirin reduces the risk of first-time myocardial infarction. The recent, highly publicized Physician's Health Study in the United States (see Steering Committee) showed a definite risk reduction from aspirin that was greater for men over 60 than for younger men. Unfortunately, fewer than 7% of the subjects in this study were over the age of 70. Disturbingly, the risk of stroke was higher in aspirin users than those taking placebo; the increase in stroke was primarily in hemorrhagic stroke, but the risk of nonhemorrhagic stroke was not reduced. The stroke figures were unfortunately not analyzed by age. This study contrasts with a British trial, in which aspirin did not prevent myocardial infarction; patients 70 years of age or older, who comprised 14% of the subjects, were not analyzed separately.

The benefits of aspirin in women with coronary artery disease are uncertain.

Recommendations

Aspirin therapy should be considered for the prevention of recurrent myocardial infarction in selected patients. The best candidates for aspirin would be those with symptomatic arteriosclerosis elsewhere, for example, the patient with a history of TIA. There is presently no reason to exclude women from this recommendation.

Patients who wish to take aspirin for the primary prevention of myocardial infarction should be fully informed of the possible increase in stroke risk. Logical candidates for this therapy would be those with a history of classic TIA or thrombotic stroke. Aspirin should not take the place of other measures to reduce coronary risk (see Chap. 17). The risks and benefits for women in this setting are uncertain for women under 65, and unknown for older women.

THE HIP FRACTURE CONTROVERSY

The incidence of deep vein thrombosis in the setting of acute hip fracture has been reported to be as high as 70%. There is a particular predeliction for proximal thrombosis, with an increased risk of pulmonary embolus. The fracture itself is thought to activate the coagulation cascade; this acts in concert with venous damage at the fracture site, which leads to platelet activation so that thrombosis is already present at the time of surgery. It is perhaps for this reason that trials of various agents have not consistently demonstrated a substantial risk reduction of postoperative thromboembolic complications. However, fatal pulmonary embolus is a dreaded complication of hip fracture in the elderly and it is common though not universal practice for the orthopedic surgeon to anticoagulate the patient if there is no contraindication to doing so. The risk of intra- and postoperative bleeding complications is low if anticoagulation is moderate and probably does not outweigh the risk of thromboembolism.

In joint replacement surgery, the risk of thromboembolism is also high and studies of antithrombotic therapy appear to show somewhat greater benefit than in hip fracture. However, unlike surgery for fracture, joint replacement is an elective procedure that is performed in a well-controlled setting, so that results of these studies should not necessarily be applied to the setting of emergency repair of hip fracture.

It is not known what form of anticoagulation is superior in controlling thromboembolic complications associated with hip fracture and the choice of agent seems to be dependent on the experience of the local operating team. Warfarin, miniheparin, aspirin, and dextran have all been used with varying success but good comparative studies are needed. A recent study demonstrated a selective reduction by aspirin of proximal deep vein thrombosis, but an overall superiority of warfarin in reducing thromboembolic events (see Powers et al.). Bleeding complications were uncommon. In general, dextran is avoided in very elderly or debilitated patients because of the risk of fluid overload and congestive heart failure.

Likewise, the ideal dose of the antithrombotic agent has not been determined. A dose of warfarin that produces a prothrombin time (PT) higher than 1.5 times control may increase the risk of bleeding. The dosage of heparin in this setting has not been well studied but heparin doses of 10,000 units or less per day appear to be ineffective; indirect evidence from joint replacement studies suggests that the dose should be adjusted to maintain the activated partial thromboplastin time (aPTT) in at least the high normal range. One dose of aspirin found to be effective was 650 mg twice daily; although this may be higher than necessary, the dose should be sufficient to guarantee antiplatelet activity early on in treatment.

Dosing of antithrombotic agents is discussed further in sections on individual agents.

There is no consensus as to whether the agent should be instituted before or after surgery. Low-dose antithrombotic treatment is associated with a low risk of perioperative bleeding and probably is more effective in preventing thrombotic episodes than when the agent is instituted postoperatively.

Recommendations

Prophylactic antithrombotic therapy should be given to elderly patients prior to or soon after repair of hip fracture, provided there are no contraindications. Aspirin, warfarin, or heparin should be employed according to the experience and discretion of the operating surgical team. In general, antithrombotic agents should be instituted following surgery and continued until the patient has attained maximal ambulation or function.

Warfarin dose should be adjusted to maintain the PT approximately up to 1.5 times control.

If subcutaneous heparin is used, the dose should maintain aPTT in the high normal range.

Aspirin should be instituted at 325–650 mg/day for the first 3 days. Maintenance dose probably need not exceed 325 mg/day.

Dextran should generally be avoided in very elderly, debilitated, or hemodynamically unstable patients.

Acute thromboembolic complications should be treated with full anticoagulation.

ANTICOAGULANTS

Warfarin (Coumadin, Others)

Pharmacological Considerations

MECHANISM OF ACTION. Warfarin acts by competing with vitamin K in its facilitation of the production of gamma-carboxyglutamic acid moiety on clotting factors II, VII, IX, and X. The gamma-carboxyglutamic acid moiety is essential for the binding of calcium and consequent activation of these "vitamin K factors." This moiety is also found on protein C, an endogenous substance that has intrinsic anticoagulant activity.

PHARMACOKINETICS. Warfarin is rapidly absorbed, reaching peak serum concentrations in 1 hour and having an average serum half-life of 42 hours, with wide variation. Food decreases the rate but not the extent of absorption. Warfarin is highly bound to serum proteins, primarily albumin. It is converted by hepatic microsomal enzymes to largely inactive metabolites. Commercial warfarin is a racemic mixture of two enantiomers, the S-isomer having more anticoagulant effect than the R-isomer. These isomers are metabolized at different rates, behave differently in certain drug interactions, and may account for the interindividual variation that is seen in half-life. Most, but not all, studies have demonstrated little or no decline in warfarin metabolism with age. However, the dose required to raise the prothrombin time declines somewhat with age, an observation that has not been fully explained.

The half-lives of factors VII, IX, X, and II are 6, 24, 40, and 60 hours, respectively. Warfarin begins to prolong the prothrombin time as soon as factor VII levels decline, but because of the different half-lives of newly synthesized factors in the body, the full antithrombotic effect may lag behind the early increase in prothrombin time by as long as several days after therapy begins.

The anticoagulant effect of warfarin can be reversed by the administration of vitamin K_1. Other forms of vitamin K are less effective in this regard.

Adverse Effects

The most important complication of warfarin therapy is bleeding. Although the risk of bleeding does not appear to be a function of age per se, the incidence of bleeding increases with age. This age-related increase is probably due to the increased prevalence of bleedable lesions, as well as other risk factors, including falls, dementia, and concurrent use of other medications.

Important bleeding complications in elderly patients include intracerebral hemorrhage, subdural hematoma, and gastrointestinal and retroperitoneal bleeding. Retroperitoneal bleeding may present subtly; gastrointestinal bleeding is often painless in the elderly, even when peptic ulcer is the cause. Microhematuria may occur, and although neoplastic lesions should be ruled out, benign lesions such as prostatic hyperplasia, urethral caruncle, and atrophic vaginitis are commonly the basis of this. Bruises, bleeding into large joints, epistaxis, and hematomas after needle injection are other common complications of anticoagulation. Vitamin K_1 administration cannot be expected to completely reverse the bleeding diathesis for up to 36 hours while new clotting proteins are being synthesized.

An unusual syndrome of **skin necrosis** has been described in patients with vitamin C deficiency. This severe, autosomal dominant condition, manifesting as a hypercoagulable state, is generally clinically overt by young adulthood, although less severe cases may only come to light as the result of warfarin treatment. The petechiae seen at the onset of this syndrome should not be confused as the "reddening" of hyperpigmented macules that occurs when patients with venous insufficiency receive anticoagulation. The latter may occur when anticoagulation is excessive and is indistinguishable from a petechial rash, which would otherwise be an uncommon skin manifestation of warfarin.

Drug, Nutrient, and Disease Interactions

The importance of warfarin interactions begins when a new drug is instituted and persists for several days after either drug is discontinued. It is the unanticipated change in warfarin sensitivity that is often responsible for morbidity. Because of the extensive protein binding of warfarin, many protein-bound substances can displace warfarin from its binding sites, increasing the free or active fraction of the drug. Although rapid distribution and elimination of the newly freed warfarin limits the duration of increased sensitivity, the narrow therapeutic index of the drug could make such displacement interactions important. However, for a number of drugs, even those that are highly protein-bound, other mechanisms are more likely to be responsible. Agents that reduce activity of hepatic microsomal enzymes, such as cimetidine, can enhance the anticoagulant effect of warfarin. Those that stimulate this system, such as barbiturates and rifampin, can reduce the anticoagulant effect. In addition, drugs that reduce warfarin absorption, such as cholestyramine and colestipol, may increase warfarin resistance, although these agents can also reduce vitamin K absorption, potentially increasing warfarin sensitivity.

Vitamin K deficiency may increase warfarin sensitivity and vitamin K excess can produce warfarin resistance. Causes of vitamin K deficiency include dietary insufficiency, small bowel disease with malabsorption, and, if other risk factors are present, antimicrobial killing of intestinal bacteria that produce vitamin K. Agents that reduce the absorption of vitamin K, such as mineral oil, may elevate the PT. Excessive ingestion of substances rich in vitamin K may produce warfarin resistance. Enteral formulas with a high vitamin K content have been implicated in warfarin resistance. This has prompted some manufacturers to reduce the vitamin K content of certain products. However, there is evidence that other components in enteral formulas, possibly the protein components, may bind to warfarin, reducing its absorption. These interactions are particularly important in patients who are fed by enteral tube (see Chap. 25).

Pharmacodynamic interactions with warfarin are equally important. Agents that reduce platelet function can secondarily increase the bleeding diathesis even if PT is not unduly prolonged. In addition to agents specifically prescribed for their antiplatelet function, such as aspirin, nonsteroidal anti-inflammatory agents (NSAIDs) can significantly impair platelet function. Aspirin and NSAIDs are also ulcerogenic and can increase the risk of bleeding ulcer in patients given warfarin. Other ulcerogens, such as reserpine and potassium supplements, should be used with caution.

Because of the high risk of falls in the elderly, any agent that increases the risk of falls should be considered as one that participates in a warfarin-drug interaction in this age group since the fall can lead to traumatic bleeding.

There are many reports of warfarin-drug interactions in the literature, but not all have been well documented and others are inconsistent. Important drug interactions are summarized in Table 15-1. For a complete discussion of this complex topic, the reader is referred to the Bibliography (see Hirsch).

Liver disease can increase warfarin sensitivity by reducing the production of coagulation factors, reducing the catabolism of warfarin, and impairing platelet function. Renal disease does not impair warfarin clearance significantly but severe renal disease itself can induce coagulation defects. Serum albumin is subject to relatively

Table 15-1. Some Important Drug and Nutrient Interactions with Warfarin

Pharmacodynamic Interactions

Platelet inhibitors
Ulcerogens
Anticoagulants

Pharmacokinetic Interactions

Increase Warfarin Sensitivity
Aspirin
Salicylates
Cimetidine
Quinolone antibiotics
Chloral hydrate*
Erythromycin
Sulfonamides

Decrease Warfarin Sensitivity
Barbiturates
Phenytoin
Carbamazepine
Rifampin
Estrogens
Vitamin K
Cholestyramine and colestipol*
Sucralfate*

Drugs That May Increase the Risk of Falls
Sedative-hypnotics
Antidepressants
Antihypertensive agents
Neuroleptics

*Reports inconsistent or effect variable.

rapid fluctuations in late life, so that acute and chronic illness may lead to decreased warfarin binding and increased free or active fraction of the drug. The presence of any bleedable lesion, of course, may lead to problems.

Contraindications and Precautions

Warfarin is contraindicated in bleeding disorders, in the presence of bleeding or significant bleedable lesions, if there has been recent head trauma, and in uncontrolled hypertension.

Warfarin should only be used in reliable patients. Patients with dementia or a tendency to fall should probably avoid anticoagulation unless the indication is powerful; in such cases the drug should only be used in a highly supervised or protected environment.

Geriatric patients often receive drugs from sources other than the primary care physician. Because of the vast number of drugs that interact with warfarin, the patient should be repeatedly instructed to consult the primary physician when new prescriptions are written by others or when medications are purchased over the counter. Older individuals who take warfarin should purchase a medical alert bracelet that indicates this.

Because bleeding complications may be occult, a high index of suspicion should be maintained when geriatric patients on anticoagulants develop nonspecific symptoms, such as weakness, confusion, or chest pain. Loss of blood volume, whatever the cause, is poorly tolerated in older individuals and must be diagnosed and corrected swiftly.

Indications

Warfarin is indicated for the prevention of deep vein thrombosis and its embolic complications. Common situations include the postoperative patient and acute myocardial infarction. It is suitable for use in the setting of hip fracture, but its efficacy is controversial.

Warfarin is indicated for the prevention of systemic arterial embolism in the setting of mechanical heart valve, dilated cardiomyopathy, fresh intracardiac thrombus, and elective cardioversion.

Routine use of warfarin for the prevention of arterial embolism in patients with atrial fibrillation is increasing. However, more study is needed before firm recommendations can be made for people over the age of 75 years (see The Atrial Fibrillation Controversy, above).

Warfarin may be used in an effort to prevent "breakthrough" cerebrovascular ischemic events as an alternative to aspirin in patients who do not respond to the latter; however, its efficacy in this setting is not known.

Dosing

The dose of warfarin should be determined by the level of the prothrombin time, which should be maintained in the area of 1.2 to 1.5 times the control value for all indications except recurrent systemic embolization and mechanical heart valve, in which cases the PT should be maintained at 1.5 times control. Recent evidence indicates that thromboembolism in certain clinical settings may be preventable with much less intense anticoagulation, however.

In all cases, the exact level of anticoagulation should be tailored to the patient's needs. If the patient develops important bleeding complications but no thrombosis despite PT in the "therapeutic" range, consideration should be given to "subtherapeutic" control.

The optimal PT range now recommended is significantly lower than in the past. This has to do with the change in sensitivity of the reagent used for determination of PT. In the past, a reagent comparable to the present North American reagent was already used in the United Kingdom, where many studies determining the optimum PT had been done. Thus, North American physicians were unwittingly overdosing their patients, using as a goal the British therapeutic range, which produced overly intense anticoagulation in the United States. Although the newer reagent has been in use for nearly two decades, many physicians still adhere to the older guidelines, which results in unnecessarily high doses of warfarin and an unwarranted number of bleeding episodes.

Usual starting dose: 10 mg daily for 2–3 days; thereafter, adjust dose according to PT.

Heparin

Pharmacologic Considerations

MECHANISM OF ACTION. Heparin is a polar mucopolysaccharide derived from bovine lung or porcine intestinal mucosa, which acts by accelerating the action of antithrombin III, an intrinsic anticoagulant that inhibits activated species of clotting factors XII, XI, IX, and X, and prothrombin. The enhanced activity of antithrombin III occurs when heparin binds to it and changes its conformation.

PHARMACOKINETICS. Because of its large size and polarity, heparin is poorly absorbed from the gastrointestinal tract and must be given parenterally.

In contrast to warfarin, the anticoagulant effect of heparin occurs immediately, and the action stops abruptly once it has been removed from circulation. The average serum half-life after an intravenous dose is 90 minutes. The serum half-life does not correlate with duration of anticoagulant effect. Moreover, the half-life increases with increasing dose of the drug, presumably because of saturable hepatic metabolism, and there is significant interindividual variation. Heparin is taken up by the reticuloendothelial system but may subsequently be released into the systemic circulation. A portion is converted in the liver to inactive metabolites, but the majority is thought to be excreted unchanged in the urine, particularly when a large bolus of heparin is given. The presence of renal as well as liver disease results in enhanced anticoagulant action of heparin. Although there is some evidence that antithrombin III levels decline with age, geriatric patients do not demonstrate clinical resistance to heparin. In fact, lower doses may be required to obtain the same anticoagulant effect. The reasons for this are not well understood.

In some patients, heparin progressively reduces antithrombin III activity after a few days of therapy. During therapy there are no clinical consequences of this effect since the rate at which clotting factors are inhibited continues to be accelerated. However, upon termination of heparin therapy, antithrombin levels return to normal more slowly than the clotting factors, promoting a potentially hypercoagulable state for about 3 days. There is some dispute as to the clinical importance of this phenomenon.

The anticoagulant effect of heparin can be acutely reversed by protamine, a low molecular weight protein that combines ionically with heparin to form a stable complex that is devoid of anticoagulant activity.

Adverse Effects

Bleeding is the most common side effect of heparin. As with warfarin, the risk of bleeding is increased in geriatric patients because of the increased prevalence of bleedable lesions, overt and occult. There is no evidence that this age-associated risk is due to alterations in heparin pharmacokinetics, or to differential action on the clotting system. Potential bleeding complications are similar to those seen with warfarin, as discussed above.

If bleeding occurs in the face of excessive doses of heparin, protamine should be given. However, protamine itself has intrinsic anticoagulant activity, so that for the heparin-induced anticoagulant state to be reversed, protamine must be combined with heparin on a molecule-for-molecule basis. Approximately 1 mg of protamine neutralizes 100 units of circulating heparin.

Allergy to heparin is not common. However, commercially available heparin is derived from animal tissues, and rash, pruritus, and anaphylaxis have been reported.

Thrombocytopenia occurs commonly, and may be mild or severe. Mild, transient thrombocytopenia (counts not less than $100,000/mm^3$) occurs in a minority of patients as a result of heparin-induced platelet clumping. This mild, dose-related decrease in platelet count may prolong bleeding time but does not result in serious complications. However, severe autoimmune thrombocytopenia may occur uncommonly as a result of heparin-related antiplatelet antibodies. This may happen quickly or may be delayed for up to 16 days and can result in a hypercoagulable state manifested by recurrent thromboembolic episodes, mostly in the arterial bed. The thromboembolic state is thought to be due to irreversible platelet clumping, and has not been reported in other drug-induced thrombocytopenias. It seems to occur more often with bovine than with porcine heparin and is not dose-related. Currently, the incidence of autoimmune thrombocytopenia is less than 6%, and the incidence of associated arterial thrombosis is well below 1%.

Heparin has intrinsic proteolytic activity and may cause **osteoporosis** with prolonged use. Osteoporosis has been reported at doses of 15,000 units per day after 3 to 6 months of use. This process may be accelerated in elderly patients with underlying osteoporosis. For this reason, heparin should be discontinued as soon as possible and replaced with warfarin when long-term anticoagulation is intended.

Important Drug Interactions

Aspirin and other platelet inhibitors prolong the bleeding time and should not be used with heparin.

Drugs that increase the risk of falls increase the risk of traumatic bleeding complications in ambulatory patients taking heparin and other forms of anticoagulation.

Contraindications and Precautions

Heparin is contraindicated in bleeding disorders, in the presence of bleeding or bleedable lesions, if there has been recent head trauma, and in the setting of uncontrolled hypertension. It is also contraindicated in patients with a history of heparin-related autoimmune thrombocytopenia.

Along with routine therapeutic monitoring of anticoagulant effect, platelet count should be measured every other day for 16 days.

Although there is some disagreement as to whether abrupt discontinuation of heparin produces a clinically important hypercoagulable state, some experts recommend that heparin be tapered rather than discontinued abruptly.

Other considerations are discussed in connection with warfarin (see above).

Indications

Heparin is indicated for the management of acute deep vein thrombosis, pulmonary embolus, and systemic arterial embolization.

Heparin may be used as prophylaxis against deep vein thrombosis and its complications as an alternative to warfarin in situations such as the postoperative state, acute myocardial infarction, and other high risk situations. Miniheparin may be used to prevent thromboembolism in the setting of acute hip fracture, although its efficacy is controversial.

Dosing

After a loading dose, maintenance dose of heparin is determined according to the activated partial thromboplastin time. The aPTT remains a reliable test in late life, although maintenance of recommended range for aPTT is not a guarantee against bleeding when overt or occult bleedable lesions exist. The aPTT should be maintained at 1.5 to 2.0 times the control value in acute thromboembolic disease.

There is a significant variation in the concentration of heparin on a unit per milligram basis. Bovine heparin contains 120 units and porcine 140 units per milligram, and there is individual variation among lots. Therefore, heparin is prescribed by unit.

INTRAVENOUS ROUTE. There is general, though not absolute, agreement that continuous heparin administration results in fewer bleeding episodes than does intermittent (bolus) administration, if the rate of administration can be closely monitored by infusion pump. Intravenous heparin is generally given initially in acute thromboembolic disease.

Loading dose: 5000–10,000 units.

Maintenance dose: 1000 units/hour as a continuous infusion; the dose should be adjusted by following the aPTT approximately every 6 hours for the first day or until the patient stabilizes.

SUBCUTANEOUS ROUTE. The subcutaneous route is most commonly used when miniheparin is given as prophylaxis for deep vein thrombosis in high-risk patients. The usual dose in this setting is 5000 units every 8 to 12 hours. However, when possible, the dose should be adjusted to maintain the aPTT in the high normal range.

The subcutaneous route may be also be used if intravenous access is impractical, but the onset and duration of action may be prolonged because heparin stays in the tissues longer. Full anticoagulant effect can be attained by this route.

Heparin should not be given intramuscularly because of the likelihood that local hematomas will develop.

ANTIPLATELET AGENTS

Aspirin

Pharmacologic Considerations

MECHANISM OF ACTION. Aspirin (acetylsalicylic acid) acts by acetylating and deactivating cyclooxygenase, the enzyme responsible for the conversion of arachidonic acid to thromboxane A_2 (TXA_2) in platelets, and to prostacyclin in the endothelium of the arterial intima. TXA_2 promotes platelet aggregation and local vasoconstriction, while prostacyclin inhibits platelet aggregation and promotes vasodilation. The acetylation of cyclooxygenase is a permanent effect in platelets but a temporary one in the vessel wall, so that the net effect of aspirin is to inhibit platelet aggregation, and it does so for the lifetime of the platelet. Since it takes approximately 5 to 7 days for 50% of circulating platelets to be replaced, the effect of an anti-aggregating dose of aspirin may last up to 1 week.

It is not known whether there is an age-associated alteration in the response to aspirin. There is no change in platelet count with age, and there is no strong evidence of an across-the-board change in platelet function. In vitro, there may be an enhanced tendency to platelet aggregation in elderly subjects, but the physiologic and clinical significance of this observation is not known.

PHARMACOKINETICS. Aspirin is rapidly absorbed from the stomach and upper small intestine, and reaches a peak plasma concentration in 15 to 20 minutes. Aspirin requires an acid environment for absorption. The rate and extent of absorption does not appear to be affected by age, despite the fact that gastric pH is often elevated in late life as a result of mucosal atrophy. Aspirin is bound to serum proteins, the extent increasing in a dose-dependent fashion.

Aspirin is rapidly hydrolyzed to salicylate. Part of this process takes place in the gut wall so that much of the intact drug never appears in the circulation, and it circulates in plasma primarily as salicylate. Salicylate is excreted in the kidney; the proportion of renally excreted salicylate increases with increasing doses of the drug. Aspirin and salicylate are metabolized in the liver by processes that probably do not diminish significantly with age. Regardless of dose, salicylate levels are higher in older as compared to younger adults, probably because of diminished renal excretion. Low-dose aspirin given for platelet inhibition probably is not associated with significant age-associated increases in plasma levels because at low doses renal clearance contributes to the total elimination only to a small extent.

Adverse Effects

Adverse effects of aspirin are discussed fully in Chap. 2 in conjunction with anti-inflammatory and analgesic use. At low doses now generally accepted as appropriate for antithrombotic use (325 mg daily or less), aspirin is far less likely to produce gastrointestinal problems than higher doses. Gastrointestinal symptoms can be minimized if aspirin is given in an enteric-coated preparation (Ecotrin, others). However, preexisting **gastrointestinal lesions**, whether overt or occult, may become clinically apparent at small doses, and gastrointestinal bleeding may occur. Likewise, by disrupting an important hemostatic mechanism, low doses of aspirin may increase the risk of **other bleeding complications**, such as hemorrhagic stroke. Geriatric patients may be at increased risk of subdural hematoma, epistaxis, and senile purpura.

Salicylates have a twofold effect on renal handling of urate, increasing excretion at very high doses and decreasing it at low doses. Thus, ordinary doses of aspirin may **increase serum uric acid levels.** However, gouty attacks have not been reported in large studies of low-dose aspirin.

Allergic phenomena, some severe, may occur in sensitive individuals (see Chap. 2).

It is not known if renal damage occurs with low doses of aspirin. Recent reports of an increased incidence in renal carcinoma require further study.

Important Drug Interactions

Drug interactions are discussed in Chap. 2. Although most of these interactions are significant only at analgesic and anti-inflammatory doses of aspirin, even low doses can produce bleeding when given with anticoagulants.

Contraindications

Aspirin is contraindicated in patients with bleeding disorders, bleeding lesions, and in active peptic ulcer. Aspirin should not be taken by patients who are receiving anticoagulants.

Antithrombotic Use of Aspirin

Aspirin is widely used for the prevention of thromboembolic disease. It is currently prescribed for the prevention of recurrent transient ischemic attack and stroke, restenosis of coronary artery lesions dilated by balloon angioplasty, sudden death in unstable angina, and death or reinfarction following myocardial infarction. Aspirin is one of several antithrombotic modalities used in the setting of hip fracture, but its efficacy is uncertain. It is widely used for the primary prevention of myocardial infarction but such use in the elderly is discouraged unless the patient has an additional indication, such as a history of classic TIA. Important controversies that pertain to the geriatric patient are discussed earlier in this chapter.

Dosing

The ideal antithrombotic dose of aspirin has not been determined. The lowest possible dose is desirable because gastrotoxicity is clearly dose-related. Platelet inhibition occurs with daily doses of 80 mg or less, although at doses below 325 mg/day full antiplatelet effect may not be achieved in the first 48–72 hours. The doses evaluated in clinical studies have decreased over the years. Currently, doses as low as 160 mg/day have been found effective in some settings. It is expected that the same dose will have the same effect in different diseases but this has not been proved.

Low-dose aspirin affects platelets for several days. Thus, alternate-day therapy is probably as effective as daily use.

There is some evidence that women respond less well to the antithrombotic effects of aspirin than men. It is not known if sex differences are due to qualitatively or quantitatively differing platelet responsiveness or to differing risk profiles in thromboembolic disease in general. Despite doubts as to the antithrombotic efficacy of aspirin in women, the risks of low-dose aspirin are probably not significantly greater than in men.

Usual antithrombotic dose: 80–325 mg/day. The 325-mg dose may be given on alternate days.

Dipyridamole (Persantine)

Pharmacologic Considerations

MECHANISM OF ACTION. Dipyridamole inhibits phosphodiesterase, resulting in accumulation of cyclic AMP in platelets, enhanced production of prostacyclin, and inhibition of platelet aggregation. The drug also causes the direct release of prostacyclin from the vascular endothelium and increases the concentration of adenosine at the platelet-vascular interface. All three of these effects inhibit platelet aggregation and action in a mechanism that is different from aspirin, providing the rationale that combining aspirin and dipyridamole gives an enhanced effect. However, this has not been generally supported by clinical studies.

In states of accelerated platelet turnover, dipyridamole is known to prolong platelet survival, a theoretical, indirect measure of antithrombotic action. This is the rationale for using dipyridamole in patients with artificial heart valves and dacron grafts. Dipyridamole has vasodilating action but this is generally not clinically apparent at ordinary oral doses.

PHARMACOKINETICS. The absorption of dipyridamole is highly erratic, so that orally administered drug is often not absorbed adequately for an antiplatelet effect to be achieved. Once in the system, dipyridamole is highly bound to serum proteins. It is conjugated in the liver and excreted in bile. Enterohepatic circulation occurs. Terminal half-life of dipyridamole is approximately 10 hours.

Adverse Effects

Because it is a vasodilator, dipyridamole is associated with **headaches** in certain patients, but this usually does not require cessation of therapy. It may also cause **gastrointestinal discomfort**, but this effect is often transient, and may subside with decrease in dose. Unlike aspirin and other platelet inhibitors, dipyridamole does not appear to produce gastritis or gastrointestinal bleeding, and it does not produce hypersensitivity reactions in aspirin-sensitive patients.

Combining Dipyridamole with Other Antithrombotic Agents

There is some evidence that dipyridamole reduces the number of thromboembolic episodes in patients with artificial heart valves who embolize despite warfarin therapy. Although there is a danger of enhanced bleeding with the combination of warfarin and dipyridamole, this danger is much less than with the combination of warfarin and aspirin.

Despite theoretical considerations, there is no consistent evidence that a combined regimen of dipyridamole and aspirin is clinically more effective than aspirin alone in the management of cerebrovascular or cardiovascular disease. The use of dipyridamole alone in these situations is thought to be less effective than aspirin alone. Furthermore, it is more costly and less convenient than aspirin.

Indications

The chief indication for dipyridamole is as conjoint therapy with warfarin in patients with mechanical heart valve prostheses. In this setting, it should generally be reserved for those who develop thromboembolic phenomena despite full anticoagulation with warfarin.

Although there is little or no convincing evidence that dipyridamole enhances the antithrombotic efficacy of aspirin in any clinical setting, consideration should be given to offering this agent as an alternative to aspirin for patients with aspirin allergy, particularly if warfarin is not an option. In addition, patients who fail to respond to aspirin alone should be offered the addition of dipyridamole because toxicity is low and available evidence does not completely rule out an enhanced response by a subgroup of patients.

Dosing

Usual dose range: 75–100 mg/day in 2 to 4 divided doses.

BIBLIOGRAPHY

American College of Chest Physicians. Second ACCP conference on antithrombotic therapy. *Chest* 95 Supp:1S–292S, 1989.

Antiplatelet Trialists' Collaboration. Secondary prevention of vascular disease by prolonged antiplatelet treatment. *Brit. Med. J.* 296:320–331, 1988.

The Boston Area Anticoagulation Trial for Atrial Fibrillation Investigators. The effect of low-dose warfarin on the risk of stroke in patients with nonrheumatic atrial fibrillation. *N. Engl. J. Med.* 323:1505–1511, 1990.

Cairns, J. A., Collins, R., Fuster, V., et al. Coronary thrombolysis. *Chest* 95:73S–87S, 1989.

FitzGerald, G. A. Dipyridamole. *N. Engl. J. Med.* 316:1247, 1987.

Hirsch, J. Oral anticoagulant drugs. *N. Engl. J. Med.* 324:1865–1875, 1991.

Kuhn, T. A., Garnett, W. R., Wells, B. K., and Karnes, H. T. Recovery of warfarin from an enteral nutrient formula. *Am J. Hosp Pharm.* 46:1395–1399, 1989.

Meyer, J. S., Rogers, R. L., McClintic, K., et al. Randomized clinical trial of daily aspirin therapy in multi-infarct dementia. A pilot study. *J. Amer. Geriatr. Soc.* 37:549–555, 1989.

Mungall, D. R., Ludden, T. M., and Marshall, J. Population pharmacokinetics of racemic warfarin in adult patients. *J. Pharmacokin. Biopharm.* 13:213–227, 1985.

Petersen, P. Boysen, G., Godtfredsen, J., et al. Placebo-controlled, randomised trial of warfarin and aspirin for prevention of thrombembbolic complications in chronic atrial fibrillation. The Copenhagen AFASAK study. *Lancet* 1:175–179, 1989.

Powers, P., Gent, M., Jay, R. M., et al. A randomized trial of less intense postoperative warfarin or aspirin therapy in the prevention of venous thromboembolism after surgery for fractured hip. *Arch. Intern. Med.* 149:771–774, 1989.

Shepherd, A. M. M., Hewick, D. S., Moreland, T. A., and Stevenson, I. H. Age as a determinant of sensitivity to warfarin. *Brit. J. Clin. Pharm.* 4:315–320, 1977.

Sherman, D. G., Hart, R. G., and Easton, J. D. The secondary prevention of stroke in patients with atrial fibrillation. *Arch. Neurol.* 43:68–70, 1986.

Smith, T., Viverette, F., and Adelman B. The use of antithrombotic therapy in the elderly. *Clin. Geriatr. Med.* 1(4):887–897, 1985.

Starkey, I., and Warlow, C. The secondary prevention of stroke in patients with atrial fibrillation. *Arch. Neurol.* 43:66–68, 1986.

Steering Committee of the Physicians' Health Study Research Group. Final report on the aspirin component of the ongoing Physicians' Health Study. *N. Engl. J. Med.* 321:129–135, 1989.

Stroke Prevention in Atrial Fibrillation Study Group. Preliminary report of the Stroke Prevention in Atrial Fibrillation Study. *N. Engl. J. Med.* 322:863–868, 1990.

Wessler, S., and Gitel, S. N. Warfarin. From bedside to bench. *N. Engl. J. Med.* 311:645–652, 1984.

Wittry, M. D., Thornton, T. A., and Chaitman, B. R. Safe use of thrombolysis in the elderly. Geriatrics 44(11): 28–36, 1989.

Wolf, P. A., Kannel, W. B., McGee, D. L., et al. Duration of atrial fibrillation and imminence of stroke: the Framingham Study. *Stroke* 14:664–667, 1983.

Pentoxifylline for Peripheral Vascular Disease

Intermittent claudication occurs when blood flow to the lower extremities cannot keep up with metabolic demands. In the elderly, this condition is most often associated with diffuse arteriosclerotic narrowing in the peripheral arteries, rather than isolated plaques, making surgical bypass or correction with transluminal angioplasty difficult. Consequently, a pharmacologic agent that could ameliorate this condition would be ideal. Unfortunately, a satisfactory agent may not yet exist.

PHARMACOLOGIC CONSIDERATIONS

Mechanism of Action

Pentoxifylline (Trental) is a xanthine derivative, structurally related to caffeine and theophylline.

Like other methylxanthines, pentoxifylline inhibits the enzyme phosphodiesterase, which is responsible for the conversion of cyclic AMP to AMP. Increased concentration of cAMP results in activation of protein kinase, the enzyme necessary for the breakdown of ATP.

In peripheral vascular disease normal erythrocyte deformability is diminished, presumably as a result of impaired tissue oxygenation at the microcirculatory level. Rigid blood cells pass through the microcirculation with difficulty, further reducing tissue oxygenation. Pentoxifylline is thought to act specifically on the erythrocyte membrane where it increases the amount of ATP in the erythrocyte. This increases the phosphoproteins content of the membrane, enhancing its flexibility. The drug has little vasodilating capabilities at ordinary doses in humans. However, other pathophysiologic alterations that occur as the result of microcirculatory tissue hypoxia, including increased concentrations of fibrinogen, increased platelet adhesiveness, and increased blood viscosity, are also reduced by pentoxifylline. Since intermittent claudication occurs when blood flow to the lower extremities cannot keep up with metabolic demands, symptoms should theoretically be relieved by the drug. However, the efficacy of pentoxifylline is controversial.

Pharmacokinetics

Pentoxifylline is well absorbed, with peak concentrations occurring within 3 hours. It is metabolized by the liver at least partly by oxidative processes to renally excreted metabolites, and its clearance rate is somewhat prolonged with age and in renal insufficiency. Because there is little or no short-term toxicity, age-adjusted dosing is not ordinarily required.

Pentoxifylline does not bind to plasma proteins and does not appear to accumulate in tissues.

DOES PENTOXIFYLLINE WORK?

Large controlled trials suggest that pentoxifylline improves exercise tolerance or reduces pain in some patients. Controversy regarding the drug's efficacy may be related to the fact that it could be more effective in certain subgroups than in others. Although it is impossible to predict which patients will benefit, the drug appears to be more likely to work in patients with increased blood viscosity, isolated rather than diffuse disease, and in those whose vascular disease is not related to diabetes. Since elderly patients with arteriosclerotic claudication are more likely than not to have diffuse disease, they theoretically represent a subgroup less likely to respond to pentoxifylline. In a limited open study, a small group of patients in their 70s reported significant improvement (see Crowder et al.), but no placebo-controlled study has compared young and old.

The most important parameter of response is patient satisfaction. Even a 100% improvement in walking distance may not represent a satisfactory response in a patient who is now able to walk 2 blocks instead of 1. The patient will weigh such improvements against the need to purchase and ingest a medication 3 times a day for an indefinite period.

A recent British study demonstrated that pentoxifylline was better than placebo in promoting healing of venous stasis ulcers. The patients, who were not elderly, had adequate arterial circulation to the extremities. Thus, the reported benefit could have been related to an improvement in microcirculation or a relief of stagnant venous outflow at the level of skin capillaries.

Pentoxifylline is being evaluated for use in other arteriosclerotic syndromes, including transient ischemic attack (TIA) and stroke, but there is no evidence at this time establishing its efficacy.

ADVERSE EFFECTS

Gastrointestinal symptoms were reported frequently in the past with use of an older formulation but are must less frequent since the new timed-release formulation has become available. Nausea, dyspepsia, or vomiting may be dose-related, and can be minimized when the medication is given at mealtime. Dizziness, common with the capsule form, is likewise uncommon with the tablet.

Cardiac stimulation, central nervous system excitation, bronchodilation, and diuresis, which are known effects of other xanthine derivatives, are not thought to occur with ordinary doses of pentoxifylline in humans. There have been isolated reports of angina, drops in blood pressure, and arrhythmias, which could be attributed to coexistent arterial disease expected to occur in claudication patients. Cardiac vigilance is required in any claudication patient undergoing a full therapeutic program (see Nonpharmacologic Management, below).

Long-term safety of pentoxifylline is not known, but toxicity has not been reported from other countries, where the agent has been in use since the early 1970s.

IMPORTANT DRUG INTERACTIONS

Because pentoxifylline reduces platelet adhesiveness, it has the potential to enhance the pharmacodynamic effects of anticoagulants and platelet inhibitors. However, clinical interactions have not been reported.

Hypotension has been reported to occur with pentoxifylline; therefore, a potential interaction exists between this drug and antihypertensive agents.

Cimetidine inhibits the hepatic microsomal enzyme system and increases levels of pentoxifylline. Reduced dosage of pentoxifylline may be required.

THE PLACE OF PENTOXIFYLLINE IN THERAPY

While the efficacy of pentoxifylline remains controversial, it is well accepted that older vasodilators, such as cyclandelate, niacin, isoxsuprine, and papaverine, and newer agents such as nifedipine are ineffective in intermittent claudication that is due to arteriosclerotic disease. The use of antiplatelet agents to retard atherosclerotic progression is experimental.

Because of its apparent lack of short-term toxicity, a trial of pentoxifylline may be warranted in patients with arterial claudication that is not due to vasospastic disease if they do not respond to nonpharmacologic treatment or if they are not candidates for surgical management or angioplasty.

The use of pentoxifylline in the management of venous stasis ulcers requires further study. A trial might be warranted in patients not responding to established treatments.

DOSING

Usual dose: 400 mg tid with meals. Dosage should be reduced if adverse effects occur. If no improvement has occurred at the end of an 8-week trial, the drug may be discontinued. However, stabilization of symptoms may indicate improvement so that duration of the trial should be individualized.

NONPHARMACOLOGIC MANAGEMENT

Graded aerobic exercise is considered the most effective nonsurgical treatment of claudication because it increases the formation of collateral vessels and may improve or stabilize exercise capacity. Patients are instructed to walk through the leg pain, and may be given analgesics prior to exercise in order to maximize their ability to do this. However, peripheral vascular disease is generally associated with arteriosclerosis elsewhere and increments in exercise must be made slowly. If musculoskeletal limitations prevent the patient from accomplishing an adequate walking program, cycling or swimming is a reasonable and often excellent alternative.

Certain medications may worsen arterial claudication. Beta blockers reduce blood flow to the lower extremities by producing unopposed alpha stimulation and vasoconstriction, and should be avoided if possible by patients with claudication. A possible exception to this admonition is labetolol, a beta blocker with selective alpha$_1$ blocking properties.

Medications known to reduce blood flow to the extremities should be tapered and discontinued if possible, but may be reinstituted if symptoms do not improve. Abstention from smoking is essential, because it is likely to retard progression and reduce symptoms. Individuals prone to ischemic ulcers, particularly diabetics, must undertake meticulous foot care.

It is important to remember that symptoms identical to those produced by arterial disease may be caused by lumbar stenosis, a narrowing of the lower spinal canal, which is most often seen in late life. This "pseudoclaudication" may occur because of degenerative disc disease, osteoarthritis, or spondylolisthesis, and may be present in the absence of additional neurological symptoms. Lumbar stenosis can be at fault even if pedal pulses are absent, since a significant minority of older individuals have absent pedal pulses without symptomatic peripheral vascular disease. The pain produced by spinal stenosis is sometimes relieved by maneuvers such as squatting. A neurologic history and examination should be done, while confirmation rests with appropriate radiologic examination of the lumbar spine. Other causes of claudicationlike symptoms include peripheral neuropathy, radiculopathy, osteoarthritis of the lower extremities, and venous insufficiency. Multiple pathology may coexist.

BIBLIOGRAPHY

Blombery, P. A. Intermittent claudication: an update on management. *Drugs* 34:404–410, 1987.

Colgan, M. P., Dormandy, J. A., Jones, P. W., et al. Oxpentifylline and treatment of venous ulcers of the leg. *Brit. Med. J.* 300:972–975, 1990.

Crowder, J. E., Cohn, J. B., Savitsky, J. P., et al. Efficacy and safety of pentoxifylline in geriatric patients with intermittent claudication. *Angiology* 40:795–802, 1989.

Johnson, G. Pentoxifylline and claudication. *J. Vasc. Surg.* 8:649, 1988.

Lipid-Lowering Agents

DO THE ELDERLY BENEFIT FROM CHOLESTEROL LOWERING?

It has been well established that elevated serum cholesterol is a major risk factor for coronary artery disease (CAD). More recently, it has been found that reducing serum cholesterol through diet, exercise, and pharmacologic agents reduces the incidence of myocardial ischemic events and may even lead to regression of arteriosclerotic plaques. Most of the evidence for both of these phenomena comes from studies of middle-aged men. To what extent can these findings be extrapolated to the elderly, male and female?

Cross-sectional studies reveal that serum cholesterol and low-density lipoprotein cholesterol (LDLC) increase with age, peaking about age 70 and then decreasing slightly. The increase in total cholesterol is almost entirely due to increases in LDLC. Individuals with an inherited tendency to elevated levels of high-density lipoprotein cholesterol (HDLC) can be particularly long-lived, and, although these would comprise a small proportion of the total, that proportion probably increases in older age groups. Neither the reason for the increase nor the late decline in total cholesterol is well understood, but it has been suggested that the latter is partly a survival phenomenon, those with lower cholesterol levels surviving longer. It is perhaps for this reason that total serum cholesterol is a less reliable predictor of CAD in late life than in young and middle-aged adults. However, the importance of HDLC as a predictor increases with age. Some longitudinal studies indicate moderate decreases in cholesterol over time, but this could well be due to recent society-wide changes in dietary habits.

Young and middle-aged men have higher levels of total cholesterol and LDLC than women of their age, who are probably protected by premenopausal estrogens. In contrast, elderly women have higher levels than do men of their age. This may also be a survival phenomenon, in that only those men with lower cholesterol levels were able to survive into old age, while elderly women with higher levels have not had enough time to succumb to the ravages of prolonged hypercholesterolemia. The reasons for age-related increase in LDL in both sexes may be due to a decrease in hepatic LDL receptor number or activity, or reduced intestinal cholesterol absorption, which would result in impairment of negative feedback inhibition of cholesterol synthesis.

The duration of hypercholesterolemia, and, in particular, the duration of exposure of the arterial wall to elevated levels of LDLC, are important in determining atherosclerotic risk. On the average, a cholesterol level of 200 mg/dl is unlikely to produce a critical degree of coronary atherosclerotic narrowing by age 70, but a level of 250 mg/dl produces this before age 60 and a level under 200 mg/dl is thought to delay significant disease until age 80 or beyond for individuals who survive to that age. Although the rate at which atherosclerosis develops seems to depend on exogenous factors, and varies from culture to culture, the development of atherosclerosis per se is a worldwide phenomenon. Thus, age alone is a risk factor for atherosclerosis independent of cholesterol level. The specific pathobiology of this age factor is not known, but it is thought that intrinsic aging of endothelial cells, or an age-related factor stimulating intimal smooth muscle cell proliferation, serves as an initial step or cofactor in the initiation of the atherosclerotic process. The complex relationship between lipids, aging, and atherogenesis is simply not well understood.

The diminished association of hypercholesterolemia and CAD in late life implies that lipid lowering should be less beneficial for the elderly. For example, a cholesterol level of 270 in a man under 55 is associated with a fivefold risk of CAD, while the same level in an older man less than doubles his baseline risk. Although the number of coronary events in the geriatric population as a whole is greater, and the baseline risk of an older man higher than a middle-aged man, it is valid to ask what would be gained by lowering the cholesterol. Cholesterol lowering reduces cardiac morbidity and mortality, but no primary prevention study (and only one secondary prevention study) has yet demonstrated that lowering cholesterol decreases **total** mortality. No study has included sufficient elderly subjects to reach any conclusions about that age group, and women of all ages have been poorly studied.

The beneficial effects of cholesterol lowering may accrue within 1 to 2 years in younger men, so that the shorter life expectancy of older individuals is not necessarily a strong argument against lipid lowering in late life. However, the amount of calcium in atherosclerotic plaques increases with age and it is not known at what rate or to what extent plaque regression occurs later in life. Even if a few years of life could be gained after the age of 70, the relative importance of hypercholesterolemia may well be diminished compared to other factors. The possibility of enhanced drug toxicity in older patients should also be considered part of the equation.

In short, it is not known whether the benefits of cholesterol lowering, in terms of morbidity or mortality, can be extrapolated to the elderly population, and in particular to women. In fact, there is some evidence that overall longevity is greatest in older people who have cholesterol levels between 200 and 300 mg/dl.

The link between hypercholesterolemia and thrombotic stroke is less well studied, and is thought to be weaker than for coronary heart disease. However, risk factor studies have not carefully differentiated thrombotic from hemorrhagic or cardio-embolic stroke. In the geriatric population, the ratio of hemorrhagic to thrombotic stroke decreases. It is logical to assume that reduction in cholesterol reduces atherosclerosis throughout the body. Although lipid lowering would not reduce the risk of hypertensive hemorrhagic stroke (there is some evidence that low cholesterol levels actually increase that risk), and probably would not directly reduce the risk of cardio-embolic stroke, there is no reason to assume that it would not reduce the risk of atherosclerotic stroke. Currently, however, official recommendations regarding cholesterol lowering are directed at reducing the risk of coronary artery disease, the clinical end point that has been most carefully studied.

A CRITICAL LOOK AT CORONARY RISK FACTORS IN LATE LIFE

The National Cholesterol Education Program Expert Panel on Detection, Evaluation, and Treatment of High Blood Cholesterol in

Adults has emphasized the importance of lowering LDLC levels below 160 mg/dl, or, if additional risk factors are present, below 130. The panel acknowledges that these criteria could be modified for patients over the age of 60.

Risk factors magnifying hypercholesterolemia include male sex, family history of premature coronary heart disease, hypertension, obesity, diabetes, cigarette smoking, HDLC level below 35 mg/dl, and a history of cerebrovascular or occlusive peripheral vascular disease. To what extent are these risk factors important in late life?

With age, the male-to-female ratio of coronary events approaches unity. It is not known if this narrowing of the sex ratio is related solely to the changing lipid profile of the aging female. For example, many aged men are those who have escaped premature coronary artery disease and may be at a very low risk. In fact, indirect evidence suggests that the smaller caliber of the female artery increases the woman's risk of coronary events, implying that arteriosclerotic plaques would not need to be as advanced in the female as the male, thus increasing the importance of intervention.

Family history of premature CAD may also have reduced importance in late life, since many older men from such families have eluded their genetic background and may not be susceptible to the family predilection. One could argue, however, that an elderly female with such a family history might just be arriving at the critical period of risk at age 70. Thus, family history might be a more important risk factor for an aged woman than a man.

Hypertension increases the risk of coronary events. The majority of elderly hypertensives have isolated systolic hypertension. Although systolic blood pressure above 170 mm Hg is a definite risk factor for stroke, it is not as strongly correlated with CAD. Its importance in the pathogenesis or as a marker of CAD in the elderly is not known.

Obesity, defined as 30% overweight or more, is a risk factor for CAD. Ideal body weight is difficult to determine in old age, particularly in women, who may have lost considerable height since menopause. Height-weight tables are not adjusted for this phenomenon. Frank obesity in geriatric patients may well be an important risk factor for CAD, but precise determination of what weight constitutes this risk connot be determined in late life.

Official criteria for the diagnosis of diabetes mellitus are not age-adjusted. The incidence of impaired glucose tolerance—short of frank diabetes—increases with age. There is indirect and circumstantial evidence that this modest degree of glucose intolerance is associated with micro- and macrovascular complications. It could be argued that this "glucose intolerance of aging" is a risk factor for CAD that should be considered in weighing the need for intervention.

Finally, advanced age is not considered by the Expert Panel to be a separate risk factor for CAD. This is ironic, since age is probably the greatest risk factor of all. If it were, one could argue that ideal cholesterol level should be still lower for the elderly, since it may well be the duration for which the arterial wall is exposed to moderate levels of cholesterol as much as the absolute level of cholesterol itself.

Cigarette smoking, low HDLC level, and a history of cerebrovascular or peripheral vascular disease continue to be important CAD risk factors in late life.

HYPERTRIGLYCERIDEMIA

There is controversy as to whether hypertriglyceridemia in the absence of hypercholesterolemia is an independent risk factor for CAD. Triglycerides do not exist in atheromas, and have not been epidemiologically linked to atherogenesis, in the absence of other risk factors. Studies that do indicate a link fail to take into account the fact that measurements of triglyceride generally depend on measurements of very low-density lipoprotein (VLDL), which is rich in triglyceride but which also contains cholesterol. Severe elevations of triglyceride do, of course, increase the risk of pancreatitis. In making decisions to treat hyperlipidemia, one should have as a goal lowering LDL cholesterol, while preventing increase of triglyceride above 800 mg/dl, a level at which the risk of pancreatitis is high. An attempt should be made to identify and reverse secondary hypertriglyceridemia, which can be due to obesity, alcohol, beta blockers, diuretics, and estrogens, even the bile acid resin group of cholesterol-lowering agents (see below).

RECOMMENDATIONS

Geriatric hypercholesterolemia should be treated in patients who are highly motivated and functional, and in whom such intervention would not pose a burden that would deflect attention from medical problems of greater or more certain importance. Having selected the patients for intervention, recommendations of the Expert Panel may be extrapolated to patients over the age of 70. However, risk factors such as male sex, family history, obesity, and possibly hypertension should be given less weight and "glucose intolerance of aging" more weight in decisions to treat high levels of LDL. Goal cholesterol need not be modified in late life. However, the exact level to be attained should be strictly individualized, depending on the patient's function, motivation, and ability to participate in a cholesterol-lowering regimen. In particular, the presence of additional risk factors should not mandate that pharmacologic means be used to lower LDLC to 130 mg/dl if those risk factors are of questionable importance in advanced age.

Hypertriglyceridemia in the absence of hypercholesterolemia should not be treated pharmacologically unless the level poses a risk of pancreatitis.

If nonpharmacologic treatment fails to lower LDLC to goal levels, bile acid resins may be given. Use of these agents can be justified in an age group for whom the benefits of cholesterol lowering are not known, because they are rarely if ever associated with severe adverse effects. Other agents should be considered second line and should generally be reserved for highly motivated patients with symptomatic coronary artery disease.

NONPHARMACOLOGIC MANAGEMENT

Diet, exercise, cessation of smoking, and correction of hyperglycemia should be undertaken or attempted before resorting to pharmacologic treatment. Dietary modifications should be geared to weight loss if the patient is obese, and should include reduction in intake of cholesterol and saturated fat. Dietary information is available from the American Heart Association, the National Heart, Lung, and Blood Institute, and other professional organizations. Patients may do well by following sensible popular diets such as that recommended by Weight Watchers, with few if any modifications. Dietary goals may differ in the elderly. Severe dietary modification should be avoided if it places the patient at risk of nutritional deficiencies. Quality of life considerations must always be taken into account. Complaints that food or smoking is the "only remaining pleasure" should be taken seriously and addressed.

The importance of dietary fiber is controversial. Addition of soluble fiber such as psyllium (Metamucil) and oat bran produces additional but minor lowering of cholesterol. This effect has been attributed to reduction in dietary cholesterol absorption, enhanced bile acid excretion, or the mere fact that the patient concurrently reduces fat intake. Although a high-fiber diet should be encouraged, soluble-fiber supplements should be given along with realistic expectations. Some experts suggest mixing psyllium with bile acid resins as a means of normalizing bowel function when the latter are prescribed.

Fish consumption should be encouraged because it may well confer the advantages of omega-3 fatty acids without the disadvantages and unknowns involved in consumption of concentrated fish oils (see below).

Exercise may have to be seriously modified because of musculoskeletal limitations. Because of transportation problems, the elderly often do not have access to exercise centers, and because of fear of muggings, they may resist walking programs. With these limitations in mind, walking programs, swimming, or, for the nonswimmer, water exercises are ideal. Stationary bicycling is generally safe and well accepted.

Cholesterol-elevating drugs should be discontinued if possible. Drugs that may increase serum cholesterol include thiazide diuretics and nonselective beta blockers. Although estrogen can also raise serum cholesterol, this is due to an increase in the beneficial HDL subfraction and it should not be discontinued for this reason.

Modifiable coronary risk factors, such as hyperglycemia and smoking, should be corrected, since they are cofactors with hyperlipidemia in the development of CAD. Abnormal glucose tolerance without frank diabetes should not be treated pharmacologically because the consequences of hypoglycemia can be severe in the elderly.

FIRST-LINE AGENTS: THE BILE ACID SEQUESTRANTS, CHOLESTYRAMINE AND COLESTIPOL

Pharmacologic Considerations

Cholestyramine (Questran) and colestipol (Colestid) are anionic exchange resins that sequester bile acids in the intestine, interrupting their enterohepatic circulation. Bile acids are produced by the liver as oxidation products of cholesterol, and secreted by the liver during digestion in order to emulsify fats, enhancing their absorption. In the intestine, cholestyramine and colestipol bind and sequester bile acids, increasing their fecal excretion. Since less bile acid is returned by the portal vein to the liver, more cholesterol is converted to bile acid in the liver, reducing the cholesterol pool. In addition, since bile acid is required for the intestinal absorption of cholesterol, sequestrants ultimately increase fecal loss of cholesterol. As a result of these changes, there is a compensatory increase in hepatic LDL receptor number, plasma clearance of LDL is enhanced, and plasma levels of LDL decline. At the same time, hepatic production of 3-

hydroxy-3-methylglutaryl-coenzyme A (HMG-CoA) reductase, the rate-limiting enzyme for cholesterol synthesis, is increased. More cholesterol is ultimately synthesized by the liver in response to this, although there is a net decrease in blood levels. VLDL synthesis likewise increases. Since VLDL consists of 50%–60% triglyceride, this increase will be reflected in increased serum triglyceride levels. The rise in triglycerides may be transient, returning to baseline after about 4 weeks of treatment, or may not occur at all. However, patients with significant hypertriglyceridemia at baseline may experience substantial elevations in triglyceride levels. HDL levels generally do not change, but may increase.

Cholestyramine or Colestipol?

Although structurally different, cholestyramine and colestipol share the same mechanism of action. At the appropriate dosage, these agents lower cholesterol to the same degree. Choice of agent should depend on relative cost and patient preference. Cholestyramine has a sandy consistency, while colestipol is granular, odorless, and tasteless. Cholestyramine is also available in a "candy bar" form (Cholybar), while colestipol can be purchased as a premixed liquid. Since compliance is expected to be poorer with these agents than with tablet medications, considerations such as cost, individual palatability, and vehicle options should be discussed with the patient.

Since the structures of cholestyramine and colestipol differ, their relative abilities to bind to various substances may differ.

The dosages of cholestyramine and colestipol are not equivalent (see Dosing).

Adverse Effects

Bile acid resins are insoluble and are neither digested nor absorbed by the normal intestine. Thus, direct systemic effects do not occur. However, anion exchange may result in enhanced systemic reabsorption of chloride ion and hyperchloremic acidosis has been reported with cholestyramine, which is a chloride salt. This effect has not been reported in adults, but electrolytes should be periodically monitored.

There are hardly any reports of clinical nutrient deficiencies in the literature associated with bile acid resin treatment in adults, although this does not rule out the possibility of subclinical deficiency states. Bleeding diathesis due to vitamin K deficiency has been reported, but this effect is probably exceedingly rare in adults with normal digestion.

Earlier preparations of cholestyramine (Questran) contained tartrazine, which can produce allergic reactions. Tartrazine has been eliminated from the preparation.

Although bile acid resins do not invariably elevate serum triglyceride, **hypertriglyceridemia** may be exacerbated in some patients and may be severe in patients at risk. Patients with baseline triglyceride levels over 500 mg/dl who also require LDL lowering generally should be treated with agents other than bile acid sequestrants or should receive concurrent treatment with triglyceride-lowering agents, such as gemfibrozil.

The claim that the elderly cannot tolerate the constipating tendency of bile acid sequestrants has been overstated. These substances do alter the consistency of the feces and may cause **constipation, bloating,** and **nausea. Intestinal obstruction** has been reported. However, the gut seems to adjust well to the agents when initial doses are low and dose increases are made gradually. Some patients may respond well to initial small doses and increases may not even be necessary. At all times, bile acid resins must be given with adequate liquid. If constipation develops, a laxative may be given. One approach is to administer bulk-forming laxatives mixed with the sequestrant powder itself. If loose stools develop in conjunction with bile acid resins, it is conceivable that steatorrhea may have been precipitated by impaired absorption of fat-soluble vitamins, perhaps indicating a preexisting, subclinical small intestinal dysfunction.

Elevated alkaline phosphatase levels have been reported, but frank hepatic disease has not. The significance of these isolated reports is not known.

Drug and Nutrient Interactions

Anionic resins are capable of binding with a variety of substances in the intestine and cholestyramine or colestipol have been reported to reduce the absorption of a number of cationic agents, and may decrease enterohepatic circulation of others. This phenomenon has been harnessed in the treatment of digitoxin intoxication and pseudomembranous colitis.

Potential drug-drug interactions are listed in Table 17–1. Most drugs compete quite well with these agents for intestinal absorption. However, it is best to advise that cholestyramine and colestipol be taken at least 1 hour before or 4 hours after other drugs are ingested.

Table 17–1. Some Agents Whose Levels May Be Reduced by Bile Acid Resins

Digitalis preparations
Thiazide diuretics
Warfarin
Propranolol
L-thyroxine
Tetracycline
Cephalexin
Penicillin
Naproxen
Acetaminophen
Vitamins A,D,E,K, folate
Vitamin B_{12} intrinsic factor complex
Methotrexate
Phenylbutazone
Piroxicam
Ursodiol
Corticosteroids?
Phenobarbital?

Fat-soluble vitamins may be sequestered by bile acid resins and deficiency of vitamins A, D, E, and K may occur. Folic acid and B_{12} intrinsic factor complex may also be bound. Clinical deficiency manifesting as osteomalacia, steatorrhea, or hemorrhagic diathesis may be more theoretical than real in adults with normal intestinal function. Alterations in the metabolism of cations such as calcium, magnesium, iron, and zinc may occur,but this has not been well studied and frank deficiency has not been reported.

Contraindications

Bile acid resins are contraindicated in patients with known hypersensitivity to the agents or their constituents, in biliary obstruction, and in bowel obstruction. They should be used cautiously in patients with constipation. Immobilized patients should generally not receive these agents because of the high risk of fecal impaction in this setting. Patients with fasting triglyceride levels over 500 mg/dl should generally not receive bile acid resins as initial therapy unless triglyceride-lowering agents are given concurrently.

Precautions

If bile acid resins are taken in conjunction with a drug whose absorption is reduced by these agents, discontinuation of the resins should prompt careful reevaluation of the other agent, particularly if it is a drug with a narrow therapeutic-to-toxic ratio, such as warfarin or digoxin.

Bile acid resins should not be ingested in their dry powder form, which can be inadvertently inhaled or can produce intestinal obstruction.

Patients on long-term treatment with bile acid resins should receive a daily multivitamin. This recommendation is based on theoretical considerations and not on widespread clinical observations that these agents produce vitamin deficiency.

Indications

Bile acid sequestrants are indicated as adjunctive treatment of elevated levels of LDL cholesterol, unless significant hypertriglyceridemia is present. These agents are unlikely to be effective in the rare cases of homozygous familial hypercholesterolemia. However, such patients represent fewer than 2% of hypercholesterolemic subjects, and would be expected to represent a still smaller proportion of affected elderly.

Because they are far safer than other lipid-lowering agents, and because the risk-benefit ratio of pharmacologic treatment of hypercholesterolemia in the elderly is not known, bile acid resins are the agents of choice for that age group. A 2-month trial of these agents should be completed before any other agent is even considered.

Other Uses

Bile acid sequestrants may relieve pruritus due to cholestasis. Cholestasis results in elevated plasma bile acids, which produce pruritus when they enter the skin. Bile acid sequestrants may also be effective in pruritus due to renal failure. Although the specific agent producing pruritus in this condition is not known, it has been suggested that cholestyramine sequesters "middle molecules" not excreted by hemodialysis.

Cholestyramine has been used as adjunctive treatment of enterocolitis due to *Clostridium difficile* because the bile acid resin is believed to bind the toxin produced by the organism. Further study of its efficacy in this condition is required.

Dosing and Preparation

Cholestyramine

Initial dose: 4 g (9 g powder) in 6 oz of vehicle just before or during the meal, once daily. The dose should not be increased until a 1-month trial has been completed and further lipid lowering is indicated.
Monthly dose increment: 4 g/day.
Usual dose range: 4 g bid-qid.

Cholestyramine is also available in a candy-bar form (Cholybar), which can be chewed but should also be taken with sufficient liquid.

Colestipol

Initial dose: 5 g granules mixed in 6 oz liquid shortly before the meal, once daily. Guidelines for incremental doses are as for cholestyramine.
Usual dose range: 5 g bid-qid.

SUGGESTED VEHICLES FOR POWDERED BILE ACID RESINS. Fruit juice, apple sauce or other fruit puree, flavored low-fat yogurt, thin soups, water.

ALTERNATIVE AND ADJUNCTIVE AGENTS

Lovastatin (formerly mevinolin; Mevacor)

Pharmacologic Considerations

MECHANISM OF ACTION. Lovastatin is structurally similar to and acts as a competitive inhibitor of 3-hydroxy-3-methylglutaryl-coenzyme A (HMG-CoA) reductase, the rate-limiting enzyme in the synthesis of cholesterol. Although overall cholesterol synthesis is not significantly altered, reduction in cholesterol synthesis results in compensatory increase in the activity of hepatic LDL receptors and enhanced removal of LDL from plasma. LDL levels are also lowered as a result of increased clearance of VLDL and VLDL remnants, which are precursors of LDL. Direct reduction in LDL synthesis does not appear to be as important a process in the lowering of plasma levels. HDL levels remain unchanged or increase, for reasons that are not well understood.

There is a diurnal variation in the action of HMG-CoA, with enhanced activity and increased rate of cholesterol synthesis occurring at night. Thus, it is thought that evening dosing of lovastatin produces maximal cholesterol lowering.

Monotherapy with lovastatin may lower LDL levels by as much as 40%, and, as with other cholesterol-lowering agents, it is assumed that cardiac benefits will accrue as well. However, lovastatin itself has not been studied long enough to establish its efficacy in reducing coronary heart disease or to confirm its long-term safety.

PHARMACOKINETICS. Lovastatin is incompletely absorbed from the gastrointestinal tract and undergoes extensive hepatic extraction, with less than 10% being excreted in the urine and less than 5%

entering the systemic circulation. It is a pro-drug and is converted to its active form in the liver, along with an active metabolite with a half-life of 1 to 2 hours. Levels of lovastatin peak in the plasma in 2–4 hours. Lovastatin is highly bound to serum proteins.

Little pharmacokinetic data are available on this agent, and it has apparently not been well studied in the elderly. Serum half-life would be expected to be somewhat prolonged in the elderly, owing to its extensive hepatic extraction. Although the action of the drug is primarily in the liver, as yet unknown systemic effects could theoretically be enhanced by higher blood levels of the unmetabolized drug.

Adverse Effects and Concerns

Lovastatin is generally well tolerated. A small number of patients have reported side effects such as **headache, rash, pruritus,** and **gastrointestinal symptoms** such as nausea, diarrhea, constipation, and dyspepsia. **Reversible elevations in liver function tests** may occur, but serious toxicity has not yet been reported. More troubling are reports of **myalgia** and frank **myositis** with elevations in creatine kinase. Although disastrous consequences may not occur as the result of monotherapy with lovastatin, rhabdomyolysis with renal failure has been reported when the drug was given in conjunction with other agents known to reduce its metabolism, and in the presence of hepatic failure.

Because of limited experience with this agent, long-term toxicity is not yet known. Theoretical concerns about progressive hepatic disease should be heeded. In the 1960s, lipid-lowering agents that interfered with cholesterol synthesis were found to produce cataracts, and this has raised concerns about lovastatin. Lovastatin in high doses has been found to produce cataracts in animals. The cataractogenic agents of the 1960s interfered with cholesterol biosynthesis at a later step in the synthetic process, leading to the buildup of toxic intermediates, but lovastatin does not lead to the production of these substances. Fears that lovastatin itself, either through a direct toxic effect or as a result of impaired cholesterol synthesis, could lead to cataract formation have not been borne out to date.

The consequences of long-term suppression of cholesterol biosynthesis on cell membranes or steroid hormones are not known. Nor is there any information on the consequences of inhibiting HMG-CoA reductase, which is involved in other important functions pertaining to electron transport and glycoprotein synthesis.

Important Drug Interactions

Gemfibrizol and cyclosporine may enhance potential toxicity of lovastatin by interfering with metabolic clearance mechanisms. Lovastatin has no apparent effect on hepatic microsomal enzymes and no drug-drug interactions have been reported on that basis. However, because of reports of myositis, and because of the limited experience with this agent in the U.S. population, caution should be observed when combining lovastatin with other drugs, particularly those that can affect hepatic function. Other lipid-lowering agents, such as nicotinic acid and gemfibrizol, are to be used with caution. Likewise, lovastatin and chronic alcohol ingestion are considered a bad combination because of the potential of additive hepatotoxicity.

Contraindications

Lovastatin is contraindicated in the presence of hepatic disease or myositis.

Precautions

Because long-term ocular safety of lovastatin has not been firmly established, the manufacturer currently recommends baseline and annual ophthalmologic evaluation to observe for the development or progression of lens opacities. Results of these examinations, however, should be interpreted in the light of the fact that older patients not taking lovastatin are at high risk of developing cataracts.

Liver function tests and creatine kinase should be periodically monitored, and patients should be observed for the possible development of clinical myositis.

The Place of Lovastatin in Therapy

Becaue there is insufficient direct experience with this drug in elderly patients, lovastatin is not generally recommended for the management of hyperlipidemia in that age group. It should be used only in patients with symptomatic coronary artery disease who fail to tolerate or respond to an appropriate trial of bile acid sequestrants. As an alternative to gemfibrizol, lovastatin may also be used as an adjunct to bile acid sequestrants if the latter produce unacceptable hypertriglyceridemia.

Because the action of lovastatin depends on the presence of adequate LDL receptors, it is not as effective in homozygous familial hypercholesterolemia, which is characterized by absent LDL receptors. However, these patients are particularly rare in the geriatric population.

Dosing

Initial dose: 20 mg given in the evening.
Monthly dose increment: 10 mg/day.
Maximum dose: 40 mg bid. Daily dosages higher than 60 mg should be divided.

Gemfibrizol (Lopid)

Pharmacologic Considerations

MECHANISM OF ACTION. Gemfibrizol is a fibric acid derivative, structurally related to clofibrate. It enhances the activity of lipoprotein lipase, decreasing the production of triglyceride and VLDL, and enhancing the removal of VLDL from plasma. Total cholesterol and LDL levels are moderately reduced with therapy, while HDL levels are increased, the latter by an unknown mechanism. Reductions in LDL levels are probably related to reduction in VLDL levels. The major lipid alteration that occurs is a sizable decrease in levels of plasma triglyceride.

In the Helsinki Heart Study of asymptomatic 40- to 55-year-old hyperlipidemic men (see Manninen et al.), gemfibrizol was shown to reduce the risk of coronary heart disease independently of its triglyceride-lowering effect and in conjunction with only modest decreases in LDL. The cardioprotective effect was noted after only 2 years but was not accompanied by a reduction in total mortality. The exact reason for the beneficial cardiac effect is not known, but subtle changes in coagulation parameters and fibrinolysis may occur. The clinical effects of gemfibrizol have not been well studied in the elderly, in women, or in multi-ethnic Americans.

PHARMACOKINETICS. Gemfibrizol is well absorbed, peak plasma levels occurring within 1–2 hours. It is extensively protein-bound and undergoes enterohepatic circulation, but is ultimately conjugated and excreted in the urine. Limited pharmacokinetic information indicates that its average 8–hour serum half-life remains unchanged in the elderly.

Adverse Effects

Mild gastrointestinal symptoms may occur. Like its cousin clofibrate, gemfibrizol increases bile lithogenicity and may increase the formation of **gallstones**. This effect may be less severe than with clofibrate, however, and further study is required to determine the overall significance of this effect.

Mild **anemia** and **leukopenia** have occurred, and are thought to be due to bone marrow suppression. **Rash, eosinophilia, myalgia, elevations in liver enzymes**, and **blurred vision** have been reported.

Gemfibrizol has produced tumors in animals, but the drug has not been in use long enough to determine whether it is carcinogenic in humans, a problem that was of concern with clofibrate (see below).

Important Drug Interactions

Like clofibrate, gemfibrizol displaces warfarin from protein-binding sites and has been shown to increase the anticoagulant effect. A potential interaction with oral hypoglycemic agents requires further exploration.

The combination of gemfibrizol and another lipid-lowering agent, lovastatin (see above), has been reported to cause severe myositis, by an effect that may be related to reduced lovastatin metabolism.

Contraindications and Precautions

Because of its ability to increase bile lithogenicity, gemfibrizol should not be given to patients with known gallbladder disease. This is a particularly important consideration in the elderly population where silent gallstones occur with great frequency.

Liver function tests and blood count should be periodically monitored.

The Place of Gemfibrizol in Therapy

The efficacy and toxicity of gemfibrizol have not been well studied in elderly patients. It is not known, for example, whether the production of gallbladder disease would outweigh cardiac benefits. The drug should therefore be reserved for patients with symptomatic coronary artery disease when elevated LDLC is complicated by severe hypertriglyceridemia, a condition in which it is best to avoid bile acid sequestrants. However, gemfibrizol is also suitable for use alone or in combination with bile acid sequestrants when elevated LDLC is accompanied by low HDLC.

Gemfibrizol is indicated for the prevention of pancreatitis in the presence of marked (over 800 mg/dl) hypertriglyceridemia. It is not, however, effective in familial chylomicronemia associated with lipoprotein lipase deficiency.

Dosing

Initial dose: 300 mg bid.
Monthly dose increment: 300 mg/day.
Maximum dose: 600 mg bid.

Nicotinic Acid (Niacin)

Pharmacologic Considerations

Nicotinic acid (niacin) is a water-soluble vitamin belonging to the *B complex*. It is present in meats, liver, grains, and legumes. Tryptophan is a precursor of nicotinic acid, and dietary sources of tryptophan may be a partial, though incomplete, source of the vitamin. Niacin deficiency results in pellagra.

Nicotinic acid is rapidly and completely absorbed, and is converted in the liver to nicotinamide (niacinamide). This amide form is the source of nicotinamide adenosine dinucleotide (NAD) and its phosphate (NADP), the important coenzymes in intermediary metabolism. When high doses are given, the amidation capacity of the liver is exceeded and sufficient free nicotinic acid circulates, only small concentrations being required for pharmacologic effects to occur.

Although only 15 mg/day need be ingested to prevent overt deficiency, the pharmacologic actions of nicotinic acid are produced only at high doses. In addition to lipid lowering, pharmacologic actions include fibrinolysis and vasodilation.

Nicotinic acid exerts its lipid-lowering effect by inhibiting hepatic production of VLDL, which is the parent compound and primary source of LDL. Decreased production of VLDL is thought to occur because nicotinic acid inhibits lipolysis, resulting in decreased delivery of free fatty acids to the liver for triglyceride production. HDL levels generally increase but triglyceride levels do not.

Free nicotinic acid is excreted by the kidney. The pharmacokinetics have not been studied in the elderly.

The serum half-life of nicotinic acid is only about 1 hour, so that traditional dosage recommendations have called for frequent administration to maintain adequate plasma levels of the active nicotinic acid. However, there is evidence that aggressive, frequent dosing may not be needed for long-term clinical benefit to occur.

Vitamin preparations contain nicotinamide, which is pharmacologically distinct from nicotinic acid, has no lipid-lowering effect, and no adverse systemic effects at ordinary doses.

Adverse Effects

Nicotinic acid increases the production of prostacyclin, producing **cutaneous flushing** of the face, neck, and trunk, generally within 15 minutes of ingestion. Since prostacyclin production may fall to pretreatment levels over time, the flush can be minimized by starting with a low dose of nicotinic acid. Daily use of aspirin or other prostaglandin inhibitors reduces and may eliminate this adverse effect.

Hepatic dysfunction may occur when high doses (more than 3 g/day) are ingested, but is rare at low doses. Fulminant hepatic failure has been reported. Abnormalities in liver enzymes are common and appear to be dose-related. Mild, stable elevations in liver function tests are practically universal when lipid-lowering doses are given; it has been suggested that this is a required concomitant of therapy. However, significant transaminase elevations necessitate discontinuation of treatment. Nicotinic acid may produce **gastrointestinal symptoms** such as nausea, diarrhea, and abdominal discomfort, and may activate **peptic ulcer. Hyperuricemia** may also occur. Less commonly, nicotinic acid results in **impaired glucose tolerance.** Reversible cystoid **maculopathy** occurs in a very small number of cases and is thought to be due to a disruption in the metabolism of retinal neuronal tissue with accumulation of intracellular fluid. Other reported side effects include **hyperpigmentation** and **acanthosis nigricans.**

There is indirect evidence that nicotinic acid has **arrhythmogenic potential,** but this has not been proved nor is it well understood.

Important Drug Interactions

Concurrent use of alpha adrenergic blocking agents may exacerbate flushing or produce hypotension. Nicotinic acid may reverse the effects of uricosuric agents.

Contraindications

Pharmacologic doses of nicotinic acid should not be given in the presence of liver disease, cardiac arrhythmia, gout, peptic ulcer, or inflammatory bowel disease.

Precautions

If nicotinic acid is to be given to elderly patients, liver function, uric acid level, blood glucose, and cardiac rhythm should be monitored during treatment. The recommendation to scrutinize cardiac rhythm is based on indirect evidence that nicotinic acid is arrhythmogenic; however, a strong association between this agent and arrhythmias has been established.

The Place of Nicotinic Acid in Therapy

Nicotinic acid is often used to lower LDLC if bile acid sequestrants are ineffective or not tolerated, and is used in conjunction with those agents to enhance their cholesterol-lowering effect. It is preferred to bile acid sequestrants in patients with significant hypertriglyceridemia and is also more effective in increasing HDL cholesterol. Compliance with nicotinic acid may be poor because of side effects, but there is some evidence that lower than traditionally recommended doses may be effective.

The arrhythmogenic potential of nicotinic acid is not well understood, but is a clinical observation that must be respected. The long-term Coronary Drug Project (see Canner et al.) demonstrated that nicotinic acid reduces nonfatal myocardial infarction in nonelderly men without reducing total mortality. Subsequent follow-up of survivors from the original study demonstrated a decrease in total mortality but with a long lag time of 6 years after the drug had been discontinued. During the study, patients treated with nicotinic acid had a higher incidence of cardiac arrhythmias than those on placebo, which could theoretically account for the incomplete benefit to patients while they were taking the drug. These results suggest the troubling possibility that the drug might only be useful to those who survive it. Since an overall beneficial effect was not demonstrated for 15 years, it is difficult to know what the risk-benefit ratio to aged men might be. However, any fears as to the safety of nicotinic acid must be set against the fact that even less is known about the long-term effects of newer drugs, such as lovastatin and gemfibrizol.

Nicotinic acid is a useful adjunct to treatment in patients whose hypercholesterolemia is accompanied by low levels of HDL or high levels of triglyceride, and is probably superior to bile acid resins in this regard. However, it should be prescribed to elderly patients only when pharmacologic treatment is urgently desired.

Preparations

Generic preparations may vary in their bioavailability and efficacy. If inadequate lipid-lowering occurs with one brand, a dose increase or trial of another brand may prove effective. Sustained-release tablets have been associated with enhanced hepatotoxicity and other adverse effects, but this may be related to the fact that patients comply better with the regimen and are exposed to higher total doses of the drug.

Dosing

Initial dose: 50–100 mg tid with meals. This low dose may be sufficient for some people.
Monthly dose increment: No more than 500 mg/day.
Maximum dose: 500 mg tid.
Note: Although doses as high as 6–8 g/day have been used, these doses cannot be justified in the elderly.

OTHER AVAILABLE AGENTS

Clofibrate (Atromid)

Clofibrate, closely related in structure to gemfibrizol, has been in use longer, but is uncommonly used today because of fears regarding toxicity inferred from long-term clinical trials, and because of questions as to its clinical efficacy. In one trial, clofibrate use produced increased overall mortality and this was attributed to gallbladder disease and gastrointestinal malignancies. Although there is controversy regarding these toxicities, agents are available that are equally or more effective. Gemfibrizol is more effective than clofibrate in lowering triglycerides, and has not yet been associated with significant increases in malignancies. Clofibrate also causes a myopathy associated with elevations in muscle enzymes. Another disadvantage of clofibrate is that it participates in a number of pharmacokinetic drug interactions, a problem that may well be shared by gemfibrizol. Clofibrate is not presently recommended for the geriatric patient.

Probucol (Lorelco)

Probucol is a sulfur-containing phenolic compound that is structurally dissimilar to other cholesterol-lowering agents. It increases the catabolism of LDL and increases biliary excretion of cholesterol, thereby lowering plasma levels of LDL. Probucol also reduces the synthesis of apolipoprotein A_1, and reduces lipoprotein lipase, resulting in significant lowering of HDL cholesterol. HDL cholesterol is often lowered out of proportion to the lowering of LDL levels, a fact that is of theoretical concern since HDL is thought to prevent arteriosclerosis by transporting cholesterol away from the arterial wall to extra-arterial tissue depots. Xanthomas have been noted to disappear with probucol treatment, an apparent paradox if one accepts the traditional hyperlipidemic model of atherogenesis. However, probucol has properties that prevent oxidative transformation of LDL to an atherogenic substance and may promote HDL transport to the liver, enhancing the "reverse cholesterol transport" system that removes lipids from the vessel wall to safe tissue depots. According to this model, probucol could theoretically prevent and perhaps reverse arterial disease by mechanisms other than altering serum lipid levels.

The drug has not been adequately studied in controlled trials to determine its effect on clinical heart disease. It has no significant effect on levels of triglyceride.

Probucol is poorly absorbed and excreted primarily in the feces. However, its hydrophobic properties cause it to be stored in fat to such an extent that it persists in the body for many months after treatment is stopped. Although probucol has not been well studied in geriatric patients, its volume of distribution would be expected to be higher in the elderly, with levels persisting even longer.

Probucol may prolong the QT interval and has produced ventricular tachycardia in animals. It has also been associated with eosinophilia, angioneurotic edema, and paresthesias. Long-term toxicity is not known.

The theoretic possibility that probucol could produce regression of atherosclerosis would make it potentially useful in the elderly. However, the drug cannot yet be recommended in geriatric patients because of its arrhythmogenic potential, its protracted tissue deposition, and its as yet unproven clinical efficacy.

Fish Oils

Omega-3 polyunsaturated fatty acids, including eicosapentaenoic acid (EPA) and docosahexaenoic acid (DHA), have been shown to cause lipid alterations and impair platelet function to the degree that they have been promoted for use in the prevention and treatment of atherosclerotic disease. Interest in fish oils has recently increased because of epidemiologic evidence and observations regarding atherosclerotic disease in populations who consume diets high in fish.

Mechanism of Action

Whereas the lipid-altering effects of omega-3 fatty acids is not fully understood, EPA is thought to exert its antiplatelet effect by competing with arachidonic acid (AA) for cyclooxygenase. In platelets, AA is converted to thromboxane A_2 (TBX) under the direction of cyclooxygenase. TBX is a powerful platelet aggregant and vasoconstrictor that normally balances the opposite effects of prostaglandin PGI_2 (prostacyclin). Diet high in EPA increases EPA content of platelets, reducing the production of TBX. EPA also is converted to PGI_3, which has an additional antiaggregant effect, and may inhibit endothelial cell production of platelet-derived growth factor. DHA alters platelet function by different mechanisms, and is itself converted to EPA. Omega-3 fatty acids also have been shown to reduce experimental atherosclerosis in animals, which may be partly related to an anti-inflammatory effect such as altered leukotriene production.

Some studies have demonstrated that fish-oil supplements reduce plasma levels of LDL and VLDL, without altering levels of HDL, and are even more potent in lowering levels of triglyceride (TG). However, they may have little or no cholesterol-lowering effect in people who have normal TG levels. Clinical trials have not yet honed in on the precise nature of their effect and toxicity. As is the case for conventional lipid-lowering agents, almost no studies have included elderly patients. Studies that have demonstrated lipid-lowering effects have used 5–20 grams of fish oil, doses that can be attained only by taking 15–30 capsules per day. For comparison, the equivalent of 5 g of fish oil is contained in 0.5 lb of certain types of salmon, 2.5 lb of cod, or 6 lb of swordfish. Five grams of fish oil adds nearly 600 kcal per day to the diet; 10 g nearly 1200 kcal.

Adverse Effects

Fish-oil supplements in high doses can cause **vitamin E deficiency, bloating, increased bleeding time,** and, on account of increased calorie intake, **weight gain.** Environmental pollutants, such as mercury and pesticides, which have been known to contaminate fish, could theoretically be found in commercial fish-oil capsules, but could be removed during appropriate purification processes.

Precautions

Fish-oil supplements should not be taken by patients who are taking anticoagulants.

Preparations

Fish-oil supplements are available without prescription in 500- and 1000-mg capsules, containing between 300 and 500 mg of fish oil per 1000-mg capsule. Depending on the preparation, there may be other constituents, such as small amounts of vitamin A, D, B, and E, calcium, or iron.

Fish versus Fish Oil

Fish itself may be cardioprotective, for reasons unrelated to lipid-lowering effects, and in amounts containing far less omega-3 fatty acids than that promoted by fish-oil advocates. Fish containing the highest amount of omega-3 fatty acids include herring, salmon, blue fish, lake trout, and mackerel. Certain shell fish, such as lobster and shrimp, also contain these fatty acids, and, despite their relatively high cholesterol content, are thought by some investigators to be cardioprotective in and of themselves.

The amount of omega-3 fatty acids contained in the fish in question ranges from 400 to 3200 mg per 8-oz serving.

Recommendations

Fish consumption is an accepted part of a cardioprotective diet. At least 3 meals per week should be fish meals, but these meals are intended to replace foods high in atherogenic substances, and are not intended as a supplement, so that additional fat should not be used in their preparation. Patients who are interested in increasing the content of omega-3 fatty acids in the diet can be advised to ingest fish high in these substances (see above).

There is no evidence that sporadic use of fish-oil supplements has any benefit. When a substance is available without prescription, and, moreover, is a "natural" dietary component, it is tempting to recommend it for the elderly, in whom one wishes to maximize nonpharmacologic treatment. However, a fish-oil supplement in the experimentally determined doses of 5–10 g/day, delivered in the absence of its natural vehicle (the fish), must be considered a pharmacologic agent. The risk-benefit ratio of these doses is not known, can only be achieved by the addition of substantial calories to the diet, and have not been studied at all in the elderly.

BIBLIOGRAPHY

Bierman, E. L., Arteriosclerosis and aging. In C. E. Finch and E. L. Schneider (eds.), *Handbook of the Biology of Aging* (2nd ed.). New York: Van Nostrand Reinhold, 1985. Pp. 842–858.

Brensike, J. F., Levy, R. I., Kelsey, S. F., et al. Effects of therapy with cholestyramine on progression of coronary atherosclerosis: results of NHLBI Type II Coronary Intervention Study. *Circulation* 69:313–324, 1984.

Canner, P. L., Berge, K. G., Wenger, N. K., et al. Fifteen year mortality in Coronary Drug Project patients: long-term benefit with niacin. *J. Amer. Coll. Cardiol.* 8:1245–1255, 1986.

Castelli, W. P., Garrison, R. J., Wilson, P. W. F., et al. Incidence of coronary artery disease and lipoprotein cholesterol levels: the Framingham study. *JAMA* 256:2835–2838, 1986.

Consensus conference. Treatment of hypertriglyceridemia. *JAMA* 251:1196–1200, 1984.

Crouse, J. R. Hypertriglyceridemia: a contraindication to the use of bile acid binding resins. *Amer. J. Med* 83:243–248, 1987.

Gordon, T., Castelli, W. P., Hjortland, M. C., et al. High density lipoprotein as a protective factor against coronary heart disease: the Framingham Study. *Am. J. Med.* 62:707–714, 1979.

Grundy, S. M. HMG-CoA reductase inhibitors for treatment of hypercholesterolemia. *N. Engl. J. Med.* 319:24–33, 1988.

Grundy, S. M. Cholesterol and coronary heart disease. A new era. *JAMA* 256:2849–2858, 1986.

Hazzard, W. R. Biological basis of the sex differential in longevity. *J. Amer. Geriatr. Soc.* 34:455–471, 1986.

Heel, R. C., Brogden, R. N., Pakes, G. E., Speight, T. M., and Avery, G. S. Colestipol: a review of its pharmacological properties and therapeutic efficacy in patients with hypercholesterolaemia. *Drugs* 19:161–180, 1980.

Herold, P. M., and Kinsella, J. E. Fish oil consumption and decreased risk of cardiovascular disease: a comparison of findings from animal and human feeding trials. *Am J Clin Nutr.* 43:566–598, 1986.

Hershcopf, R. J., Elahi, D., Andres, R., et al. Longitudinal changes in serum cholesterol in man: an epidemiologic search for an etiology. *J. Chron. Dis.* 35:101–114, 1982.

Hotz, W. Nicotonic acid and its derivatives: a short survey. *Adv. Lipid Res.* 20:195–217, 1983.

Hunninghake, D.B., Miller, V.T., Goldberg, I., et al. Lovastatin: follow-up opthalmologic data. *JAMA* 259:354–355, 1988 (letter).

Iso, H., Jacobs, D. R., Wentworth D., et al. Serum cholesterol levels and six-year mortality from stroke in 350,977 men screened for the multiple risk factor intervention trial. *N. Engl. J. Med.* 320:904–910, 1989.

Kaiser, F. E., and Morley, J. E. Cholesterol can be lowered in older persons. Should we care? *J. Amer. Geriatr. Soc.* 38:84–85, 1990.

Lavie, C. J., Gau, G. T., Squires, R. W., and Kottke, B. A. Management of lipids in primary and secondary prevention of cardiovascular diseases. *Mayo. Clin. Proc.* 63:605–621, 1988.

Leaf, A., and Weber, P. C. Cardiovascular effects of n-3 fatty acids. *N. Engl. J. Med.* 318:549–557, 1988.

Lovastatin Study Group II. Therapeutic response to lovastatin (mevinolin) in nonfamilial hypercholesterolemia. A multicenter trial. *JAMA* 256:2829–2834, 1986.

Manninen, V., Elo, M. O., Fric, M. H., et al. Lipid alterations and decline in the incidence of coronary heart disease in the Helsinki Heart Study. *JAMA* 260:641–651, 1988.

Miller, N. E. Aging and plasma lipoproteins. In W. R. Hazzard, R. Andres, E. L. Bierman, et al. (eds.), *Principles of Geriatric Medicine and Gerontology.* New York: McGraw-Hill, 1990. Pp. 767–776.

Morisaki, N., Mori, S., Kobayashi, J., et al. Effects of long-term treatment with probucol on serum lipoproteins in cases of familial hypercholesterolemia in the elderly. *J. Amer. Geriatr. Soc.* 38:15–18, 1990.

National Cholesterol Education Program Expert Panel. Report of the National Cholesterol Education Program Expert Panel on Detection, Evaluation, and Treatment of High Blood Cholesterol in Adults. *Arch. Intern. Med.* 148:36–69, 1988.

Palumbo, P. J. Cholesterol lowering for all: a closer look. *J.A.M.A.* 262:91–92, 1989.

Schaefer, E. J., and Levy, R. I. Pathogenesis and management of lipoprotein disorders. *N. Engl. J. Med.* 312:1300–1310, 1985.

Hypoglycemic Agents

DIABETES IN THE ELDERLY

The most common form of diabetes affecting the elderly is type II, or non-insulin-dependent diabetes mellitus (NIDDM), accounting for at least 90% of cases in people over the age of 65. Type II diabetes is a disorder of unknown etiology, but genetic factors as well as the aging process are felt to be important. Serum insulin levels may be low, but more often normal or inappropriately high basal levels are seen. Hyperglycemia occurs as a result of delayed release of insulin from the pancreas and variable degrees of peripheral insulin resistance.

Only a small minority of elderly diabetics have type I, or insulin-dependent diabetes mellitus (IDDM). Type I diabetes is thought to occur as an autoimmune response to viral infection, which results in pancreatic beta-cell depletion and insulinopenia, and a high rate of microvascular and macrovascular complications. Most, if not all, of the elderly who have this type of disease belong to the small category of individuals who have contracted IDDM after the age of 40 and have managed to survive into old age. They tend to differ clinically from elderly patients with type II diabetes, who require insulin because they do not respond adequately to oral hypoglycemic agents or to diet. The need for insulin in the latter group of patients may be temporary, because of intercurrent illness, weight gain, or use of drugs that impair glucose tolerance, or it may be permanent because oral hypoglycemic agents fail to work or cease to be efficacious.

Although there is abundant evidence that "tight control" of blood glucose and maintenance of a perfect euglycemic state is desirable and lowers the risk of microvascular complications, such an approach cannot be applied to all elderly patients. Robust elderly are likely to feel better when euglycemia has been attained, and, depending on their longevity, they may be protected from long-term complications. Frail or extremely aged patients, however, may have little to gain from tight control, which furthermore may be impractical and in some cases unwise. Hypoglycemia may be more severe and prolonged in elderly individuals and is more likely to result in stroke or myocardial infarction than in younger patients. Symptoms of hypoglycemia may be less obvious in some elderly because of autonomic neuropathy or dementia. Because of the frequent coexistence of dementia, visual disorders, and reduced manual dexterity, strict adherence to a medical regimen may be difficult or even unsafe. Finally, urine glucose monitoring, which is less sensitive than blood glucose monitoring, is even less precise in the elderly. Renal glucose threshold increases with age so that blood glucose may have to be significantly elevated (often over 200 mg/dl) before glycosuria occurs.

For all of these reasons, it is prudent to adopt a conservative approach in the management of hyperglycemia in selected elderly. Serum glucose may need to be maintained at 30–40 mg/dl above the usual recommended level as a buffer against hypoglycemia. In robust patients, or in those with competent caregivers, diabetes can often be managed more precisely.

As many as 10% of people over 65 in the United States have impaired glucose tolerance without fulfilling official criteria for diabetes mellitus. Such patients commonly are found to have random blood sugars in the 160–170 mg/dl range while maintaining fasting blood sugar of 140 mg/dl or less. This is considered to be a mild form of the insulin resistance that is seen in frank type II diabetes mellitus. This "glucose intolerance of aging" is **not** considered a normal age-related phenomenon since it is an independent risk factor for myocardial infarction, and is associated with an increased risk of developing overt diabetes mellitus. It is not known whether treatment reduces long-term risk of vascular disease, but certain of these patients may be at risk of presenting with hyperosmolar coma if severe stress or illness occurs. Because of the particular dangers of hypoglycemia to the elderly, mild glucose intolerance should not be treated pharmacologically. Blood sugar should be monitored periodically and acute illness should be treated promptly.

ORAL HYPOGLYCEMIC AGENTS

Pharmacologic Considerations

Mechanism of Action

Sulfonylurea agents are structurally related to the sulfonamide antibiotics, having been discovered during research on that group of agents. They lower blood glucose by increasing pancreatic insulin secretion on the short term, and by increasing the sensitivity of target tissues to endogenous insulin on the long term. The exact site of action in the latter mechanism is not known. Sulfonylurea agents may also act by decreasing hepatic glucose synthesis, which is accelerated in NIDDM.

Sulfonylurea agents are ineffective in the absence of functioning pancreatic tissue, as in chronic pancreatitis and pancreatectomy, and are ineffective in type I diabetes mellitus.

Pharmacokinetics

The sulfonylurea agents are readily absorbed from the gastrointestinal tract. They are metabolized in the liver to renally excreted metabolites that have varying degrees of hypoglycemic activity. The difference in the activity of these metabolites has an impact on the duration of biologic actions exhibited by individual agents. Because of age-related changes in renal function, the contribution of these metabolites to hypoglycemic effect could be even more significant in many elderly patients. In addition, the biologic action of certain oral hypoglycemic agents outlasts the presence of drug and metabolites in serum.

Adverse Effects

All hypoglycemic agents can cause **hypoglycemia**. Sulfonylurea-induced hypoglycemia differs from that caused by insulin in that it may be unpredictably delayed (up to 1 week from initiation of therapy), or prolonged (up to 2 weeks), depending on the agent used and the underlying clinical condition of the patient. In these cases, the patient should be hospitalized until euglycemia has been firmly established.

In the past, **prolonged hypoglycemia** was reported most often with chlorpropamide and acetohexamide, which have the longest half-lives. It has also been reported fairly frequently with tolbutamide and with glyburide, however. The frequency of these reports may only partly reflect prescribing patterns. Hypoglycemia outlasting the putative biologic half-life of the intermediate and short-acting agents is not well explained, but underlying renal or hepatic disease and concurrent use of interacting drugs is often implicated. In the case of glyburide, accumulation of drug and prolonged pharmacodynamic action in islet cells has been demonstrated. The risk of prolonged hypoglycemia increases steadily with age but is unusual in patients who are otherwise well.

Certain oral hypoglycemic agents reversibly impair urinary clearance of free water and may produce **hyponatremia.** Chlorpropamide has been implicated in the syndrome of inappropriate ADH secretion (SIADH), an association seen most often in elderly women; coma and death have occurred. Tolbutamide has also been reported to cause hyponatremia, but far less commonly. Other agents appear to be devoid of this effect. Tolazamide, glyburide, and acetohexamide actually have a weak diuretic effect.

Skin rashes and other **allergic phenomena** may occur. Because of their similarity in structure to the sulfonamides, cross-reactivity may occur.

Sulfonylurea agents have been reported to produce **cholestatic jaundice.** Although this effect is unusual, hepatic necrosis and death have occurred.

There is long-standing controversy surrounding **cardiovascular effects** of oral hypoglycemic agents. Animal studies on the chronotropic effects of tolbutamide and glyburide have been contradictory and long-term effects on the human heart are unknown. The oral hypoglycemic agents do not have an adverse effect on the lipid profile; in fact, lipid levels may improve as blood glucose comes under control. The cardiovascular controversy stems from the 10-year multicenter University Group Diabetes Program (UGDP) study of blood glucose control (see Scientific Advisory Panel). This study initially concluded that oral hypoglycemic agents were not sufficiently efficacious and were associated with increased cardiovascular death as compared to diet, insulin, or placebo. The only oral agents studied were phenformin (a nonsulfonylurea) and tolbutamide. The ensuing decade-long controversy culminated in disavowal of the study's conclusions, and ultimate repudiation of the results by the American Diabetes Association. However, a lingering effect of the controversy is that the FDA still requires a package insert warning of increased cardiovascular risk. Despite this, sulfonylurea agents are widely used in North America and Europe, and remain a practical and effective method of managing diabetes in the elderly. Phenformin, a biguanide, is no longer on the market in the United States.

Loss or Lack of Efficacy (Primary and Secondary Failures)

Primary failure of an oral hypoglycemic agent is defined as the inability to ever develop adequate control of blood sugar despite maximum doses. This occurs in 15%–20% of subjects. The more carefully a patient is selected, the less likely primary treatment failure will occur. *Secondary failure* is defined as the loss of efficacy after an apparently adequate response. This occurs at a rate of approximately 5%–10% of treated patients per year in the absence of modifiable factors such as weight gain, intercurrent illness, or drug-induced hyperglycemia. Although these failures are not completely understood, baseline or progressive insulinopenia may be an important factor. A small number of patients with apparent NIDDM actually have slowly progressive type I diabetes as demonstrated by the presence of islet cell antibodies.

Oral hypoglycemics are most likely to be efficacious in patients with no history of acidosis, previous control on no insulin or less than 40 units per day, no prior failure of an oral agent, duration of diabetes less than 5 years, onset of the disease after age 40, absence of additional pancreatic disease, mild to moderate obesity, and no acute or chronic illness. However, there are many exceptions to this, so that a trial of an oral agent is justified in most elderly diabetics.

Important Drug Interactions

Drug interactions may occur with oral hypoglycemic agents in several ways. However, it is not known to what extent all agents of this class participate in all interactions.

The risk of sulfonylurea-induced hypoglycemia may be increased by agents that themselves have hypoglycemic action, such as salicylates, alcohol, or disopyramide. The risk of hypoglycemia in these circumstances is greatest in patients with hepatic or renal disease, or inanition. The effects of beta blockers on glucose metabolism are variable, but these drugs should generally be avoided in medically treated diabetics because they may mask the symptoms of hypoglycemia. In this regard, it should be pointed out that symptoms of hypoglycemia may be blunted with age independent of beta blocker use, as counterregulatory systems are altered.

Metabolism of the sulfonylurea agents can be affected by drugs that inhibit (e.g., cimetidine) or stimulate (e.g., barbiturates, rifampin) hepatic microsomal enzymes. Other agents can reduce the urinary elimination of sulfonylurea agents or their active metabolites, enhancing their hypoglycemic effect. Finally, all sulfonylurea agents are highly protein-bound and are able to displace similarly bound drugs from protein-binding sites or be displaced by them, temporarily altering the effects of either agent. The second-generation agents differ in the nature of their binding, making them theoretically less susceptible to displacement interactions than earlier agents. The role of displacement from protein binding sites is uncertain; however, drug interactions may still occur via other mechanisms.

Agents that impair glucose tolerance, such as corticosteroids, phenytoin, and thiazides, may counteract the hypoglycemic effects of the sulfanylurea agents.

When taken with alcohol, chlorpropamide frequently produces flushing, palpitations, or nausea, and, occasionally, wheezing in susceptible individuals ("disulfiram reaction"). This interaction is not due to the production of hypoglycemia but appears to be caused by an alteration of alcohol metabolism that results in the accumulation of the toxic metabolite acetaldehyde. Other sulfonylurea agents have rarely been implicated in this reaction.

Important drug interactions are summarized in Table 18–1.

Contraindications and Precautions

Oral hypoglycemic agents should not be used in IDDM or in hyperglycemia due to serious infections and other acute exacerbating factors. They should generally be avoided in liver or renal disease. If

Table 18–1. Potential Drug Interactions with Oral Hypoglycemic Agents

Increased Hypoglycemic Effect	Reduced Hypoglycemic Effect
Alcohol	Thiazide diuretics
Salicylates	Corticosteroids
Disopyramide	Rifampin
Beta blockers	Estrogen
Sulfonamides	Gemfibrizol
Chloramphenicol	Barbiturates
Allopurinol	Beta blockers
Probenecid	Phenytoin
Phenylbutazone	
Sulfonamides	
Monoamine oxidase inhibitors	
Cimetidine and ranitidine	
ACE inhibitors?	

there are no suitable alternatives in patients with mild to moderate renal insufficiency, glipizide, tolbutamide, and possibly tolazamide are the preferred agents.

Oral hypoglycemic agents should be used cautiously in patients with known sensitivity to sulfonamides and related agents.

Indications

Oral hypoglycemic agents are indicated in the treatment of NIDDM when euglycemia cannot be attained by exercise or diet alone.

Oral agents are **not** indicated in the treatment of mild glucose intolerance in the elderly if official criteria for diabetes mellitus are not met. They are not indicated in the treatment of type I, insulin-dependent diabetes.

Dosing

Dosages are summarized in Table 18–2.

Specific Agents

First-Generation Agents

Tolbutamide (Orinase) is a useful agent that has been eclipsed by the second-generation agents. Because its short duration of action tends to be somewhat prolonged in older patients, it may occasionally provide satisfactory control when given once daily. This is a potentially useful property in the easily controlled patient who might be at risk for nocturnal hypoglycemia. Tolbutamide is metabolized to inactive metabolites and there is some advantage to using it in mild renal insufficiency in patients who are unable to administer insulin. Hyponatremia has been reported, however, and caution should be observed.

Tolbutamide is available in many generic forms; bioavailability may vary among the different brands.

Tolazamide (Tolinase) is a highly satisfactory but underused

Table 18–2. Commonly Used Oral Hypoglycemic Agents

Agent	Brand	Duration of Hypoglycemic Action (hr)	Usual Dose Range (mg)*
Tolbutamide	Orinase	6–12	500–2000 mg in 2 to 4 divided doses
Chlorpropamide	Diabenese	24–72	100–500 mg
Tolazamide	Tolinase	12–18	100–500 mg at once or in 2 divided doses
Glyburide	Diabeta Micronase	Up to 24	1.25 mg once daily to 10 mg bid
Glipizide	Glucotrol	Up to 24	2.5 mg once daily to 15 mg bid

*Some patients may respond to smaller doses.

agent. It has an intermediate duration of action comparable to the second-generation agents and can be used with relative safety on a once-daily basis. It has been reported less often than the newer agents to produce severe hypoglycemia, although it is not known if the infrequency of those reports reflects prescribing patterns. Tolazamide has not been reported to cause hyponatremia; rather, it has a mild diuretic action that is probably not clinically significant. Its chief theoretical disadvantage over the newer agents is that, like other first-generation agents, its protein-binding characteristics should lead to displacement interactions; however, this has not been substantiated.

Chlorpropamide (Diabinese) has an extremely long duration of action. A portion of this drug is excreted unchanged in the urine and its duration of action tends to be further prolonged in the elderly. Because of this, and because of its ability to produce hyponatremia in older individuals, it should generally be avoided. However, there appears to be no particular advantage to discontinuing this drug in someone who has been managed safely on it for a long period of time, as long as the person remains well. Chlorpropamide has been used to salvage secondary treatment failures. However, its success rate in this regard is dubious.

An additional disadvantage to chlorpropamide is its ability to produce a disulfiramlike reaction when taken with alcohol (see above).

Acetohexamide (Dymelor) has a potentially long duration of action due to the production of a metabolite with greater hypoglycemic action than the parent compound. It has diuretic and uricosuric action.

Although it has fewer potential disadvantages than chlorpropamide, acetohexamide is seldom used, and there is not enough clinical experience with it to make specific recommendations. It has no known advantages over other oral hypoglycemic agents.

Second-Generation Agents

The second-generation sulfonylurea agents, glipizide and glyburide, have a few potential advantages over tolbutamide and tolazamide, but should not be considered as perfect alternatives. They have been used to salvage secondary failures to the first-generation agents, but their successful salvage rate is nonetheless very low and may not be higher than that demonstrated with chlorpropamide. Glipizide and glyburide may participate in fewer drug displacement interactions than the older agents because they have different protein-binding properties. However, they may still participate in drug interactions by other mechanisms.

Glipizide (Glucotrol) is metabolized in the liver to inactive metabolites and is therefore theoretically useful in patients with impaired renal function. Elimination seems to be unimpaired with age, so that its duration of action should be more predictable. Overall, it should be one of the safer sulfonylurea agents to use in the elderly and its intermediate duration of action makes it well suited to once-a-day dosing. More cases of severe hypoglycemia have been reported with glipizide than with either tolbutamide or tolazamide, but these agents have not been directly compared in controlled studies.

Glyburide (DiaBeta, Micronase) has an intermediate duration of action, and, like glipizide, is suitable for once-a-day dosing. One of its hepatic metabolites is slightly active. This feature has not been shown to be particularly problematic in elderly patients without overt renal insufficiency and it is generally well suited for geriatric use. However, glyburide has been implicated more often than most of the other agents in prolonged hypoglycemia (see Adverse Effects, above).

Like glipizide and tolazamide, glyburide does not produce hyponatremia. Like tolazamide, it has slight diuretic action.

USE OF INSULIN IN THE ELDERLY

Many elderly diabetics will require insulin at some time, either temporarily or permanently. Insulin is required in severe hyperglycemia, diabetic hyperosmolar coma, or diabetic ketoacidosis. Severe hyperglycemia and hyperosmolar coma are common presentations of diabetes in the elderly or may complicate the otherwise stable course of patients with mild diabetes. In these cases, the need for insulin may be only temporary; these patients frequently can be managed on oral hypoglycemic agents or diet alone once the precipitating factor has been eradicated.

Many diabetics who have been well managed on diet or oral agents will develop deterioration of diabetes itself, most likely because pancreatic reserve has been exhausted, and will ultimately require insulin for control of blood glucose. However, in these cases as well, modifiable factors may be present and the need for insulin may be temporary.

Many late-onset diabetics in today's geriatric population are currently being managed with insulin but have never received an adequate trial of oral agents. A number of these patients can be weaned from insulin and managed with oral agents or on diet alone.

In elderly diabetics, even those who have had episodes of severe hyperglycemia or nonketotic coma, it is not uncommon for the maintenance insulin requirement to be quite low. Type II elderly diabetics who "escape" from the effects of oral hypoglycemic agents can frequently be managed on no more than 20 units of insulin per day, suggesting that there are other factors involved in this disease besides insulin resistance. In other cases, insulin requirements will be significantly higher.

There is no particular type or preparation of insulin that is more effective in the elderly diabetic. Selection of insulin preparation should be based on considerations such as glucose control, cost, and ease of administration. Insulin allergy occurs among the elderly and this too may guide the selection of a particular agent.

PRACTICAL CONSIDERATIONS

The physician must anticipate the impediments to care of the elderly diabetic who requires insulin. Very frequently the limiting factor is the inability of the patient to administer insulin because of dementia, poor manual dexterity, or poor vision. Noninstitutionalized elderly frequently cannot obtain caregivers. Payment for home-care workers is generally not reimbursed by third-party payers. These workers are usually not permitted by vendors to administer insulin.

Auxiliary appliances can be employed by visually or physically impaired individuals in order to self-administer insulin. Unfortunately, elderly diabetics frequently have more than one impairment and may be unable to use these devices correctly. A local visiting nurse service can draw up a week's supply of insulin to be stored in the refrigerator and administered by patient or caregiver on a daily basis. If regular- and intermediate-acting insulin are mixed in prefilled syringes, regular insulin gradually binds to the protamine-zinc components of NPH insulin and becomes converted to an intermediate-acting agent. A commercially available product (Mixtard) can circumvent this difficulty. This product consists of 30% regular and 70% NPH insulin in a fixed, stable combination, and can be used if this ratio is appropriate for the patient. It is also a useful product for patients who are unable to figure out the more complicated process of drawing up two types of insulin.

Home blood glucose monitoring is far more accurate and useful than urine monitoring and should be employed if it can be ascertained that the patient or caregiver can perform this correctly. If urine glucose measurements are the only option, the limitations of this method should be recognized.

PRECAUTIONS

Age changes in counterregulatory mechanisms may mask the expression of hypoglycemic symptoms, such as sweating and tachycardia. This problem is analogous to that which exists in diabetes complicated by autonomic neuropathy. For this and other reasons, patient reporting of symptoms may not be a reliable indicator of significant hypoglycemia. Frequent monitoring of blood glucose is essential in patients at risk.

NONPHARMACOLOGIC TREATMENT

Whenever possible, nonpharmacologic treatment should be maximized. Important approaches include diet, sensible exercise, timely management of intercurrent illness, and avoidance of medications known to impair glucose tolerance. Other modifiable risk factors for vascular and cardiac disease should be attended to. These include hypertension, obesity, smoking, and hyperlipidemia.

BIBLIOGRAPHY

Bantle, J. P. The dietary treatment of diabetes mellitus. *Med. Clin. N. Amer.* 72:1285–1299, 1988.

Gerich, J. E. Oral hypoglycemic agents. *N. Engl. J. Med.* 321:1231–1245, 1989.

Harris, M. I., Hadden, W. C., Knowler, W. C., et al. International criteria for the diagnosis of diabetes and impaired glucose tolerance. *Diabetes Care* 8:562–567, 1985.

Kilvert, A., Fitzgerald, M. G., Wright, A. D., and Nattrass, M. Clinical characteristics and aetiological classification of insulin-dependent diabetes in the elderly. *Q. J. Med.* 60:865–872, 1986.

Meneilly, G. S., Greenspan, S. L., Rowe, J. W., and Minaker, K. L. Endocrine systems. In J. W. Rowe, and R. W. Besdine (eds.), *Geriatric Medicine* (2nd ed.). Boston: Little Brown, 1988. Pp. 408–413.

Scientific Advisory Panel of the Executive Committee, American Diabetes Association. Policy Statement. The UGDP Controversy. *Diabetes* 28:168–170, 1979.

Seltzer, H. S. Drug-induced hypoglycemia. *Endocrinol. Metab. Clin. N. Amer.* 18(1): 163–183, 1989.

Thyroid Hormones

Classic symptoms of hypothyroidism, such as dry skin, coarsening of the voice, hair loss, constipation, lethargy, and confusion, are common concomitants of old age. Thus, when these symptoms appear, they may be mistaken for normal aging or for pathological conditions that occur commonly in late life, and the diagnosis of hypothyroidism may be missed. Conversely, the patient is sometimes treated for hypothyroidism when he or she is actually euthyroid, or has mild chemical hypothyroidism that has not actually produced the symptoms. The diagnosis of primary hypothyroidism rests on the demonstration of low thyroid hormone levels in conjunction with clearly elevated levels of thyroid stimulating hormone (TSH).

The fact that a patient is taking thyroid hormone replacement does not necessarily mean that he or she has ever been hypothyroid. Some elderly patients have been taking thyroid hormone for many years, occasionally for so long that the diagnosis might have been made on the basis of tests no longer considered to be specific, such as basal metabolism rate or protein-bound iodine. Patients who come to the physician with a remote or uncertain diagnosis of hypothyroidism should have thyroid medication reduced temporarily while appropriate thyroid function tests are performed.

Thyroid function tests must be interpreted with caution in the elderly. The most sensitive test for the diagnosis is a TSH level, which is unequivocally elevated in primary hypothyroidism. Clinically important pituitary hypothyroidism associated with a low TSH level is exceedingly rare and will not be considered here. Serum thyroxine (T_4) level may be altered by a variety of factors, particularly affecting binding of thyroxine to serum proteins. Acute and chronic illness are among the many things that readily lower thyroid binding proteins in elderly patients, so that total T_4 is frequently reduced although the patient is euthyroid. Less often, T_4 is misleadingly elevated, on account of such factors as hormone administration. T_4 level should be corrected for alterations in binding proteins by using a confirmatory test such as the T_3 resin uptake. Levels of triiodothyronine (T_3) are also frequently reduced in euthyroid elderly patients. This may be because of age- and disease-associated decreased peripheral conversion of T_4 to T_3, with enhanced conversion to inactive reverse T_3 (RT_3). Despite the fact that T_3 is biologically more active than T_4, patients with sole reductions in serum T_3 are, strictly speaking, euthyroid. This has been attributed to a possible intracellular conversion to T_3 or subcellular action of T_4, but this explanation is speculative.

TSH is elevated in over 10% of geriatric patients. The presence of a normal or near normal corrected T_4 level in conjunction with a mildly elevated TSH level is referred to as the *failing thyroid syndrome*. Some investigators advise treatment of all patients in this category in the hopes of preventing clinical hypothyroidism. Others feel that this is ill-advised because there is no good evidence that treating such mild chemical hypothyroidism has clinical benefit; they hesitate further because thyroid hormone may accelerate osteoporosis and promote cardiac symptoms in elderly patients. It is probably sensible to treat these cases on an individual basis. Although the presence of symptoms in conjunction with mild chemical hypothyroidism merits attention, rarely if ever does treatment of such patients eradicate symptoms such as confusion, constipation, bradycardia, or weight gain. In geriatric patients with mild hypothyroidism, these symptoms are generally due to nonthyroidal disease. The significance of mild hypothyroidism in depression is controversial.

Because hypothyroidism in the elderly is so prevalent and subtle in presentation, all patients over 65 should be screened for this condition. If the diagnosis of primary hypothyroidism is made, thyroid hormone replacement should be undertaken. An asymptomatic patient with the failing thyroid syndrome should receive follow-up thyroid function testing once or twice a year.

PHARMACOKINETICS

Thyroid hormone is variably absorbed. Standardization of preparations has minimized but not eliminated variability of absorption, an imperfection that is probably not clinically important in most situations. Approximately one third of endogenous T_4 is converted to T_3 by deiodination in several organ systems, primarily the liver and the kidney. Depending on clinical conditions, varying proportions of T_4 are converted to RT_3. T_3 and RT_3 are further deiodinated to inactive metabolites. T_4 is bound avidly, and T_3 less avidly, to serum proteins, mainly thyroid binding globulin (TBG).

Thyroid hormones are conjugated in the liver and excreted in the bile. Enterohepatic circulation occurs. The metabolic clearance rate of endogenous T_4 declines with age, so that the half-life increases from roughly 6.4–7 days in young adults to 8.4–10 days by age 80. The half-life of T_4 is further prolonged in hypothyroidism. However, it is not possible to predict when exogenous hormone will produce the euthyroid state because this depends on how long it takes to saturate available binding sites of TBG.

TSH measurements remain the most reliable and practical means of determining the response to treatment. Pituitary response to change in thyroid status is not immediate, so that 4–6 weeks may elapse after adequate thyroid replacement before TSH is completely normal. These factors, combined with the possible cardiac vulnerability of the geriatric patient, demand that initial thyroid replacement doses be kept low and dose increments made slowly.

The half-life of T_3 is less than one third that of T_4. The half-life of thyroid hormones is shorter than normal in hyperthyroidism.

Eighty percent of circulating T_3 is derived from extrathyroidal enzymatic degradation of T_4, a process that declines with age. Despite this, thyroid hormone replacement, even with pure levothyroxine (T_4), produces adequate levels of T_3 and a euthyroid state.

WHICH AGENT?

The physician is currently faced with a choice of many forms of thyroid replacement. These are summarized in Table 19-1.

Levothyroxine (Synthroid, Levothroid, others) is synthetic T_4, which is the major form of thyroid hormone produced by the thyroid gland. In the body, endogenous and exogenous T_4 is converted to active T_3 outside of the thyroid gland. While peripheral conversion of T_4 to T_3 is thought to be slightly impaired with age, replacement with levothyroxine is associated with adequate levels of T_3 in elderly

Table 19–1. Available Thyroid Preparations

Preparation	Brand	Constituents	Equivalent Dose
Levothyroxine	Synthroid Levothroid	T_4	0.025 mg (25 μg)
Liothyronine	Cytomel	T_3	5 μg
Desiccated Thyroid	Various	$T_4 + T_3$	¼ grain
Liotrix	Thyrolar Euthroid*	$T_4 + T_3$	"¼"
Thyroglobulin	Proloid*	$T_4 + T_3$	*

* Smallest available dose is equivalent to 50 μg levothyroxine.

patients, and relatively constant serum levels of T_4 and T_3 are maintained throughout the day, once a steady state is reached. In all age groups, replacement with levothyroxine produces a serum ratio of T_4 to T_3 that roughly corresponds to that found in euthyroid patients. This is not the case with other agents (see below).

Levothyroxine is the formulation of choice for geriatric patients, as for other age groups.

Liothyronine (Cytomel, others) is synthetic T_3. This agent gained acceptance because of the theoretical advantage of giving the active form of the hormone, but it has not been demonstrated that there is any clinical advantage to giving active hormone rather than a precursor (T_4). Rather, daily doses of T_3 are rapidly absorbed and rapidly eliminated from the body, producing a "rush" of hormone. Unlike the constant levels of thyroid hormone produced by levothyroxine, administration of compounds containing T_3 produces an early marked rise in serum T_3, often to thyrotoxic levels, followed by a relatively rapid decline, and may produce symptoms of hyperthyroidism in a significant minority of patients. This could be particularly harmful to elderly patients, many of whom have subclinical or overt cardiac disease.

Use of preparations containing T_3 in the treatment of hypothyroidism is discouraged by geriatricians. There are probably more patients in the older age group taking these preparations simply because they were placed on them long ago, before their routine use was discouraged.

It has been suggested that the rapid onset and short duration of action of T_3 might be advantageous in the treatment of myxedema coma. However, this is controversial, with many physicians recommending parenteral levothyroxine instead. A practical consideration is the fact that parenteral levothyroxine is much more widely available than parenteral liothyronine in pharmacies in the United States.

If a patient is taking liothyronine, confirmatory thyroid testing must be interpreted very cautiously. If the dose is "appropriate," serum levels of T_4 will be extremely low, while T_3 levels will fluctuate during the day. Blood should be tested at least 6 hours after the daily dose. Unfortunately, interindividual variability in timing makes blood testing an unreliable indicator of dosing adequacy.

Desiccated thyroid is prepared from animal glands, usually pork or beef. T_4 and T_3 are present in their naturally occurring intrathyroidal ratio, which is variable. Standardization of the various brands available is thought to provide sufficiently uniform concentrations of thyroid hormone from batch to batch, although uniformity is probably not as good as with the synthetic preparations. Whether or not this variability is of clinical significance in a medically stable patient is not known.

Desiccated thyroid, like other preparations that combine T_4 and T_3 in one tablet, provides these hormones in a ratio that resembles that in the thyroid gland, rather than in the serum. This T_4-to-T_3 ratio is much lower than the ratio that is present in serum in the euthyroid state.

The disadvantages of giving active T_3 occur with desiccated thyroid, as with pure T_3 (see liothyronine, above). In contrast to liothyronine, however, administration of desiccated thyroid and other combination agents leads to an increase in serum levels of T_4. These levels are nonetheless lower than the levels produced by replacement with levothyroxine. Low or low-normal T_4 levels may prompt the physician to further increase the dose, which may produce even higher T_3 levels. Thyrotoxic symptoms can be produced by daily surges in T_3 levels with this preparation.

Liotrix (Euthroid, Thyrolar) is a combination of synthetic T_4 and T_3 in a fixed ratio of 4:1. The disadvantages of preparations containing T_3 have been discussed above. Euthroid is not available in doses lower than the equivalent of 0.05 mg levothyroxine and therefore cannot be adequately titrated in geriatric patients.

Thyroglobulin (Proloid) is prepared from hog thyroid gland and contains T_4 and T_3. It has no advantages over other agents in use. A major disadvantage of this preparation is that it is not available in doses lower than the equivalent of 0.05 mg levothyroxine and therefore cannot be adequately titrated in geriatric patients.

ADVERSE EFFECTS

Thyroid hormone can exacerbate **cardiac arrhythmias, symptoms of ischemic heart disease,** and **silent ischemia.** The risk of these effects is greatest in patients with underlying cardiac disease, and when excessive thyroid hormone is given.

Thyroid hormone enhances the absorption of dietary carbohydrates and enhances metabolic clearance of insulin. Thus, thyroid replacement may elevate blood sugar in some diabetics until a steady state is achieved. Glucose should be carefully followed during initial thyroid replacement.

Overtreatment may produce symptoms of hyperthyroidism, including tachyarrhythmias, angina, nervousness, palpitations, sweating, tremor, and changes in bowel habits. Symptoms of hyperthyroidism are frequently atypical, masked, or absent in elderly patients.

CONTRAINDICATIONS

Thyroid hormone is contraindicated in hyperthyroidism. It should not be used in the euthyroid state except for purposes of suppressing nonfunctioning nodules.

PRECAUTIONS

Because of the frequent coexistence of overt or subclinical cardiac disease, the initial dose of thyroid hormone should be very low and dose increments should be made slowly in elderly patients. Periodic electrocardiogram should be performed until full dosing is achieved. Unstable cardiac status may require temporary discontinuation of thyroid hormone and subsequent resumption of a lower dosage. Although myxedema itself may produce cardiac symptoms, which may actually be improved by the institution of thyroid hormone, extreme caution is required in this setting.

Full replacement doses tend to be approximately 30% lower in aged patients than younger adults, probably because of decreased metabolic disposal. Clinical end points are unreliable, and determination of optimum dose rests on periodic thyroid function testing.

Over the years, it is possible that the patient's optimum replacement dose could further decline, as metabolic clearance of hormone continues to decline with advancing age. However, because hypothyroidism in the elderly is often due to subclinical thyroiditis, thyroid function may decline further, necessitating an increase in dose. Thyroid status should be monitored in the long term using appropriate thyroid function tests.

INDICATIONS

Thyroid hormone is indicated in the treatment of hypothyroidism. It may be used in euthyroid individuals for purposes of suppressing nonfunctioning solitary thyroid nodules. These nodules must first, however, be evaluated for the presence of carcinoma. This is particularly important in late life when thyroid carcinoma tends to be more aggressive.

DOSING IN PRIMARY HYPOTHYROIDISM

Initial dose: 0.025 mg levothyroxine per day.
Dose increment: 0.025 mg added to daily dose every 4 weeks, until TSH is lowered to normal range.
Note: Patients with cardiac disease may require lower initial and incremental doses. There may be a lag phase of several weeks before the TSH normalizes, so that when normal TSH is approached, further dose increases should not be made until a few weeks have elapsed and the TSH can be rechecked.

Dosage equivalents of the various preparations are given in Table 19-1.

BIBLIOGRAPHY

Gambert, S. R., and Tsitouras, P. D. Effect of age on thyroid hormone physiology and function. *J. Am. Geriatr. Soc.* 33:360–365, 1985.

Hodkinson, H. M., and Irvine, R. E. The endocrine system—thyroid disease in the elderly. In J. C. Brocklehurst, *Textbook of Geriatric Medicine and Gerontology* (3rd ed.). Edinburgh: Churchill Livingstone, 1985. Pp. 686–714.

Jackson, I. M. D., and Cobb, W. E. Why does anyone still use desiccated thyroid USP? *Am. J. Med.* 64:284, 1978.

Livingston, E. H., Herschman, J. M., Sawin, C. T., et al. Prevalence of thyroid disease and abnormal thyroid tests in older hospitalized and elderly persons. *J. Amer. Geriatr. Soc.* 35:109–114, 1987.

Sex Hormones and Related Agents

ESTROGEN
Because of dramatic changes in the hormonal environment that occur at the time of menopause, a functional estrogen deficiency exists in late life. The clinical manifestations that have traditionally been attributed to these hormonal changes in women include osteoporosis, pelvic relaxation, atrophic vaginitis, and urinary stress incontinence. It is not always clear to what extent estrogen deficiency alone is to blame for these problems when they occur. Nonetheless, estrogen replacement appears to offer some degree of clinical benefit. Unfortunately, the older the patient, the less benefit is likely to occur.

Postmenopausal hot flushes, which are clearly suppressed by estrogen replacement therapy, probably do not persist into late life. Only rarely do women continue to have such menopausal symptoms more than 10 years after the last menstrual period; in 80% of cases, these symptoms subside within 2 years. Flushes and related symptoms that begin years after the menopause are likely to be due to other problems and should be approached as such.

The effects of estrogen on skin and hair are less well defined and will not be considered here.

Hormonal Changes in Women
At the time of menopause, ovarian synthesis of estradiol, the most potent form of estrogen, declines by 85%. In the postmenopausal woman, estrone becomes the most abundant source of estrogen, but it is only one sixth as active as estradiol. Postmenopausal estrone is largely derived from peripheral conversion of nonovarian androgens, primarily androstenedione, in the adrenal gland, adipose tissue, and liver. The production of estrone doubles after the menopause, but this accelerated conversion rate does not make up for loss of ovarian estradiol. In addition, levels of androgenic precursors decline.

Progesterone levels become noncyclical and are maintained at low levels found in the secretory phase of the premenopause.

These hormonal changes occur largely at the time of the menopause and do not progress significantly with age thereafter. However, the severity of osteoporosis, urinary dysfunction, and pelvic relaxation continues to increase with time.

Pharmacologic Considerations
Mechanism of Action
Estrogen acts on the cellular level where it binds to specific nuclear receptors and initiates a series of events leading to increased protein synthesis in target tissues. Among the effects of estrogen is reversal of postmenopausal cellular atrophy of estrogen-sensitive tissues, including stratified squamous tissue lining the vagina and the distal urethra. In nongeriatric subjects, estrogen appears to reverse age-related thinning of the epidermis in general, probably by increasing collagen synthesis. However, this effect reaches a plateau, with no increase in collagen occurring after a finite period of time, and the

276

effect has not been successfully applied to the treatment of skin aging.

Estrogen is thought to reduce the sensitivity of the osteoclast to parathyroid hormone, thereby reducing the increased bone resorption that occurs in osteoporosis. Recent work indicates that estrogen receptors are found in bone itself, so that the therapeutic effect of the hormone could be a direct one. The subject of estrogen treatment of osteoporosis is fully discussed in Chap. 22.

Clinically, estrogen is administered as estradiol, estriol, estrone, or as conjugated estrogens. There is no strong evidence that one form produces a better therapeutic effect than another.

Other Actions

In the liver, estrogen stimulates protein synthesis. When estrogen is administered orally, the amount of hormone delivered to the liver is great and protein synthesis is markedly enhanced. Important proteins that are affected include fibrinogen, renin substrate, coagulation factors, hormone binding globulins, and apolipoproteins A_1 and A_2, the key protein constituents of high-density lipoprotein (HDL) cholesterol. Estrogen decreases production of the intrinsic anticoagulant antithrombin III, enhancing coagulability, and decreases production of hepatic triglyceride lipase, increasing triglyceride levels.

Pharmacokinetics

Estrogens are available in preparations that enable the hormone to be rapidly and completely absorbed through the gastrointestinal tract, mucous membranes, and the skin. Estrone, estradiol, and inactive estrone sulfate are all reversibly interconverted in the liver and other peripheral sites, and ultimately oxidized to steroids with varying estrogenic potency. For this reason, the administered estrogen may be present in the serum in different forms. When given orally, potent estradiol still yields only a small increase in serum estradiol, but a large increase in estrone, thus failing to approximate the premenopausal hormonal environment in the serum. At the cellular level, this ratio is reversed, which may in part explain the observation that there is little therapeutic difference among the various preparations.

In its first pass through the liver, roughly 30% of oral estrogen is inactivated to renally excreted conjugates. A portion of estrogen and its metabolites undergoes enterohepatic circulation. This pathway may be particularly important when exogenous estrogens are administered by the oral route.

Like endogenous estrogens, exogenous estrogens are bound to serum albumin and sex hormone binding globulin (SHBG). Estrogen itself increases production of SHBG, reducing the unbound, free fraction of estrogen that is able to cross cell membranes and exert its pharmacologic action.

Routes of Delivery

Estrogen is available for oral, vaginal, and transdermal use. Parenteral routes of delivery, namely, transdermal and intravaginal, circumvent the liver on the "first pass," and minimize the production of hepatic by-products. This may reduce side effects that are mediated by the liver, but more study is needed to ascertain whether therapeutic effects are altered in any way.

Like the oral route, **vaginal** application of conjugated estrogen produces a low ratio of estradiol to estrone in serum. In contrast, micronized 17-beta estradiol produces a high ratio, approximating that seen in the premenopause. However, because of cellular metabolism and action, it is possible that the youthful ratio in serum does not confer a therapeutic advantage to the postmenopausal woman.

Absorption of estrogen through the vagina is significant, but may vary from patient to patient. It is most rapidly absorbed through atrophic vaginal mucosa, and this absorption may diminish somewhat with use as the mucosa cornifies in response to the estrogen. The amount absorbed is generally attenuated after 3 to 4 months of use, theoretically reducing its systemic efficacy. However, the vaginal route appears to be more effective than oral estrogen in reversing vaginal mucosal atrophy.

Transdermal estradiol is available in a skin patch that produces constant serum levels of estrone and estradiol for 3 days. Again the ratio of estradiol to estrone is high, but the advantages of this are unknown. Production of hepatic by-products is low. While this reduces the incidence of adverse effects, it could theoretically eliminate cardioprotective effects of estrogen by failing to increase hepatic production of apolipoproteins. More study is needed to know whether this is in fact the case.

Transdermal estradiol has proliferative effects on the endometrium, reduces the severity of postmenopausal hot flushes, and increases the maturational index of vaginal cytology. There is only limited information on the effects of transdermal systems on bone mineral density, but there is no reason to believe it would be less effective than oral hormone for the prevention of osteoporosis.

Available Forms of Estrogen

Conjugated equine estrogen (Premarin, others) consists of a mixture of estrone sulfate and renally excreted sulfates of equine estrogens that produce estrogenic effects in humans. When administered orally, it appears to have somewhat greater ability to form hepatic by-products than oral estrone or micronized (orally available) 17–beta estradiol. This may be because the equine estrogen, equilin, has greater potency.

17-beta estradiol is available in a micronized form that is well absorbed orally (Estrace) or vaginally. It is also available as a transdermal preparation (Estraderm). Although endogenously more potent than estrone, there is no evidence that estradiol preparations are therapeutically superior to other exogenous estrogens in postmenopausal women.

Estrone is given orally as the sulfate (Ogen). It is thought to be therapeutically equivalent to conjugated estrogens and estradiol, but has not gained popularity in the United States. **Estriol** is not generally available in the United States, although it is arguably as effective and safe as other forms.

Ethinyl estradiol and mestranol are potent preparations that are used primarily in oral contraceptives. They are metabolized very slowly by the liver and have very long half-lives, resulting in great potency. Furthermore, their ability to produce hepatic by-products is greatly exaggerated as compared to their estrogenic effects, even in low doses, so there is no rationale for using them in postmenopausal replacement therapy.

Adverse Effects

The effects of postmenopausal estrogen on women over the age of 75 probably differ from those seen in younger patients. This is related not only to the pharmacology of preparations used, but also to physiologic differences in older women. Side effects of postmenopausal estrogens have been determined from studies that include primarily middle-aged subjects.

Estrogen stimulates the endometrium and produces hyperplasia. **Breakthrough bleeding** may occur. **Withdrawal bleeding** is more likely if progestogen is added to the regimen. Age-related atrophy of the endometrium does not necessarily prevent this because the endometrium remains sensitive to hormonal stimulation. Bleeding may be the reason for an elderly patient not to accept hormonal treatment because it is perceived as the resumption of menses. Continuous daily administration may eliminate withdrawal bleeding.

Exogenous estrogens are associated with a 2- to 15-fold increased risk of **endometrial carcinoma.** These levels of risk should be viewed in light of the fact that endometrial cancer is uncommon. The risk increases with increasing doses and with duration of hormone use. The risk of endometrial carcinoma in general increases with age, but it is not known if older women are at increased risk of estrogen-associated adenocarcinoma.

Unopposed estrogen produces **endometrial hyperplasia** in a large proportion of women. The adenomatous or atypical histologic types are precursors to endometrial carcinoma. Fortunately, estrogen more commonly produces cystic hyperplasia, which is considered benign. No chemical form of estrogen that is therapeutically effective has been shown to be safer than any other in this regard.

The risk of developing endometrial carcinoma or its precursors can be significantly reduced by the addition of progestational agents to the regimen (see below). However, individual patients may still be at risk for developing cancer despite the addition of progestational agents. Baseline and periodic endometrial biopsy are recommended in patients on long-term estrogen. Unfortunately, this medically benign procedure may be difficult to perform in elderly women, in whom the cervix is often stenotic. Estrogen therapy itself may facilitate the procedure, but patient acceptance is nonetheless low.

Many of the adverse effects to be discussed in the following paragraphs have been noted in young women on oral contraceptive agents, and it is not known to what extent the risk can be extrapolated to women in the geriatric age group. Combination oral contraceptive agents contain potent synthetic estrogens, whereas the postmenopausal woman is most often treated with forms of estrogen that appear to have less effect on hepatic protein synthesis. Also, combination oral contraceptives contain progestational agents and it is often difficult to know which side effect is due to these, which to estrogen, and which to the combination. Finally, oral contraceptives contain the synthetic androgenic progestins, whereas the conventional postmenopausal agent, medroxyprogesterone, differs significantly in its metabolic effects. Although these hormones are active substances, and were not intended by nature to circulate in the elderly woman, another important difference is that postmenopausal treatment involves replacement, whereas oral contraceptives constitute a hormonal supplement.

Thrombophlebitis is a recognized risk of estrogen therapy. Estrogen increases the production of hepatic coagulation factors and is associated with decreased antithrombin-III activity. Coagulability may also be enhanced by actions on platelets and on lower extremity hemodynamics. Although no increase in the incidence of clotting has been reported with postmenopausal estrogen use (Premarin), it is prudent to avoid all estrogen products in women with a history of thrombophlebitis during pregnancy or prior hormonal treatment. This type of history suggests the possibility of a subclinical hypercoagulable state that could be unmasked by pharmacologic influences. A remote history of phlebitis in association with a risk factor such as prolonged bed rest, hip fracture, or surgery theoretically should not proscribe the use of estrogen if the indication is a strong one. Unfortunately, there is not enough data to guarantee its absolute safety in these patients.

By stimulating the production of hepatic triglyceride lipase, estrogen may result in **elevation of serum triglycerides.** The clinical consequences of this are uncertain.

Estrogen **increases bile lithogenicity** and gallstone size may be increased. This is presumed to be due to alterations in hepatic cholesterol metabolism leading to increased cholesterol synthesis and increase in the cholesterol fraction of bile. There is some evidence that transdermal estrogen is less likely to do this than oral preparations.

Approximately 5% of patients treated with estrogen develop reversible **elevations of blood pressure.** This has been attributed to hepatic production of renin substrate and theoretically could be avoided if the non-oral route is used. However, postmenopausal replacement therapy has generally been associated with maintenance or even lowering of blood pressure, the reasons for which are unclear. Hypertension probably is not a major problem in the elderly patient treated with estrogen, but periodic blood pressure monitoring is recommended, particularly in those who have diastolic hypertension.

Impaired glucose tolerance has been reported with oral contraceptive use, and is probably related to the progesterone component, which decreases binding of insulin to its tissue receptors. Unopposed estrogen may actually reduce this insulin resistance and has occasionally been reported to improve glucose tolerance in diabetics. Medroxyprogesterone has not been shown to impair glucose tolerance. Nonetheless, because of the high prevalence of impaired glucose tolerance in the elderly, periodic checks of glucose are warranted.

Other effects attributed to estrogen include migraine headache, edema, breast swelling and tenderness, nausea, and weight gain. Liver disease has been associated with oral contraceptive use but the importance of this problem in postmenopausal replacement therapy is not known.

Estrogens, Lipids, and Arterial Disease

Estrogens increase the serum levels of HDL cholesterol, in particular the subfraction (HDL_2) most strongly associated with decreased atherogenic risk. Low-density lipoprotein cholesterol (LDL) levels are decreased by estrogens. Studies of postmenopausal women have in fact generally demonstrated a decreased cardiac mortality in those on estrogen replacement compared to those not using estrogen. Estrogen may elevate triglyceride levels; however, hypertriglyceridemia in the absence of hypercholesterolemia may not increase cardiac risk (see Chap. 17).

Non-oral estrogens are less likely to stimulate hepatic production of apolipoproteins and do not as readily increase levels of HDL. LDL levels may decline, however. More study is required to ascertain whether non-oral estrogen retains the putative cardioprotective effect attributed to oral estrogen.

The cardiac consequences of added progestins are not known (see Progestational Agents, below).

Although the cardiac effects of postmenopausal hormones are not perfectly understood, the importance of hyperlipidemia itself in the elderly is the subject of controversy (see Chap. 17). Maintenance of a cardioprotective lipid profile must be weighed against other risks and benefits of these hormones in elderly women.

Estrogen and Breast Cancer

There is considerable controversy as to whether exogenous estrogens increase the risk of breast cancer. Most studies show that estrogen users have no increased risk of developing breast cancer, but there is not unanimous agreement. Part of the disagreement is probably due to the fact that these are not prospective studies in which high-risk patients were identified by baseline mammogram or exhaustive family history. It is logical to conclude that there is a subgroup of patients who harbor subclinical tumors that, if not initiated by exogenous estrogen, are accelerated by it.

One recently published study in Sweden (see Bergkvist et al.) demonstrated that long-term postmenopausal estrogen therapy increased the risk of breast cancer. Too few women in that study used conjugated estrogens (the most commonly used preparation in the United States) to know precisely, but no increased risk could be demonstrated in that subgroup. As in most estrogen studies, the patients were not in the geriatric age group. Although the risk of breast cancer increases with age, it is not known if elderly women would be at higher or lower risk than others exposed to hormones.

In contrast to the risk of estrogen-induced endometrial cancer, in which the addition of progesterone is clearly beneficial, the role of progesterone in the development or prevention of breast cancer is not well defined. The Swedish study suggested that the addition of a progestational agent might actually increase the risk. This is in contrast to previous studies.

In summary, the link of estrogen and breast cancer remains unresolved. However, it is likely that careful patient selection and baseline mammogram will keep the risk at bay. Progestational agents do not necessarily reduce the risk of developing breast cancer and may increase the risk in certain women.

Effects on Laboratory Values

Exogenous estrogens increase the hepatic synthesis of many proteins, including cortisol-binding globulin (CBG), thyroid-binding globulin (TBG), and transferrin. Increase in these particular proteins is probably unimportant medically, but will alter laboratory parameters. Increased TBG falsely elevates total T_4 levels; confirmatory assessment of TBG with resin uptake test (T_3RU) should be done to rule out true hyperthyroidism. Increased transferrin may confuse the differential diagnosis of anemia. Increased CBG may falsely elevate serum cortisol levels.

Important Drug Interactions

Although there is little clinical information on drug interactions with postmenopausal hormone therapy, there is abundant information on interactions with oral contraceptive agents. These drugs may lose their efficacy when hepatic enzyme-inducing drugs are given, producing clinically obvious end points, such as pregnancy or breakthrough menstrual bleeding. Clinical consequences of these interactions would be more difficult to judge in the patient being treated for geriatric disorders such as osteoporosis. Important enzyme inducers include rifampin, anticonvulsants, and meprobamate. Theoretically, enzyme inducers should interfere less with nonoral than with oral estrogens.

Hormones can also influence the metabolism of other drugs. Oral contraceptives have been reported to inhibit the metabolism of tricyclic antidepressants, barbiturates, meperidine, methyldopa, and diazepam. Potential interactions occur with other benzodiazepines, phenytoin, theophylline, and prednisone. However, estrogen can reduce the sensitivity of warfarin by increasing the production of clotting factors.

Although reports of clinical interactions with postmenopausal hormones are sparse, it is prudent to observe precautions when drugs with narrow therapeutic-to-toxic ratio are being given. Likewise, potent enzyme inducers should be expected, on theoretical grounds, to reduce the efficacy of postmenopausal hormones.

Contraindications

Estrogen is contraindicated in patients with a history of breast or endometrial cancer. It is also contraindicated when there is a history of thrombophlebitis related to pregnancy or hormone treatment. It is relatively contraindicated in those with a history of thrombophlebitis in other settings, such as prolonged bed rest or hip fracture.

Estrogen is contraindicated in patients with symptomatic gallbladder disease or liver disease. Those with "silent" gallstones should only take estrogen if the indication is extremely strong, and in these cases periodic ultrasound monitoring should be performed. Estrogen is contraindicated in patients with serum triglyceride levels approaching 500 mg/dl.

Precautions

Patients on estrogen treatment should have baseline and periodic monitoring of blood pressure, blood glucose, and serum triglyceride.

Baseline mammogram should be performed on patients prior to the institution of hormone replacement therapy. Annual mammogram is recommended thereafter.

Endometrial sampling for the presence of carcinoma or hyperplasia should be offered to patients at baseline and annually. This procedure may be made more difficult in elderly women if there is cervical stenosis. Cervical pap smear should be performed at baseline and annually; sample should include the endocervix, as well as the posterior fornix where extruded endometrial cells may sometimes be found.

The Place of Estrogen Therapy in Geriatrics

Estrogen is indicated for the treatment of dyspareunia, dryness, discharge, or pruritus due to atrophic vaginitis. If vaginal bleeding occurs in association with atrophic vaginitis, serious pathology of the genitourinary system should be ruled out before bleeding is attributed to atrophic vaginitis and estrogen therapy is instituted.

Urinary stress incontinence in geriatric patients responds variably to estrogen treatment (see Chap. 23).

Estrogen is indicated for the prevention of postmenopausal osteoporosis, but its use in women over the age of 75 years is controversial. This topic is discussed in detail in Chap. 22.

In contrast to perimenopausal hot flushes, flushes that present late in life, after the cessation of earlier menopausal symptoms, should not be treated with estrogens. Such symptoms are related to other medical problems or to medications, and the cause should be investigated.

Estrogen is not indicated for the prevention or treatment of age-related changes such as sagging skin, photoaging (dermatoheliosis), or hair loss. Although some investigators have demonstrated anti-aging effects on collagen in vitro, clinical efficacy of estrogen for these indications is anecdotal and has not been substantiated.

PROGESTATIONAL AGENTS IN POSTMENOPAUSAL ESTROGEN REPLACEMENT THERAPY

It is widely accepted that the addition of a progestational agent to postmenopausal estrogen therapy reduces the risk of endometrial carcinoma. However, the addition of a progestin may not be without its pitfalls.

In the United States, the most widely prescribed agent for this purpose is medroxyprogesterone, which resembles native progesterone biologically more so than other progestins.

Mechanism of Action

Progesterones are thought to prevent estrogen-induced endometrial hyperplasia by antagonizing the stimulatory effects of estrogen on epithelial DNA synthesis. This may come about via a reduction in uterine estrogen receptors or by a direct antagonism of estrogen-induced cell division. This view replaces the traditional explanation that progesterone promotes shedding of the stimulated endometrium. The older view is questionable because the continuous (as opposed to cyclical) addition of progestins leads to hypoplastic or atrophic changes of the endometrium.

Progesterone may also antagonize the effects of estrogen in other tissues, including the breast and brain. However, progesterone may have a direct effect on bone, acting synergistically with estrogen to maintain bone mass.

Synthetic progestins used clinically differ from native progesterone in some of their pharmacologic effects.

Medroxyprogesterone (Provera) is presently the progestational agent most commonly prescribed to postmenopausal women in the United States. Unlike the 19-norprogesterones, which are used in oral contraceptive therapy and certain endocrine disorders, medroxyprogesterone, a 17-acetoxyprogesterone, has very low androgenic activity while maintaining adequate antagonistic effects on estrogen in the endometrium. A related agent, megestrol (Megace), is used primarily in the treatment of endometrial carcinoma.

Medroxyprogesterone is absorbed orally. Unabsorbed medroxyprogesterone may be partly metabolized in the gastrointestinal mucosa itself. Its biologic half-life is approximately 40–60 hours. Formulations differ in their bioavailability. It has been suggested that preparations that are better absorbed may have more potent and possibly more undesirable metabolic effects than demonstrated in oft-quoted studies, but this remains to be clarified.

Adverse Effects

Synthetic progestins **raise serum levels of LDL cholesterol** and lower HDL cholesterol. When added to a postmenopausal estrogen regimen, this is thought to negate the beneficial lipid profile produced by the latter. It has been argued that medroxyprogesterone has a less adverse effect in this regard than the 19–norprogesterones, but this has been disputed. Lack of lipid alterations demonstrated in early studies may have been due to poor bioavailability of the medroxyprogesterone preparation tested, and metabolic effects may change with dose and duration of therapy. There is some evidence that cyclic administration of progestin has less adverse effect on lipids than continuous. Native progesterone appears to be devoid of adverse effects on lipids, but orally absorbed preparations are not yet available in the United States.

Further study is needed to determine what progesterone regimen can best maintain the cardioprotective lipid profile produced by estrogen.

While most, but not all, evidence suggests that exogenous estrogens do not increase the risk of breast cancer, the effects of added progestin have been less well studied. Progesterone antagonizes the effects of estrogen in normal breast tissue but there is conflicting evidence of the effects of progestins in estrogen-associated breast cancer.

The addition of a progestational agent to an estrogen regimen increases the likelihood of **withdrawal bleeding**, which may be associated with cramping and related menstrual discomforts. Breakthrough or irregular bleeding may also occur. Resumption of menstrual-like bleeding late in life may produce annoyance, dismay, fear, or bemusement. The patient should be forewarned about the possibility of bleeding. Continuous progesterone therapy is less likely than cyclic to produce bleeding.

In the doses used to treat postmenopausal women, medroxyprogesterone is generally well tolerated. Symptoms such as acne, hirsutism, and weight gain seen with 19-norprogesterones are not an important problem in postmenopausal regimens using medroxyprogesterone. Medroxyprogesterone does not appear to produce elevations in blood pressure, alterations in clotting factors, or impairment in glucose tolerance.

Nonetheless, one must carefully assess the risk-benefit ratio of adding a progestational agent. The incidence of endometrial cancer is low, even in women given unopposed estrogen. The addition of progestin does not reduce and may increase the risk of breast cancer, and there is reason to believe that it reverses the cardioprotective effect of estrogens.

Precautions

Patients should have baseline and periodic monitoring of blood pressure, blood sugar, and cholesterol subfractions.

Indications

Addition of a progestational agent, medroxyprogesterone, is indicated in women on long-term estrogen replacement therapy if the uterus is present, in order to prevent the development of endometrial cancer. Periodic endometrial biopsy is not a substitute, but may be an alternative for women in whom the addition of progesterone is not desirable.

CYCLIC OR CONTINUOUS THERAPY?

Estrogen has traditionally been prescribed in a cyclic regimen for 3 weeks of the month, withdrawing treatment for the last week. This method is based on the assumption that it is best to mimic the natural menstrual cycle and allow the stimulated endometrium to rest or to shed. It will also reduce the absolute exposure to the exogenous hormone. However, continuous estrogen is theoretically more physiologic for the postmenopausal woman because it produces sustained youthful levels throughout the month. Potential advantages of continuous progestin include a lower incidence of withdrawal bleeding and a less complicated regimen.

There is no evidence that cyclic administration of unopposed estrogen is safer for the endometrium than continuous treatment. Animal studies indicate that with continuous treatment the stimulatory effects of estrogen ultimately wane. Cyclic estrogen as well as continuous estrogen may be associated with vaginal bleeding. There is some evidence that cyclic progestins are less harmful to the lipid profile than continuous treatment, but this point requires further study.

DOSING

There is no reason to be confident that the currently recommended doses of estrogen and progestins are appropriate for all women. However, there are no convenient, inexpensive, or well-accepted methods by which to gauge the most effective or safest dose. Endometrial biopsy is the definitive method of judging whether progestin dose is adequate. Vaginal bleeding may respond to lowering of the estrogen dose or raising of the dose or duration of progesterone. Bone mineral density study may gauge the adequacy of the estrogen dose in osteoporosis, but is relatively inaccurate for short-term (less than 2-year) dose adjustments. Metabolic parameters such as urinary hydroxyproline and urinary calcium are nonspecific and may be expensive.

Therefore, dose guidelines given below represent the average recommended dose. Equivalent doses of various preparations are given in Table 20–1.

For Osteoporosis

Average daily dose: conjugated estrogen 0.625 mg/day.
This topic is covered in more detail in Chap. 22.

Table 20-1. Estrogen Preparations: Dosage Equivalents

Estrogen Dose Equivalents*
Equine estrogen (Premarin, others) 0.625 mg
Estradiol (Estrace) 1 mg
Estrone (Ogen) 1.25 mg
Transdermal estradiol (Estraderm) 0.05 mg (10 cm²) given every 3rd day

*Equivalent to 0.625 mg equine estrogen.

For Stress Urinary Incontinence

Daily: topical application of estrogen cream to urethra. If no response in 1 month, 0.3–0.625 mg conjugated estrogen cream per vagina.

Maximum daily dose: 1.25 mg; if no response in 3 months, discontinue use.

Other routes of administration may be preferred by some patients.

This topic is covered in more detail in Chap. 23.

For Atrophic Vaginitis

Daily: 0.3–0.625 mg conjugated estrogen cream per vagina for 3 months. Upon resolution of symptoms, dose may be reduced to thrice weekly, or periodic courses of treatment may be given as needed. Other routes of administration may be preferred by some patients.

Maximum daily dose: 1.25 mg.

Cyclic Regimen

Daily estrogen for days 1–25 of cycle; no estrogen for remainder of the calendar month. If uterus is intact, add medroxyprogesterone 5–10 mg on days 12–25 of cycle.

Continuous Regimen

Conjugated estrogen 0.3–1.25 mg/day. If uterus is intact, add medroxyprogesterone 2.5–5.0 mg/day.

TAMOXIFEN

Tamoxifen is a nonsteroid with antiestrogenic properties. Its major use in geriatrics is in the treatment of breast cancer.

Pharmacologic Considerations

Mechanism of Action

Tamoxifen is structurally related to diethylstilbesterol. It is thought to act by binding competitively to estrogen receptors (ER) and inhibiting binding of estrogen. Tamoxifen has little or no estrogenic activity in breast tissues, but the presence of the tamoxifen-ER complex results in compensatory increase in the production of ER, so that estrogenic activity can then take place over time. It has thus been suggested that tamoxifen may exert at least part of its antitumor effect independent of its interaction with the ER; indirect evidence for this is that it appears to have some effect on certain ER-negative breast tumors. In fact, tamoxifen is species- and tissue-specific, acting as an estrogen antagonist in some species or tissues and an agonist in others. There may be interindividual variation as well.

The new view of tamoxifen's mechanism of action has led to an extension of its application. It is still primarily used against breast tumors in women over the age of 50, who tend to have tumors rich in ER, but who also tend to have a better prognosis than younger women with breast cancer in general. It is generally believed that ER-rich tumors are more responsive to tamoxifen than those tumors with lower concentrations of ER or with ER-negative tumors, but it is currently not possible to accurately predict which category of patient is most likely to respond.

Other Actions

Like estrogen, tamoxifen or its metabolites may have a variety of effects on the liver, although few have been well defined. Tamoxifen stimulates hepatic production of sex hormone binding globulin, suggesting that it could influence production of other hepatic proteins. In contrast, it has been associated with moderate reductions in levels of antithrombin III, an endogenous anticoagulant. A few reports that tamoxifen affects levels of serum lipids are contradictory.

In accordance with its tissue-specific effects, tamoxifen may behave as an estrogen agonist with respect to bone. Limited study has revealed that tamoxifen has no adverse effect on and may even act to preserve bone mass. It is thought to block bone resorption mediated by parathyroid hormone. Its effects on bone have not been studied in women without breast disease, who may have lower baseline bone mineral content than those prone to breast disease; thus, it is not known if it has applicability in the treatment of osteoporosis.

Pharmacokinetics

Tamoxifen is well absorbed, reaching peak levels in the serum after 4 or more hours. It is extensively metabolized in the liver to several active metabolites, the function of which have not been precisely defined. It is possible that one or more of these is responsible for both pharmacodynamic and pharmacokinetic effects.

Tamoxifen and its metabolites are eliminated very slowly, which may be partly because of enterohepatic circulation. Biologic half-life is more than 2 weeks. Steady-state plasma concentrations are not achieved for up to 4 weeks.

Tamoxifen is highly bound to serum albumin.

Adverse Effects

Tamoxifen is better tolerated than other hormonal treatments for breast cancer and important immediate side effects are unusual.

Nausea and vomiting may occur in some patients; it is not known if this is due to gastric irritation or a central mechanism.

"Tumor flare" may occur when tamoxifen is first initiated, and is thought to be due to temporary enhancement of tumor. This can be characterized by a transient increase in pain, erythema, or swelling at the site of the primary tumor or a soft tissue metastasis. **Transient hypercalcemia** may be associated with this phenomenon if tumor has metastasized to bone. Tumor flare and associated effects are generally benign.

Central nervous system (CNS) symptoms are unusual, but **depression** has occurred. Less commonly reported effects include **headache** and **irritability**. CNS symptoms are explained by the fact that there are estrogen receptors in the brain.

Tamoxifen is thought to have **estrogen agonist effects on genital tissues** of postmenopausal women. These effects could be beneficial in women with atrophic vaginitis, but discharge, bleeding, and vaginitis have also been reported. Effects on other estrogen-sensitive urogenital tissues have not been well documented. Reports that tamoxifen increases the risk of endometrial carcinoma are confounded by the fact that patients with breast cancer are at higher risk of developing endometrial cancer in general.

Thromboembolic phenomena have been reported rarely. Although the cancer setting itself could predispose to these events, it is possible that they could be related to tamoxifen's ability to reduce antithrombin-III levels; individuals with hereditary antithrombin-III deficiency would be more prone to this problem.

A form of **retinopathy** has been associated with tamoxifen but is thought to be exceedingly rare at ordinary doses.

Hot flushes are reported in a significant minority of premenopausal women, but are unlikely to occur in geriatric patients because baseline estrogen status is low.

As mentioned above, tamoxifen appears to preserve rather than reduce bone mass. There is thus no evidence that this "anti-estrogen" would be harmful to women with osteoporosis.

Important Drug Interactions

Tamoxifen has been reported to increase warfarin sensitivity leading to bleeding episodes. It has been speculated that this is due either to a protein displacement reaction or to the competition between warfarin and tamoxifen for hepatic microsomal enzymes, resulting in decreased warfarin metabolism. In the latter mechanism, a reduction in tamoxifen metabolism could also occur; any resulting change in antitumor efficacy of tamoxifen would depend on the extent to which tamoxifen or its active metabolites were responsible for the antitumor effect. It would be difficult to document such effects, which have not yet been reported in patients on tamoxifen who are exposed to other drugs affecting hepatic microsomal enzymes.

Tamoxifen has also been associated with increases in serum levels of digitoxin, possibly because of the same mechanism. An interaction with digoxin would not be expected.

There is some evidence that tamoxifen and chemotherapeutic agents given together each counteract the antitumor effect of the other.

Is Tamoxifen an Alternative to Surgery in Elderly Women?

The place of tamoxifen as adjuvant treatment in postmenopausal women with node-positive, ER-positive breast cancer has been well established. When tamoxifen is added to the primary treatment regimen, it improves disease-free survival. It may not affect overall survival, however, and its value as adjuvant treatment in nonmetastatic breast cancer is controversial.

If tamoxifen were found to be equal in efficacy to surgery for primary breast cancer, it would be a very useful treatment modality in geriatrics, particularly in the very aged, debilitated patient. Limited study indicates that tamoxifen given alone may be no worse than mastectomy alone in preventing death from breast cancer. However, patients receiving tamoxifen alone appear to have a higher local recurrence rate than those treated by mastectomy alone, and may eventually require surgery to eradicate primary (as opposed to metastatic) disease. Although tamoxifen would have served to postpone surgery for some women treated in this way, in other cases postponement of surgery might have the result that the tumor would become inoperable. Thus, limited study suggests that tamoxifen cannot be relied on to eradicate tumor but, by slowing tumor growth, it could be sufficient treatment in someone with projected short life expectancy.

A disadvantage of tamoxifen is that it may need to be taken indefinitely, whereas surgery, if curative, is a definitive procedure. Thus, noncompliance with tamoxifen therapy could lead to treatment failure. This could be an important disadvantage in the very patients for whom tamoxifen alone might be considered, such as those with dementia or those with multiple medical problems requiring a complicated drug regimen.

An obvious advantage of tamoxifen over mastectomy is cosmetic acceptability. However, it is not known how tamoxifen alone compares in efficacy to modified surgery such as lumpectomy or quadrantectomy, or how it compares to no treatment. There is limited evidence that tamoxifen alone is roughly comparable to radiation therapy in prolonging survival of women with locally invasive tumors. Until more is known, tamoxifen should be given as sole therapy only to patients unwilling or unable to undergo mastectomy or other established treatments.

The goal of tamoxifen given alone is to reduce the risk of developing metastatic disease, which may prove lifesaving or life-prolonging in certain patients, despite the fact that it does not necessarily prevent local disease progression. This may be an acceptable alternative to women of very advanced age or those who are medically unstable, whose life expectancy is more likely to be curtailed by nonneoplastic disease.

Indications

Tamoxifen is indicated in elderly women with metastatic cancer of the breast and may be used if ER status is unknown. The use of adjuvant tamoxifen in patients with localized (node-negative) resected tumor is controversial.

Tamoxifen may be used as sole therapy in women unable or unwilling to undergo surgery or radiation therapy for resectable tumor. Used in this way, it is not considered definitive treatment and may only postpone rather than eliminate the need for surgery.

Tamoxifen has a place in the management of male breast cancer as well, and currently is used as adjuvant therapy. Breast cancer in men is unusual but occurs largely among the elderly. Because of the infrequency of this problem, the precise indications for tamoxifen in men have not been well delineated.

The role for tamoxifen in the premenopausal woman with breast cancer is expanding but has not been well defined. Its use in benign conditions, such as mastalgia, is under investigation.

Dosing

Usual dose: 10 mg bid. The entire dose probably can be given once a day because of the long biologic half-life, but this method of administration has not been tested. Further study is needed to establish the optimal duration for the various indications.

HORMONAL TREATENT OF ADVANCED PROSTATE CANCER

The incidence of prostate cancer increases dramatically with age, with as many as 70% of men over the age of 80 harboring at least small foci of cancerous cells in the prostate, as demonstrated at autopsy. Although the high prevalence of these foci is not matched by a high rate of symptomatic disease, advanced prostate cancer remains an important clinical problem in older men. Hormonal manipulation is the hallmark of treating advanced prostate cancer. For a complete discussion of prostate cancer treatment, the reader is referred to the Bibliography readings (see Surya & Provet).

The purpose of hormonal treatment is to reduce androgenic stimulation of prostate cancer cells. The various modalities available are bilateral orchiectomy, the exogenous estrogen congener diethylstilbesterol (DES), the gonadotropin-releasing hormone-agonist leuprolide, and the antiandrogen flutamide.

Diethylstilbesterol (DES)

DES is a nonsteroid, which, in one of its steric configurations, is structurally similar to estrogen and has potent estrogenic action. It is taken orally and reduces serum testosterone levels by suppressing pituitary release of luteinizing hormone and possibly by a direct action on the Leydig cell. DES has not been shown to be more effective than bilateral orchiectomy in reducing symptoms and prolonging life in patients with metastatic prostate cancer. Although it is more acceptable to some men than orchiectomy, DES is medically less suitable because of its toxicity.

Adverse Effects

DES may produce **fluid retention**, painful **gynecomastia**, and **thromboembolic phenomena.** In contrast to the cardioprotective effects that exogenous estrogens produce in postmenopausal women, men with prostatic carcinoma who take DES have an **increased rate of mortality due to cardiovascular and cerebrovascular disease** over men who are treated with other methods. Although it is not surprising that there might be sex differences in response to exogenous estrogens, the cardiovascular and related toxicity of DES may be due to the fact that it is a long-acting substance and has greater potency than preparations commonly used in postmenopausal women.

Like estrogen, DES confounds thyroid function testing by increasing synthesis of thyroid binding globulin and other hepatic proteins.

Dosing

The usual recommended dose is 1 mg tid. However, there is evidence that smaller doses may be equally effective while producing fewer adverse effects.

Leuprolide (Lupron)

Leuprolide is an analog of gonadotropin releasing hormone, which acts by suppressing testicular function and testosterone release. This comes about after an initial stimulation of testicular function, which may actually produce a temporary disease flare. Ultimately, leuprolide produces a down-regulation of pituitary receptors and symptoms regress. The addition of the antiandrogen flutamide reduces the likelihood of disease flare (see below).

Leuprolide is as effective as DES and its efficacy is enhanced by concurrent administration of flutamide. Unlike DES, leuprolide does not appear to produce cardiovascular complications. Hot flushes, impotence, and decreased libido occur, and correlate with reductions in serum testosterone levels. Some of these problems may be less noticeable to men of advanced age but should be anticipated nonetheless. Another disadvantage of leuprolide is that it must be given by injection. The medication is also very expensive.

Leuprolide should be dispensed according to the directions of the oncology or urology consultant.

Flutamide (Eulexin)

Flutamide is a nonsteroid with antiandrogen effects. It prevents the binding of testicular and adrenal androgens to tissue receptors, and appears to be as effective as DES in the management of advanced prostate cancer. Although it commonly produces gynecomastia, it is less likely than DES to produce thromboembolic problems. Mild diarrhea may occur. Since it can be given orally, flutamide is more convenient than leuprolide. However, at present, flutamide tends to be given together with leuprolide to enhance the efficacy of the latter.

Flutamide should be dispensed according to the instructions of the oncology or urology consultant.

BIBLIOGRAPHY

Barrett-Connor, E. Postmenopausal estrogen replacement and breast cancer. *N. Engl J.* Med 321:319–320, 1989.

Bergkvist, L., Adami, H., Persson, I., et al. The risk of breast cancer after estrogen and estrogen-progestin replacement. *N. Engl. J. Med.* 321:293–297, 1989.

Bush, T. L., and Miller, V. T. Effects of pharmacologic agents used during menopause: impact on lipids and lipoproteins. In D. R. Mishell (ed.), *Menopause: Physiology and pharmacology.* Chicago: Year Book Medical Publishers, 1987. Pp. 187–208.

Chetkowski, R. J., Meldrum, D. R., Steingold, K. A., et al. Biologic effects of transdermal estradiol. *N. Engl. J. Med.* 314:1615–1620, 1986.

Gazet, J. C., Markopoulos, C., Ford, H. T., et al. Prospective randomised trial of tamoxifen versus surgery in elderly patients with breast cancer. *Lancet* 1:679–681, 1988.

Hirvonen, E., Malkonen, M., and Manninen, V. Effects of different progestogens on lipoproteins during postmenopausal replacement therapy. *N. Engl. J. Med.* 304:560–562, 1981.

Legha, S. S. Tamoxifen in the treatment of breast cancer. *Ann. Intern. Med.* 109:219–228, 1988.

Lufkin, E. G., Carpenter, P. C., Ory, S. J., Malkasian, G. D., and Edmonson, J. H. Estrogen replacement therapy: current recommendations. *Mayo Clin. Proc.* 63:453–460, 1988.

Mandel, F. P., Geola, F. L., Meldrum, D. R., Lu, J. H. K., Eggena, P.,

Sambhi, M. H., et al. Biological effects of various doses of vaginally administered conjugated equine estrogens in postmenopausal women. *J. Clin. Endocrinol. Metab.* 57:133–139, 1983.

Robertson, J. F., Todd, J. H., Ellis, I. O., et al. Comparison of mastectomy with tamoxifen for treating elderly patients with operable breast cancer. *Brit. Med. J.* 297:511–514, 1988.

Surya, B. V., and Provet, J. A. Manifestations of advanced prostate cancer: prognosis and treatment. *J. Urol.* 142:921–928, 1989.

Tenni, P., Lalich, D. L., and Byrne, M. J. Life threatening interaction between tamoxifen and warfarin. *Brit. Med. J.* 298:93, 1989.

Turken, S., Siris, E., Seldin, D., et al. Effects of tamoxifen on spinal bone density in women with breast cancer. *J. Natl. Cancer Inst.* 81:1086–1088, 1989.

Weinstein, L. Efficacy of a continuous estrogen-progestin regimen in the menopausal patient. *Obstet. Gyn.* 6:929–932, 1987.

Pharmacologic Approaches to Erectile Dysfunction

Sexual dysfunction is common in elderly men, with more than 50% suffering from impotence or erectile difficulties after the age of 75. In the majority of cases, organic causes such as vascular disease, neuropathic disorders, or a combination of medical problems may be at fault. Impotence is more likely to be multifactorial in the older man, and although psychogenic factors account for a smaller proportion of problems in this age group, they are frequently present. Important psychological factors in late life include depression and fear of or anxiety over a permanent involutional decline in sexual performance.

Many drugs may affect sexual function adversely, including sedatives, alcohol, antidepressants, cimetidine, estrogens, antiandrogens, anticholinergic agents, and antihypertensives, notably methyldopa, clonidine, reserpine, and guanethidine. The actual contribution of these drugs to impotence must be evaluated on a case-by-case basis because of the powerful effect of psychogenic factors.

Endocrinologic problems, such as hyperprolactinemia and primary or central hypogonadism, may be contributory, but it is important to emphasize that age alone is not associated with endocrinologic or gonadal failure. There is some evidence that androgen metabolism becomes impaired with advancing age leading to a decline in the production of the more potent androgenic hormones. Serum testosterone levels seem to decline with age, as do the number of sexual events, but no age-adjusted standards for testosterone have been determined and many very aged men have been found to have levels that are clearly in the normal range. Finally, the correlation between testosterone levels and sexuality is far from perfect.

The approach to the elderly man with impotence differs mainly in that expectations of sexual performance should take into account the normal physiologic changes that occur with age. The number of sexual events declines, the duration and firmness of erection may decline, and the time required to achieve an erection may be prolonged. These age changes occur with great interindividual variability and should always be evaluated in light of the patient's previous sexual performance.

A sensible search should be made for potentially reversible causes of sexual dysfunction. Counseling is an important component of treatment. Surgical approaches may be considered in selected, highly motivated patients (see Krane et al.).

The use of pharmacologic agents is controversial. A recent pharmaceutical mailing promoted Virilon (methyltestosterone capsules) and Aphrodyne (yohimbine) for "sexual retirement." A discussion of androgens and yohimbine is being included in this book because of this kind of publicity and because of patient inquiries.

SHOULD ANDROGENS BE USED?

The use of androgens has not been systematically studied in the setting of geriatric impotence. Androgens are unlikely to be effective except in conditions that are clearly related to hypogonadism, and in the elderly male the diagnosis of physiologic hypogonadism should not be made purely on the basis of a low serum testosterone level. Low serum testosterone levels do not correlate well with impotence in late life, and more often than not reflect the presence of underlying disease rather than hypogonadism. In addition, when interpreting serum levels, it is important to remember that testosterone is bound to sex hormone binding globulin, which increases somewhat with age. This leads to a decrease in the free or active fraction of serum testosterone, so that measurements of total rather than free hormone can be very misleading. Perhaps more important, serum levels do not measure androgenic activity at the tissue level.

Treatment with **oral androgens** may produce **edema, hepatic cholestasis,** and other forms of **liver disease.** Hepatic complications are largely related to the 17-alpha ethyl moiety of certain preparations (methyltestosterone, danazole, others) and have not been linked to parenteral testosterone esters. However, **all forms** of testosterone are capable of **stimulating the growth of prostatic tumors.** Although the exact risk has not been well delineated, the potential risk of empiric treatment with androgens might well outweigh the benefits in elderly men, in whom overt and subclinical prostatic pathology is extremely common.

Testosterone administration **may increase libido without improving erectile function.** While some investigators claim that androgen therapy may be effective in restoring potency in older men, the efficacy and risk-to-benefit ratio have not been studied in a controlled fashion.

Contraindications

Androgens are contraindicated in patients with prostatic carcinoma and should generally be avoided in those with benign prostatic hyperplasia and poorly controlled fluid-retaining states.

Recommendations

Until placebo-controlled study demonstrates that androgens are effective in subgroups of eugonadal elderly, indiscriminate use in such patients is discouraged, and androgen use should generally be confined to patients with sexual dysfunction that is clearly associated with hypogonadism. However, its potential usefulness should not be entirely discounted. A trial may be warranted in selected elderly men who are sexually active and highly motivated, if there is low free serum testosterone, and if there is no contraindication. These recommendations are not based on controlled study.

Dosing

Testosterone enanthate or cypionate 200 mg IM once a month for 3–4 months. If response occurs, continue for 6 months. This is considered a trial. Therapy should be discontinued at 6-month intervals in order to evaluate the effect.

YOHIMBINE (APHRODYNE, OTHERS)

Pharmacologic Considerations

Mechanism of Action

Yohimbine is an indole amine alkaloid, chemically related to reserpine. It is derived from the bark of yohimbine (Corynanthe yohimbe), which was considered an aphrodisiac before the modern medical era. The drug is a selective alpha$_2$ adrenergic blocking agent that acts presynaptically and has little blocking effect on postsynaptic alpha$_1$ receptors. Alpha$_2$ stimulation inhibits release of norepinephrine from nerve terminals and produces peripheral vasodilation. Central alpha$_2$ stimulation raises blood pressure. Yohimbine blocks the central alpha$_2$ activating action produced by clonidine.

The penis is richly implanted with alpha$_2$ receptors, although the distribution of these receptors has not been well delineated. Since alpha$_2$ stimulation inhibits the release of norepinephrine from nerve terminals, yohimbine increases the local concentration of norepinephrine. The effect of this should be to produce arteriolar and sinusoidal vasoconstriction and **produce** impotence rather than alleviate it, however, so that other explanations for its putative action must be invoked. Yohimbine does produce certain central excitatory effects at high doses so that a central mechanism could be invoked.

Although studies of yohimbine have included men as old as 70 years of age, there is no data on the older age group as a whole. In general, evaluations of drugs for impotence have demonstrated less benefit for older subjects than younger ones. The authors of a recent study assert that yohimbine may be effective in the treatment of psychogenic impotence even if some organic factors are present (see Reid et al.).

Pharmacokinetics

There is very limited pharmacologic data on yohimbine. It appears to be well absorbed orally and is completely metabolized, none being recovered unchanged in the urine. The serum half-life is only 35 minutes in young men. There is no pharmacokinetic information available in elderly men. Behavioral changes related to this agent may not be temporally related to its serum levels; some investigators report that its sexual effect in humans occurs in a delayed fashion, perhaps 2–3 weeks after therapy is instituted.

Adverse Effects

Yohimbine has been reported to produce **dizziness, nervousness, insomnia,** and **nausea,** but limited study suggests that the drug is generally well tolerated. Theoretically, this drug could produce fluid retention, tremor, central excitation, tachycardia, and exacerbation of hypertension, effects that have been observed in experimental conditions. Therefore, until more is known, caution is advised in the elderly.

Contraindications

Until more is known about the effects of currently recommended doses of yohimbine, it is prudent to avoid this agent in poorly controlled hypertension, tachycardia, cardiac arrhythmias, and anxiety states.

THE PLACE OF YOHIMBINE IN SEXUAL DYSFUNCTION

Until more is known about its risks, yohimbine should be dispensed cautiously and sparingly in elderly men; and until more is known about its efficacy, it should not be touted as an aphrodisiac. However, it may be counterproductive for the physician to denigrate the efficacy of an agent that is about to be prescribed for a condition so fraught with psychogenic input. Because of the importance of psychologic factors in the treatment of impotence, response to yohimbine does not rule out a placebo effect. A placebo-controlled trial of yohimbine, with informed consent, may be warranted in selected, highly motivated patients.

Dosing

The usual recommended dose is 6 mg tid. However, until more is known about this agent in elderly men, the starting dose should be 3 mg tid. If no adverse effects develop, and if desired efficacy does not occur within 2–3 weeks, the dose may be increased to 6 mg tid.

BIBLIOGRAPHY

Korenman, S. G. Impotence. In W. R. Hazzard, R. Andres, E. L. Bierman, and J. P. Blass (eds.), *Principles of Geriatric Medicine and Gerontology.* New York: McGraw-Hill, 1990. Pp. 1146–1154.

Krane, R. J., Goldstein, I., and Saenz de Tejada, I. Impotence. *N. Engl. J. Med.* 321:1648–1659, 1989.

Malloy, T. R., and Malkowicz, B. Pharmacologic treatment of impotence. *Urol. Clin. N. Amer.* 14:297–305, 1987.

Morales, A., Condra, M., Owen, J. A., et al. Is yohimbine effective in the treatment of organic impotence? Results of a controlled trial. *J. Urol.* 137:1168–1172, 1987.

Mulligan, T., and Katz, P. G. Erectile failure in the aged: evaluation and treatment. *J. Amer. Geriatr. Soc.* 36:54–62, 1988.

Reid, K., Surridge, D. H., Morales, A., et al. Double-blind trial of yohimbine in treatment of psychogenic impotence. *Lancet* 2: 421–423, 1987.

Medical Treatment of Osteoporosis

OSTEOPOROSIS IN THE ELDERLY

Osteoporosis is the loss of bone predisposing to fracture. After peaking in young adulthood, bone mass declines linearly with age in both men and women. In women, this process accelerates for several years after the menopause, leveling off to the previous age-related linear decline. At all ages, the average man has greater bone mass than the average woman. Because of these sex differences, osteoporotic fractures are much more common in women than in men. A variety of factors protect and impair bone integrity and result in wide interindividual variation in bone mass. Risk factors for osteoporosis are listed in Table 22–1.

Two clinical syndromes of osteoporosis have been described—*involutional* ("senile") and postmenopausal osteoporosis. Involutional osteoporosis is thought to result from the age-related linear decline in bone mass affecting both sexes and involving primarily compact bone of the proximal extremities (hip and proximal humerus). Postmenopausal osteoporosis has been attributed to the self-limited but accelerated process that takes place in certain women, affecting primarily trabecular bone (spine and wrist). There is significant overlap in the two syndromes with regard to their clinical expression, and probably their pathophysiology as well. Presently recognized treatment modalities are applied to both syndromes in women, but the controversial agent fluoride may produce different effects in trabecular and cortical bone.

The geriatric patient with osteoporosis differs from her middle-aged counterpart in important ways. Bone loss is generally well advanced by the age of 75 and there is no known treatment that reverses the process. Thus, the elderly patient has established osteoporosis and the fracture threshold has most likely already been attained. In addition, some elderly patients with osteoporosis have a component of superimposed osteomalacia due to vitamin D deficiency. Whereas osteoporosis involves the proportional loss of organic bone matrix and mineral, osteomalacia involves a disproportional loss of mineral. This mixed bone pathology is clinically indistinguishable from pure osteoporosis, but is likely to be present if vitamin D levels are low. Histologic osteomalacia is common in climates with a short sunny season, especially in home-bound elderly, and probably contributes to the fracture rate. Although osteoporosis is not reversible, it is possible to improve the mineralization defect that characterizes the osteomalacia component of the disease. It is probable that improvements in vitamin D status can reduce the risk of fractures.

Another important difference between the elderly and the middle-aged patient with osteoporosis is that the older patient may have more risk factors predisposing to falls, further increasing the likelihood of fracture and dramatically increasing the risk of hip fracture. This is an obvious problem but is often neglected in treatment regimens directed towards that age group. Any fall should be carefully evaluated and preventive measures taken. For a discussion of this important topic, the reader is referred to the readings in the Bibliography (see Tinetti & Speechley).

Table 22-1. Risk Factors of Bone Fragility

Advanced age
Female sex
Family history
Nonblack race
Early menopause
Slight body habitus
Non-obesity
Lack of physical activity; immobilization
Low calcium diet
Lactose intolerance
Cigarette smoking
Lack of sunlight exposure

Gastric surgery
Small bowel resection
Hyperthyroidism
Medications
   Corticosteroids
   Heparin
   Phenytoin
   Phenobarbital
Disease states
   Hyperparathyroidism
   Inflammatory bowel disease
   Renal failure
   Liver failure
Ultra high protein diet*
High caffeine intake*
Furosemide*

*Increases urinary calcium loss; effect on bone not known.

Pharmacologic treatment of established osteoporosis is of limited value since most modalities retard bone loss but fail to increase bone mass. Possible exceptions to this are fluoride and the diphosphonates, but these are not currently recommended (see below). At present, treatment should be directed toward retarding further bone loss, preventing falls, and ruling out other diseases or factors that can impair bone integrity, such as hyperparathyroidism, osteomalacia, myeloma, and Cushing's syndrome. For an exhaustive discussion of this issue, the reader is referred to the Bibliography readings (see Riggs & Melton).

ESTROGEN
Estrogen is the most effective medical means of preventing bone loss and is discussed more fully in Chap. 20. Unlike other agents in use, and with the possible exception of calcium, estrogen is the only agent that has been unequivocally demonstrated to reduce the risk

of fractures. Other agents have achieved their place in therapy because radiographic evidence shows they retard loss of bone mineral, which is not incontrovertible proof of bone integrity or diminished fracture risk.

Mechanism of Action

Estrogen retards but does not completely prevent age-related and postmenopausal bone loss. It is thought to act by decreasing the sensitivity of the osteoclast to parathyroid hormone, and may have direct effects on bone via estrogen receptors found in osteoblasts. In most women, estrogen produces little or no restoration of osteoporotic bone and therefore has limited utility in established osteoporosis.

When estrogen is instituted soon after the menopause, it reduces the accelerated rate of bone loss that occurs in the first 7 or 8 years after the menopause. This accelerated rate is thought to be in some way related to the hormonal alterations that take place at the time of menopause and it has been argued that estrogen has no effect later on. However, there is some theoretical basis for treating elderly patients with estrogen. Parathyroid hormone (PTH) levels increase with age in subsets of women, possibly because PTH is excreted by the kidney, or because age-related decline in calcium balance results in secondary elevations of PTH. Estrogen is known to stabilize bone disease in young and elderly women with primary hyperparathyroidism, suggesting that the effect of estrogen is not lost in late life. To date, limited clinical study directed at the patient over 70 years of age shows that there might be a beneficial effect of estrogen on maintenance of bone mineral density.

When to Use Estrogen in the Elderly

The use of estrogens in the woman 75 years of age or older is controversial. Some physicians feel that estrogen treatment at this age is never indicated. However, the claim that estrogen is ineffective when instituted late in life comes from lack of adequate data in the geriatric patient. If the patient with symptomatic osteoporosis is otherwise healthy, with projected long life expectancy, is highly motivated, is expected to receive regular follow-up, and if there are no contraindications, estrogen should be strongly considered. Estrogen may be particularly suitable in the patient with primary hyperparathyroidism, or if other estrogen-deficient symptoms exist, such as atrophic vaginitis or urinary stress incontinence.

It is likewise controversial whether estrogen should be instituted solely for the prevention of osteoporosis in the woman in late life, as compared to the woman in late middle age, if there are no signs or symptoms of the disease, or if the woman happens to have "failed" a radiologic test of bone mineral density. This controversy too derives from lack of data, and this group may well benefit. However, estrogen should rarely if ever be given to black women for this indication because they are at low risk of postmenopausal osteoporosis and develop involutional osteoporosis much later in life. Estrogen has no place in the management of male osteoporosis.

The ideal duration of estrogen therapy is not known. There is some evidence that when estrogen is discontinued accelerated bone loss occurs, suggesting that it should be continued indefinitely. However, it is not known if the protective action of estrogen persists for an indefinite period of time. Elderly patients who have taken estrogen since the menopause may continue to take the hormone if they have tolerated it well and if they are followed carefully. However, the physician should carefully review the indications for estrogen if it was instituted at the time of menopause.

The recommendations and controversy regarding the place of progesterone in an estrogen regimen are discussed in Chap. 20.

Choice of Agent

The most widely prescribed estrogen in the United States is conjugated equine estrogen (Premarin). Of the various **oral** estrogen compounds available, this preparation is also the most widely used. The more potent synthetic estrogens, such as mestranol and ethinyl estradiol, have no advantages in this condition and may be more toxic.

Estrogen delivered by the non-oral route avoids first-pass hepatic metabolism, reducing the likelihood of adverse reactions that are mediated by the liver. It is not known whether non-oral estrogen is more or less cardioprotective than oral estrogen; non-oral administration may produce fewer cardioprotective lipoproteins but also fewer clotting proteins. **Vaginal** preparations of conjugated estrogen are well absorbed initially, but may not be adequately absorbed on the long term to achieve a full effect on bone. **Transdermal estradiol** is quite effective in combatting menopausal symptoms such as hot flushes, and although its antiosteoporosis efficacy as compared to oral estrogen has not yet been firmly established, there is presently no evidence that it would be ineffective.

In conclusion, oral conjugated estrogens have established efficacy in the prevention of osteoporosis, while vaginal and transdermal preparations are theoretically less likely to produce side effects mediated by the liver. The relative cardioprotective effects of oral versus non-oral preparations have not been established.

Pharmacologic considerations, adverse effects, drug-drug interactions, and contraindications are discussed in greater detail in Chap. 20.

Dosing

Although patients most likely vary considerably in their handling of and response to exogenous estrogen, there are no guidelines governing the tailoring of estrogen to individual patients. There is no easily measurable clinical end point. Metabolic measurements, such as urinary hydroxyproline, are impractical, imprecise, and expensive. Short-term radiologic monitoring is imprecise in the individual patient, and cannot be relied on for dose adjustments. The dose that is most effective in retarding early postmenopausal bone loss is 0.625 mg of equine estrogen or its equivalent. Increasing the dose further has not been found to enhance the effects. However, dose-response has not been well studied in women over 70 years of age.

By convention, estrogen is given cyclically for approximately 3 weeks per month in an effort to mimic the menstrual cycle. There is no clear-cut evidence that cyclic estrogen is safer or more effective than daily dosage. Likewise, the safest and most effective way of giving progesterone is not precisely known.

Usual Recommended Dose

IN HYSTERECTOMIZED WOMEN

Conjugated estrogen: 0.625 mg orally per day for 25 consecutive days per month. (**Dose range:** 0.3–1.25 mg/day.)

Transdermal estradiol: 0.05 mg (10 cm^2) patch applied every 3 days. Patch should be applied to rotating sites of skin of the abdomen if possible.

IF UTERUS IS INTACT

Conjugated estrogen: 0.625 mg for days 1–25 of cycle, combined with progesterone 5–10 mg/day on days 12–25 of cycle.

Transdermal estradiol: 0.05 mg as above.

CALCIUM

Calcium retards cortical bone loss and reduces the fracture rate to a degree that is intermediate between the effect of estrogen and the effect of placebo.

Pharmacologic Considerations

Calcium is the major constituent of the mineralized portion of bone, the portion that confers hardness to the skeleton. However, it is important to emphasize that bone is first and foremost a protein matrix on which calcium is stored for use in cellular function. Various hormones, particularly vitamin D, parathyroid hormone, and calcitonin, act in concert to ensure that appropriate serum levels of calcium are maintained for this purpose. Since vital physiologic processes depend on adequate calcium in the blood, bone calcium is sacrificed for this purpose, and is resorbed and laid down along with its protein matrix. Calcium deficiency stimulates the secretion of parathyroid hormone, which increases resorption of bone. Ingesting calcium does not directly enhance bone integrity. Rather, it stimulates the secretion of calcitonin and suppresses PTH secretion.

Calcium is absorbed predominantly in the upper small intestine under the direction of active vitamin D. Intestinal calcium absorption declines with age, beginning around the time of menopause in women and at approximately age 70 in men, so that calcium balance can only be maintained at intakes of calcium twice as high as recommended in younger adulthood. Calcium absorption is further reduced in the presence of vitamin D deficiency. Increased calcium needs provoke an increased stimulation of parathyroid hormone and increased bone resorption. Calcium is reabsorbed and excreted in the kidney. In healthy people, daily urinary excretion is generally maintained within a narrow range of 100–200 mg, independent of the amount ingested. A number of metabolic derangements can increase urinary calcium excretion. If daily excretion exceeds 300 mg, the risk of metabolic kidney stones increases.

Calcium is absorbed as free (ionic) calcium. The extent of absorption of various preparations of calcium differs, depending on the availability of the ion for absorption. Calcium carbonate is ionized at acid pH and therefore is absorbed best in an acid environment; it has been shown to be absorbed less well in women with age-related gastric hypochlorhydria. This malabsorption can be avoided if the preparation is taken with meals, which maximally stimulate gastric acid secretion. Unfortunately, mealtime calcium supplements can theoretically interfere with the absorption of other nutrients. Calcium citrate is probably absorbed better than calcium carbonate, but the difference in absorption may be offset by the higher amount of elemental calcium in calcium carbonate. Some experts discourage the use of calcium phosphate because phosphate increases fecal loss of calcium and increases parathyroid hormone activity. This may in turn reduce renal calcium loss, however, so calcium phosphate compounds may in fact be effective.

Adverse Effects

Calcium supplements may produce **abdominal distension, flatulence, nausea,** and **constipation.** Constipation may be a particular problem in the elderly and is sometimes alleviated by switching from calcium carbonate to the citrate. Patients with known or subclinical derangements in calcium metabolism may develop **hypercalcemia** or **hypercalciuria.**

Drug-Drug and Drug-Nutrient Interactions

Calcium interferes with the absorption of tetracycline, reducing its efficacy. Administration of the two agents should be separated by at least 2 hours, but it may be more practical to forgo calcium supplementation during treatment with the antibiotic. Phenytoin absorption may be reduced by calcium administration, requiring dose adjustments of the former. Calcium carbonate may increase urinary pH and enhance the excretion of salicylates, reducing their efficacy. Increased urinary pH may decrease the elimination of quinidine.

Calcium absorption may be impaired by concurrent administration of corticosteroids. Foods high in oxalic acid (spinach and rhubarb), and diet high in fiber, particularly phytate, are thought to impair calcium absorption, but this has not been definitively established. Calcium inhibits absorption of iron.

Thiazide diuretics increase tubular reabsorption of calcium and may produce hypercalcemia in susceptible individuals, generally by unmasking subclinical hyperparathyroidism. Co-administration of calcium supplements in such persons increases this risk. However, long-term use of thiazide diuretics may increase bone integrity, and the combination of thiazide and calcium need not be avoided, provided serium calcium level is normal (see Thiazides, below).

Contraindications

Calcium supplements are contraindicated in hypercalcemic and hypercalciuric states and in patients with a history of calcium-containing urinary tract stones.

Precautions

Blood calcium should be determined. Twenty-four hour urinary calcium excretion should be measured if practical and in any patient with a personal or family history suggesting urinary tract stones.

Which Calcium Preparation?

It is difficult to assess calcium absorption, even in sophisticated experimental conditions. The bioavailability of insoluble preparations, such as calcium carbonate and phosphate, is thought to be reduced with age because of the frequent presence of gastric hypochlorhydria. However, absorption is enhanced when these preparations are given with meals. Overall, the differences in absorption between the various preparations probably does not differ greatly.

Preparations containing phosphate increase the dietary calcium-to-phosphorus ratio, which has traditionally been thought to decrease calcium absorption, increasing the risk of bone loss. In fact, while phosphorus increases fecal calcium loss, it may reduce urinary loss. This problem has not been adequately studied in humans, but phosphate-containing calcium preparations have not been widely used. They are not likely to have metabolic advantages. Hyperphosphatemia, which can produce metastatic calcification, is probably unusual in the absence of renal failure or hyperparathyroidism.

On a practical basis, it is best to prescribe formulations containing the greatest percentage of elemental calcium, in order to minimize the number of tablets needed to attain a target dose. Since the bioavailability of calcium carbonate has been well established, and since each tablet contains a maximal amount of elemental calcium, this is currently considered the agent of choice. If calcium carbonate is poorly tolerated, calcium citrate can be given instead. Various preparations are summarized in this light in Table 22–2.

If calcium is to be given with vitamin D, it is recommended that separate rather than combination preparations be prescribed. The shelf life of calcium far exceeds that of vitamin D, which is unstable and loses strength with storage.

Indications

Calcium supplements are indicated for the prevention of osteoporosis. Calcium is ineffective alone in the treatment of osteomalacia.

Table 22–2. Some Formulations of Calcium

Tablet Dosage (mg)	Elemental Calcium per Tablet (mg)
Calcium carbonate (40% elemental calcium)	
650	260
750	300
1250	500
1500	600
Calcium citrate (21% elemental calcium)	
960	200
Calcium lactate (13% elemental calcium)	
325	42.25
650	84.5
Calcium gluconate (9% elemental calcium)	
500	45
650	58.5
975	87.75
1000	90
Calcium glubionate (6.5% elemental calcium)	
Liquid	345 mg per 15 cc

Adapted from Sewester, C. S., Olin, B. R., Hebel, S. K., et al., Drug facts and comparisons (St. Louis: Lippincott, 1990), pp. 11–11b.

Calcium supplements are also indicated in hypocalcemic states. In geriatric practice, post-thyroidectomy hypoparathyroidism is sometimes seen. This cause of hypocalcemia should be treated with a combination of calcium and vitamin D.

Dosing
Daily dose of calcium supplement plus dietary calcium should total 1500-2000 mg elemental calcium. Supplement should be given in at least 2 divided doses.

VITAMIN D
Vitamin D is a hormone required for the absorption and metabolism of calcium and for normal bone formation and mineralization. Given alone, neither vitamin D nor its metabolites have been shown to be effective in the treatment of osteoporosis. Nonetheless, other considerations in the geriatric patient make physiologic doses of vitamin D an acceptable part of the treatment regimen.

Pharmacologic Considerations
Vitamin D is obtained from dietary sources or produced in the skin where stores of 7-dehydrocholesterol (provitamin D) are converted to vitamin D in response to ultraviolet light. Animal (and human) vitamin D (cholecalciferol, vitamin D_3) is only slightly different in structure from the form used in vitamin preparations or as food supplements (ergocalciferol, vitamin D_2), which is produced by ultraviolet irradiation of plant ergosterol. Vitamin D synthesized in skin enters the systemic circulation via dermal capillaries, whereas ingested vitamin D is first incorporated into chylomicrons and absorbed through intestinal lymphatics before entering the circulation. Both forms of vitamin D are transported in the bloodstream bound to vitamin-D-binding protein, an alpha globulin, and delivered to the liver where they undergo biotransformation to 25-hydroxyvitamin D (25-OHD). The hepatic metabolite is the major circulating form of vitamin D and is the metabolite that is measured in serum for determination of vitamin D status. When levels of 25-OHD are high, conversion of vitamin D in the liver is reduced by negative feedback inhibition. The hepatic metabolite is transported to the kidney where it is converted to 1,25 dihydroxyvitamin D [1,25 $(OH)_2D$], the metabolite responsible for intestinal calcium absorption, normal bone formation and turnover. Impaired production of 1,25 $(OH)_2D$ is felt to be one of the factors involved in the pathogenesis of osteoporosis. Deficiency in vitamin D results in impaired bone mineralization and osteomalacia.

The serum half-life of vitamin D may be longer than 24 hours, and that of 25-OHD approaches 3 weeks, whereas the serum half-life of 1,25 $(OH)_2D$ is brief and its biologic half-life is approximately 6-10 hours. Vitamin D may be stored in fat deposits for many months. Vitamin D production in the skin shuts down in response to adequate levels in the serum, so that excessive sunlight exposure does not produce hypervitaminosis. This is not the case for ingested vitamin D. Although hepatic hydroxylation declines in response to high amounts, long-term ingestion of high doses of vitamin D supplements will continue to raise vitamin D levels and toxicity may occur.

Vitamin-D production is thought to decline with age. This decline is felt to be due to decreased content in aged skin of 7-dehydrocholesterol, the precursor of vitamin D, rather than to impairment of biosynthetic mechanisms. Use of sunscreen impairs vitamin-D production. Although mild malabsorption of vitamin D may occur in certain older people, there probably is no general decline in intestinal absorption with age. Hepatic hydroxylation appears to be intact, while renal hydroxylation may be impaired, due to a deficiency in renal hydroxylase enzyme. Impairment in renal hydroxylation apparently does not produce an actual vitamin-D deficiency, but may reduce the body's ability to absorb dietary calcium in the intestine or preserve calcium at the level of the kidneys at times of increased need. This sluggishness of response would leave only the bone as an immediate source of calcium, resulting in osteoporosis over time.

Age-related alterations in vitamin-D metabolism are probably only one aspect of the pathogenesis of osteoporosis. Treatment with vitamin-D metabolites has not been shown to retard the process, and at pharmacologic doses may increase bone resorption. However, lack of sunlight exposure is widely held to be an important factor leading to vitamin-D deficiency in the elderly, the clinical consequence of this being osteomalacia. The amount of sunlight required to prevent vitamin-D deficiency is probably no more than 15 minutes 3 times per week in Caucasians, but many elderly are relatively or totally house-bound, and may not make up for the lack by dietary means. A seasonal variation in hip fractures parallels seasonal variations in plasma vitamin D levels, the greatest number of fractures occurring indoors in the early spring. The increased tendency to fractures in deficient individuals may be partly due to osteomalacia superimposed on age-related bone loss. Unlike osteoporosis, osteomalacia is a reversible process.

Adverse Reactions

Vitamin-D supplementation may produce **hypercalcemia** in susceptible individuals. This is more likely to occur with prolonged high-dose therapy. **Hypervitaminosis D** is associated with hypercalcemia, hypercalciuria, soft tissue calcification, and increased bone fragility.

Drug-Induced Vitamin-D Deficiency

Anticonvulsant medications such as phenobarbital and phenytoin may lead to the development of osteomalacia by stimulating hepatic microsomal enzymes, accelerating vitamin-D metabolism. Additional mechanisms, such as accelerated vitamin-K metabolism and diminished vitamin-K-dependent bone protein (osteocalcin), have been less well characterized. The clinical consequences of these processes are the subject of dispute, but steps should be taken to ensure that vitamin-D status remains adequate in elderly patients taking these drugs. Serum concentration of 25-OH vitamin D should be measured every 1–3 years.

Contraindications

Vitamin-D supplementation should not be given in hypercalcemic states.

Precautions

Serum calcium level should be monitored periodically. High-dose formulations **are not indicated** for the prevention of vitamin-D deficiency or of age-related bone loss, except as a single annual or semiannual dose designed for long-term prophylaxis.

Indications

Vitamin-D supplementation at small (physiologic) doses is indicated for the prevention of age-related bone loss. This recommendation is largely based on theoretical considerations. The clinical goal of vitamin-D supplementation is to prevent vitamin-D-deficient osteomalacia, and, in the management of osteoporosis, is an adjunct to calcium supplementation to maximize intestinal absorption.

Larger (pharmacologic) doses of vitamin D are indicated in the treatment of vitamin-D-deficient osteomalacia and other vitamin-D-deficient states. Vitamin D is also indicated in the management of hypocalcemic hypoparathyroidism.

Dosing

Prevention of Vitamin-D Deficiency

400–800 IU daily. May be given as 50,000–100,000 **one-time** dose in the late fall, or twice a year in house-bound or institutionalized patients.

Treatment of Osteomalacia

50,000 IU 3–7 days per week until vitamin-D level normalizes.

Treatment of Hypoparathyroidism

50,000 IU 3–7 days per week, according to serum calcium level.

CALCITONIN (CALCIMAR)

Calcitonin is a naturally occurring hormone, secreted by the parafollicular "C" cells of the thyroid gland in response to hypercalcemia. The formulation available at present for therapeutic use is synthetic salmon calcitonin.

Pharmacologic Considerations

Salmon calcitonin is a peptide, whose 32 amino acids differ somewhat in sequence from the human hormone, but which is capable of reducing serum calcium and inhibiting bone resorption in humans. Salmon calcitonin has been deemed to be several times more potent than human calcitonin by its enhanced ability to reduce serum calcium in animal species. The relative antiresorptive abilities of calcitonin preparations vis-à-vis human bone in vivo is not known.

In the body, calcitonin is found in a large number of locations, including the central nervous system, and the range of its physiologic functions is probably not yet completely recognized. Its effects on bone and calcium metabolism are best understood. Acutely, calcitonin inhibits bone resorption by inhibiting the function of osteoclasts, and when given chronically, it reduces the number of functioning osteoclasts. Chronic treatment with calcitonin has been shown to retard the rate of bone mineral loss in osteoporotic subjects. However, by the end of 2 years of treatment, the antiresorptive effect seems to wane, a phenomenon known as *escape*. The resistance that develops over time to exogenous calcitonin is thought to be due to the fact that chronic treatment results in a "filling in" of the rapidly turning over resorption cavities of osteoporotic bone, so that the antiresorptive mechanism of calcitonin is no longer of any use. The longest published study examining the effect of calcitonin on bone mineral density is 2 years, so it is not known if intermittent therapy might be useful in retarding the osteoporotic process over time.

In late life, bone loss appears to result primarily from impaired osteoblast function, and theoretically, calcitonin should have little or no effect in retarding this process. Like other agents used in the treatment of osteoporosis, calcitonin has not been studied separately in elderly subjects.

Despite convincing evidence of its powerful antiresorptive effect, calcitonin has not been studied long enough to know if it actually reduces the rate of osteoporotic fractures. Its efficacy in Paget's disease has been better established. In this condition, calcitonin relieves bone pain, normalizes bone lesions, and may relieve other symptoms such as neurologic deficits and cardiac failure.

Calcitonin may have a nonspecific analgesic effect through an action involving increased secretion of beta-endorphin. Its effect in reducing pain in osteoporosis has not been well studied, but may prove to be an additional factor to be considered when deciding on a course of treatment. To date, this analgesic effect has been difficult to prove because the pain of osteoporotic fractures resolves spontaneously, and the healing of bone lesions in general would be expected to be accompanied by pain relief.

Calcitonin lowers plasma calcium and phosphorus concentration by increasing movement of calcium and phosphate into bone, and by increasing renal clearance of these ions. Calcitonin lowers serum calcium in malignant disease, but this effect is modest and transitory.

Salmon calcitonin is degraded by proteolytic enzymes in the stomach and must be given parenterally. After subcutaneous or intramuscular injection, calcitonin has a serum half-life of approximately 4 hours and a hypocalcemic effect that lasts from 6 to 12 hours. It is eliminated primarily by renal clearance.

Injectable synthetic salmon calcitonin is the only form of the hormone approved for use in the treatment of osteoporosis at the present time. Use of intranasal calcitonin is under investigation.

Adverse Reactions

Nausea occurs in about 10% of patients taking calcitonin but generally subsides with time. If **anorexia** occurs and persists, the patient's weight should be carefully monitored. **Cutaneous flushing** of the face and hands, lasting 1–2 hours, occurs in a significant minority of patients. **Urticaria** has been reported. **Erythema** at the injection site may occur. **Antibodies** to salmon calcitonin develop in at least 50% of patients after a few months; these antibodies occur at a low titer and are not associated with adverse effects. High titers occur in some patients and may rarely produce clinical resistance in patients with Paget's disease. There may be **mild, transient hypocalcemia,** but this does not appear to be of any clinical significance. **Hypercalciuria** may occur.

Secondary hyperparathyroidism may develop with prolonged treatment. This is not enough to produce significant hypercalcemia or typical symptoms of hyperparathyroidism, but is a compensatory process that counteracts the effect of calcitonin. This problem can be minimized if calcium supplementation is given along with calcitonin.

Indications

Calcitonin is indicated as adjunctive treatment in the management of osteoporosis. However, its overall efficacy in this condition remains uncertain. Calcitonin may be particularly suitable for the osteoporotic patient with associated pain, and for the patient who is unable to take estrogen.

Other Uses

Calcitonin is indicated for the management of symptomatic Paget's disease and is considered a first-line agent in the management of this disorder. Treatment should generally be directed at symptoms such as congestive heart failure, neurological symptoms, fractures, and pain due specifically to pagetic lesions. It is important to emphasize that the vast majority of individuals with pagetic lesions in bone are asymptomatic and may have pain that is due to other musculoskeletal disorders. Paget's disease is discussed in detail in the Bibliography readings (see Rosenthal et al.).

Calcitonin is used as adjunctive treatment in the management of hypercalcemia of malignancy, but its effect is modest and does not persist.

Dosing

There is not a general agreement as to the recommended dosage of calcitonin in osteoporosis. Alternate-day therapy produces a much smaller compensatory increase in PTH than does daily therapy, suggesting that long-term treatment with regular doses could produce a countereffect that would offset efficacy. This countereffect might be minimized by a smaller dose of calcitonin or by intermittent dosage, such as alternate-day therapy.

Although the official FDA approved dose of calcitonin for osteoporosis is 100 IU daily, compliance may be hindered by adhering to this recommendation. Calcitonin is costly, must be given by injection, and can produce dose-related nausea. These factors have led to the practice of initiating treatment at lower doses.

In contrast to osteoporosis, dosing in Paget's disease can be guided by observable clinical and biochemical response. Thus, higher doses are given initially in Paget's disease and the dose lowered when a response has occurred or if dose-related side effects are poorly tolerated.

In Osteoporosis

Initial dose: 50 IU IM or SQ 3 days per week.
Maximum dose: 100 IU/day.

In Paget's Disease of Bone

Initial dose: 100 IU/day.
Maintenance dose: 50 IU 3 times per week.

THIAZIDES

Thiazide diuretics increase tubular calcium reabsorption and some, but not all, studies suggest that they reduce the risk of osteoporotic fractures. Selected patients who require a diuretic for another indication may obtain some protection against bone loss. There is theoretical evidence that thiazides may be particularly suitable in the management of corticosteroid-induced osteoporosis (see Chap. 31).

It is important to emphasize that loop diuretics such as furosemide differ from thiazides in their handling of calcium. In contrast to thiazides, furosemide produces hypercalciuria. The impact of loop diuretics on fracture risk is not known.

FLUORIDE: SHOULD IT BE USED IN THE ELDERLY?

The use of fluoride in the treatment of osteoporosis is controversial, although it has been widely given for many years without having been approved for this use.

Mechanism of Action

Of the treatment modalities for osteoporosis that have been the subject of investigation, only fluoride actually stimulates bone formation and increases bone mass. Fluoride is therefore a very attractive agent from a theoretical point of view since other agents at best only retard the rate of bone loss. Fluoride would be particularly useful in the elderly patient with established osteoporosis. Unfortunately, this agent has several important disadvantages.

Fluoride increases bone mineral density but histologically the new bone is abnormal and poorly mineralized. Excessive ingestion of fluoride is associated with bone disease and enhanced bone fragility (fluorosis).

There is conflicting evidence as to the efficacy of fluoride in reducing the risk of osteoporotic vertebral crush fractures and increasing evidence that it increases the risk of nonvertebral fractures, especially at the hip. The reasons for a possible differential effect may have to do with the fact that the vertebrae and the upper femur are biomechanically distinct; fluoride increases the compression strength of bone, but may reduce its tensile strength, the latter being extremely important in the femoral neck. In addition, the mechanism of fracture of the vertebra (compression) may be quite different from that of the hip (impact or torsion). This question has not been fully worked out. However, whether or not geriatric patients with osteoporosis have symptomatic vertebral osteoporosis, they are at increased risk of hip fracture, regardless of sex. A recent status report on fluoride fails to take this important age difference into consideration (see Heaney).

Adverse Effects

Pharmacologic doses of fluoride (40–75 mg/day of sodium fluoride, equivalent to approximately 18–34 mg of fluoride ion) are poorly tolerated. Upper gastrointestinal symptoms have been reported in up to 40% of patients, depending on the type of formulation used, and bleeding may occur. Increased bone pain, especially in the lower legs, is also common. This may be due to synovitis or to the development of microfractures. Gastrointestinal symptoms and pain syndromes are dose-related and therefore manageable to a certain extent. Enteric coated or slow-release preparations may reduce the incidence of gastrointestinal symptoms, but these may not be readily available to the consumer. The risk of enhanced bone fragility is mentioned above.

It is less well understood whether long-term fluoride therapy will produce some degree of fluorosis with neurologic compression syndromes.

Recommendations

The risks and benefits of fluoride treatment to the geriatric patient with osteoporosis are not known, but there is reason to believe that the risks outweigh the benefits. Pharmacologic doses of fluoride cannot be recommended at this time and should be strictly avoided by patients with peptic ulcer or osteomalacia.

Fluoride in water and toothpaste is believed to have a topical, cariostatic effect even in late life, and use of fluoride-containing dental products is to be encouraged. The concentration of fluoride in water and dental preparations is small. Small amounts of fluoride ingested in water may also be beneficial to bone, as demonstrated in lifetime residents of locations with high concentrations of endemic fluoride, where daily ingested dose of fluoride is estimated to be from 5 to 16 mg/day. It is possible that these amounts of fluoride protect bone by suppressing parathyroid hormone rather than by becoming incorporated into bone in large amounts. Average fluoride intake in the United States ranges from 1.2 to 3.6 mg/day. These concentrations are to be contrasted with pharmacologic doses prescribed for osteoporosis.

EXPERIMENTAL THERAPY: ETIDRONATE DISODIUM (DIDRONEL)

Etidronate is a diphosphonate compound structurally related to pyrophosphate. Etidronate inhibits the action of osteoclasts, reducing bone resorption. It has been used with varying success in the management of Paget's disease of bone and a recent multicenter study of women in their sixties suggested that new, cyclical regimens could be beneficial in postmenopausal osteoporosis (see Watts et al.). This contrasted with earlier experimental findings, in which daily etidronate was shown not only to decrease resorption but also to impair mineralization of bone. The more recent trial examined the effects of cyclic treatment, based on the fact that etidronate is adsorbed onto bone and remains there for prolonged periods. Etidronate 400 mg was administered daily for 2 weeks and withheld for the remainder of a 3-month period, during which time moderate doses of calcium supplements were given. The 3-month cycle was then repeated for the duration of the trial. After 2 years, there was a significant increase in bone mineral density of the spine and a reduction in the rate of vertebral fractures, but no decrease in the rate of hip fractures was demonstrated. However, many bone experts currently feel that more study is required before this agent can be recommended for the management of osteoporosis. This may be particularly important for elderly women, for whom hip fracture is of great concern.

In the management of Paget's disease, etidronate is given on a daily basis. Because daily etidronate is known to impair bone mineralization and increase the risk of fractures, it should generally be given for no more than 6 months at a time and at a dose of 5 mg/kg. Newer experimental diphosphonates may prove safer in this regard.

OSTEOPOROSIS IN MEN

Symptomatic osteoporosis occurs in men, albeit with diminished frequency and later on in life. Vertebral fractures occur with a male-to-female ratio of 1:8 and hip fractures at a ratio of 1:2. Wrist fractures are rare in men. The reasons for this differential distribution are not known.

There is very limited information on the treatment of osteoporosis in men. A recent study failed to demonstrate a beneficial effect from calcium and vitamin-D supplementation (see Orwoll et al.). However, specific recommendations regarding medical treatment cannot be made at this time. Symptomatic osteoporosis in elderly men warrants a careful search for risk factors and secondary causes of metabolic bone disease, and a concerted effort at falls prevention.

NONPHARMACOLOGIC TREATMENT

Nonpharmacologic treatment of osteoporosis rounds out any treatment regimen, and, in the elderly, increases in importance because of the theoretical and practical limitations of giving estrogen treatment. Nonpharmacologic treatment consists of discovering and reversing modifiable risk factors (see Table 22–1), preventing falls, emphasizing erect posture, avoiding heavy lifting, and participating in a graded exercise program tailored to suit the individual patient's musculoskeletal, environmental, and cardiorespiratory limitations.

BIBLIOGRAPHY

Davis, M., Mawer, E. B., Hahn, J. J., et al. Vitamin D prophylaxis in the elderly: a simple effective method suitable for large populations. *Age Ageing* 14:349, 1985.

Fatourechi, V., and Heath, H. Salmon calcitonin in the treatment of postmenopausal osteoporosis. *Ann. Intern. Med.* 107:923–925, 1987.

Heaney, R. P. Calcium bioavailability. *Comtemp. Nutr.* 11:1–2, 1986.

Hedlund, L. R., and Gallagher, J. C. Increased incidence of hip fracture in osteoporotic women treated with sodium fluoride. *J. Bone Miner. Res.* 4:223–225, 1989.

Jensen, G. F., Christiansen, C., and Transbol, I. Treatment of postmenopausal osteoporosis. A controlled therapeutic trial comparing oestrogen/gestagen, 1,25 dihydroxy-vitamin-D_3 and calcium. *Clin. Endocrinol.* 16:515–524, 1982.

LaCroix, A. Z., Wienpahl, J., White, L. R., et al. Thiazide diuretics and the incidence of hip fracture. *N. Engl. J. Med.* 322:786–790, 1990.

Lufkin, E. G., Carpenter, P. C., Ory, S. J., Malkasian, G. D., and Edmonson, J. H. Estrogen replacement therapy: current recommendations. *Mayo Clin. Proc.* 63:453–460, 1988.

McDermott, M. T., and Kidd, G.S. The role of calcitonin in the development and treatment of osteoporosis. *Endo. Rev.* 8:377–390, 1987.

Meier, D. E., Orwall, E. S., Keenan, E. J., et al. Marked decline in trabecular bone mineral content in healthy men with age: lack of association with sex steroid levels. *J. Amer. Geriatr. Soc.* 35:189–197, 1987.

Orwoll, E. S., Oviatt, S. K., McClung, M. R., et al. The rate of bone mineral loss in normal men and the effects of calcium and cholecalciferol supplementation. *Ann. Intern. Med.* 112:29–34, 1990.

Ray, W. A. Thiazide diuretics and osteoporosis: time for a clinical trial? *Ann. Intern. Med.* 115:64–65, 1991.

Resnick, N. M., and Greenspan, S. L. 'Senile' osteoporosis reconsidered. *JAMA* 261:1025–1029, 1989.

Riggs, B. L., Hodgson, S. F., and O'Fallon, W. M. Effect of fluoride treatment on the fracture rate in postmenopausal women with osteoporosis. *N. Engl. J. Med.* 322:802–809, 1990.

Riggs, B. L., and Melton, L. J. Involutional osteoporosis. *N. Engl. J. Med.* 314:1676–1686, 1986.

Rosenthal, M. J., Hartnell, J. M., Kaiser, F. E., et al. Paget's disease of bone in older patients. *J. Amer. Geriatri. Soc.* 37:639–650, 1989.

Tinetti, M. E., and Speechley, M. Prevention of falls among the elderly. *N. Engl. J. Med.* 320:1055–1059, 1989.

Watts, N. B., Harris, S. T., Genant, H. K., et al. Intermittent cyclical etidronate treatment of postmenopausal osteoporosis. *N. Engl. J. Med.* 323:73–79, 1990.

23

Treatment of Urinary Bladder Disturbances

URINARY INCONTINENCE IN THE ELDERLY

The incidence of urinary incontinence in the elderly has been noted to be as high as 20% in the community, 35% in acutely hospitalized patients, and 50% or more in some nursing homes. Chronic urinary incontinence can lead to loss of self-esteem, social ostracism, noncompliance with diuretic medication, and, in certain patients, an increase in the risk of decubitus ulcers. Urinary incontinence can also make the difference between remaining at home with family caregivers and requiring permanent institutionalization.

Urinary incontinence in the elderly can be due to a number of factors and the specific cause must be delineated before treatment is given.

When incontinence is sudden or subacute in onset, it is either due to a reversible condition superimposed on borderline bladder function, or it may signify that serious medical illness is present. In these cases, treatment consists of managing the underlying disorder. Because acute incontinence in the elderly may be the first sign of an acute confusional state, incomplete urinary outlet obstruction, or other serious illness, it requires prompt **medical** evaluation.

Chronic urinary incontinence is often irreversible. However, attention to etiology and judicious management may prevent serious complications, can be of enormous psychological benefit to patients, and, if compared to traditional methods of keeping a patient dry, can ultimately result in decreased nursing time and cost.

For a complete discussion of the pathophysiology of bladder dysfunction, the reader is referred to the Bibliography readings (see Williams). For purposes of this discussion, bladder dysfunction can be simply classified as (1) the bladder that fails to empty, resulting in overflow incontinence, (2) the bladder that empties too often, and (3) mixed pathology. It is common for more than one cause of urinary dysfunction to exist in the elderly. In addition, symptoms such as stress leakage and urgency do not correlate exactly with specific causes of incontinence. The cause is best delineated by complete history, physical examination, urinalysis, and determination of residual urine volume. Cystoscopic or cystometric evaluation are not routine procedures but should be considered if the results would change the therapeutic plan.

Prostatic outlet obstruction due to benign prostatic hyperplasia (BPH) is the most common cause of urinary retention in elderly men. Urinary symptoms usually occur insidiously, but may be abruptly precipitated by fecal impaction, a polyuric state, or paralysis of the detrusor muscle by an anticholinergic drug. Acute urinary retention frequently occurs in such individuals when they are hospitalized. This may be caused by a combination of medication, enforced bed rest, and constipation. Diuretics can paradoxically be the offending medication in this setting when the brisk production of urine overwhelms the bladder's capacity to expel it. Prostatic carcinoma may be present in the elderly man with these symptoms, but is less often the primary cause.

Urinary retention may also occur in long-standing diabetes. This so-called "diabetic cystopathy" is a peripheral neuropathy affecting the afferent limb of the detrusor reflex; in its severe form, there is a large atonic bladder that cannot contract. The classic diabetic bladder is primarily seen in long-standing type I diabetes and is generally accompanied by other signs of autonomic neuropathy. **Most elderly diabetics with urinary dysfunction are incontinent for other reasons.** Other conditions that can cause atonic bladder are vitamin B_{12} deficiency, muscular dystrophy, and neurosyphilis, although in these diseases bladder dysfunction can be varied.

A common cause of urinary incontinence in the elderly is detrusor instability, a condition variously known as *spastic, hyperreflexic, irritable, uninhibited neurogenic,* or *unstable* bladder. This disorder is characterized by loss of central inhibition of the detrusor muscle, allowing bladder contractions to occur when the bladder is only partly filled. This often produces urinary frequency and urgency; incontinence results if the patient is unable to reach the toilet on time, which is frequently the case in older patients with musculoskeletal or other physical limitations. Although central nervous system disease can produce detrusor hyperreflexia, symptomatic unstable bladder frequently occurs in elderly patients who are neurologically normal.

Spinal cord lesions that cause paraplegia and urinary retention are unusual in the elderly, but cervical spondylosis can disrupt the cord above the sacrum causing a mixed emptying-retention syndrome called *detrusor-sphincter dyssynergy.* Afferent impulses to the central inhibitory centers are disrupted along with descending pathways that facilitate urethral sphincter relaxation. The result is an unstable bladder that cannot completely empty. Unrelated to this disorder is a newly described syndrome that also produces a mixed syndrome: *detrusor hyperactivity with impaired contractility* (DHIC) produces urgency with an inability to empty the bladder completely.

States of "pelvic relaxation" in the postmenopausal woman can lead to urinary stress incontinence, in which there is leakage of small amounts of urine when intra-abdominal pressure is increased by a cough, a sneeze, or merely standing up. The term *genuine stress incontinence* is sometimes applied to this syndrome to distinguish it from loss of urine that occurs with the same maneuvers in overflow incontinence. Although minor stress leakage often occurs in younger women, the pathophysiology of stress incontinence in peri- and postmenopausal women is thought to be related to estrogen deficiency. The distal urethra is estrogen-sensitive and has histologic maturation that corresponds to that of the vagina. Postmenopausally, it may become atrophic, avascular, and lax. If the pelvic floor itself weakens, the normal 90-degree bladder-urethral angle increases and the functional internal urethral sphincter also loses tone.

In the absence of urethral compromise, uncomplicated cystocele tends to be associated with a modest degree of urinary retention rather than incontinence.

Patients with advanced dementia almost always develop incontinence. Individuals with dementia fail to attend to matters of personal hygiene because of their confusion, but it is possible that central neurologic disease also plays a role. Normal pressure hydrocephalus, a relatively uncommon form of dementia, classically (though not always) presents as a triad of urinary incontinence, dementia, and gait apraxia. In this condition, the urinary disturbance is believed to have a central origin.

Acute urinary tract infection can precipitate incontinence by irritating the compromised bladder. However, a large proportion of elderly women have chronic asymptomatic bacteriuria, or recurrent asymptomatic urinary tract infections. Treatment of such infections in patients with established incontinence is relatively unsuccessful in restoring continence, since the bladder problem is usually due to something else.

PHARMACOLOGIC MANAGEMENT

Several agents are available for the management of bladder dysfunction. Unfortunately, few have been subjected to exhaustive or comparative study. Pharmacologic treatment may be effective in some patients and it is difficult to predict which patients will respond. Efficacy is generally greater in patients with modest degrees of incontinence; however, drug treatment can often be used to augment the effectiveness of nonpharmacologic approaches.

Antimuscarinic and Antispasmodic Agents

Mechanism of Action

The body of the bladder consists of smooth muscle, the detrusor, which contracts and expels urine in response to cholinergic stimulation. Drugs with antimuscarinic activity exert their effect by virtue of their anticholinergic activity at postganglionic receptor sites, inhibiting contraction of smooth muscle. Antispasmodic agents act by directly relaxing bladder smooth muscle and have weaker anticholinergic effect. In the unstable bladder, these agents reduce detrusor contractility and promote urine storage. They have only a fraction of the potency of atropine, the prototypic antimuscarinic agent, and, unlike atropine, do not appreciably penetrate the blood-brain barrier at ordinary doses, but exert their effect most strongly at the level of the gastrointestinal and urinary tracts. Nonetheless, agents of this class have the same potential side-effect profile of any anticholinergic agent and require vigilance in the geriatric patient. Important anticholinergic effects include **dry mouth, constipation, angle closure glaucoma, tachycardia, altered mental status,** and even **urinary retention.**

Antispasmodic agents were designed for gastrointestinal disturbances and are not all approved for bladder disturbances, but are commonly used and often well accepted by patients.

Pharmacokinetic data in the elderly is scanty for these agents.

Oxybutynin (Ditropan)

Oxybutynin is classified as an *antispasmodic* agent because of its direct effect on smooth muscle, demonstrated by its ability in vitro to inhibit detrusor contractility induced by agents other than those with cholinergic activity. This drug also possesses very mild anticholinergic activity. It is said to possess "local anesthetic" action, but its nonspecific effect on bladder pain is inconsistent and probably limited to conditions characterized by detrusor spasticity. In nongeriatric adults, the onset of action is 1 hour, peak effect in roughly 3–6 hours, and duration of action 8–10 hours.

APPLICATIONS. As an agent that promotes urinary storage, oxybutynin is used in urinary incontinence due to detrusor instability. Oxybutynin produces a low incidence of adverse effects, probably because it is only weakly anticholinergic. However, the usual precautions regarding anticholinergic effects should be observed.

DOSING

Initial dose: 5 mg bid.

Note: Some patients may respond to smaller doses. A 5-mg daily dose may be given at bedtime or other times when the problem is the most troublesome.

Maximum dose: 10 mg tid.

Flavoxate (Urispas)

Flavoxate is a tertiary amine that directly reduces detrusor contractions and has minimal anticholinergic effect. It is similar in its actions to oxybutynin, but appears to be less potent and possibly less effective.

Recent studies suggest that higher doses than previously recommended may enhance the efficacy of this agent without significantly increasing the incidence of adverse effects. However, efficacy is still limited, particularly in patients with significant, long-standing bladder problems. Like oxybutynin, flavoxate is thought to have a nonspecific effect on bladder pain unrelated to its antispasmodic properties, but this property has been demonstrated in experimental animals and does not necessarily manifest itself clinically in humans.

Flavoxate is well absorbed and undergoes extensive first-pass metabolism with little drug excreted unchanged in the urine.

APPLICATION. Flavoxate is designed for use in the management of detrusor instability but is rarely used because it is thought to be less effective than oxybutynin. It is theoretically useful in the syndrome of DHIC (see above), but has not been evaluated in that setting.

DOSING

Initial dose: 200 mg tid.

Maximum dose: A total daily amount of 1200 mg (in 3 to 4 divided doses) has been recommended by some investigators but has not been studied extensively in the older patient.

Propantheline (Pro-Banthine, Others)

Propantheline is an analogue of atropine. It is a quarternary ammonium compound and is incompletely and erratically absorbed when taken orally. It does not penetrate the blood-brain barrier at ordinary doses, but despite this it has been reported to cause confusional states. Unlike atropine, propantheline possesses significant **antinicotinic (ganglionic blocking) effect** in addition to the antimuscarinic effect. Blockade at sympathetic postganglionic sites interferes with the release of norepinephrine, decreasing urethral resistance, and possibly limiting the usefulness of the drug in patients whose unstable bladder is complicated by urethral laxity. Other important antinicotinic effects are **orthostatic hypotension** and **impotence.**

Atropinelike side effects may occur as with other agents of this class.

The onset of action of propantheline is 30 minutes and the duration of action is roughly 4 hours.

APPLICATION. Propantheline is used for detrusor instability. It may worsen stress urinary incontinence due to outlet weakness. It should be used cautiously in older patients because of its ability to produce orthostatic hypotension.

DOSING

Initial dose: 7.5 mg bid.

Maximum dose: 30 mg tid.

Sympathomimetic Agents

The adrenergic responses of the bladder are governed largely by beta receptor activity in the body of the bladder and alpha activity in the outlet. Beta stimulation causes smooth muscle relaxation while alpha stimulation causes muscle contraction; this combined effect promotes urine storage. Estrogen enhances the effects of sympathetic stimulation. When used alone, sympathomimetic agents have been shown to be clinically useful mostly for their alpha-agonist effects, restoring continence to patients with mild to moderate outlet weakness. A clinical effect on the detrusor muscle is less well established so that modification of the sympathetic nervous system is not a common approach in the management of unstable bladder.

Sympathomimetic drugs cause **excitability, insomnia, nervousness, tremor, cardiac arrhythmias,** and **elevation of blood pressure.** Patients with subclinical BPH may develop **urinary retention** from the increased outlet resistance produced by these agents.

Phenylpropanolamine is an indirect sympathomimetic agent with both alpha and beta agonist properties. Ephedrine and its stereoisomer pseudoephedrine have similar pharmacologic properties and efficacy, but have a greater tendency to produce central stimulation and generally are not used for bladder problems.

Applications

Phenylpropanolamine is sometimes used in the management of incontinence due to weakness of the bladder outlet. In women, sympathomimetic agents are often combined with estrogen for enhanced effect. Phenylpropanolamine is also prescribed in combination with anticholinergic agents if there is detrusor instability (see below).

Imipramine (Tofranil, Others)

The tricyclic antidepressant (TCA) imipramine possesses both anticholinergic and alpha-agonist properties. It also possesses calcium-antagonist properties that may result in reduced contractility of the detrusor muscle. Imipramine also has ganglionic blocking action. The relative importance of these actions is not known, but the drug has been shown to reduce bladder contractility and increase outlet resistance, and has been used in the management of both unstable bladder and stress incontinence.

Imipramine penetrates the central nervous system readily, and it has been postulated that its actions on the bladder are partly centrally mediated. Likewise, it can produce **sedation** and is more likely to cause **confusion** than other drugs used for incontinence. Other side effects include **urinary retention, dry mouth, constipation, angle closure glaucoma,** and **orthostatic hypotension.** Like other TCAs, imipramine **depresses cardiac conduction** and should not be used in patients with conduction system disease. In general, it is less well tolerated than the other urinary agents in the elderly, but it may be a logical choice in the incontinent patient who requires a TCA for another reason, such as depression or a chronic pain syndrome.

Imipramine has a long duration of action and theoretically should be effective when the total dose is given only once a day. However, the few studies of this agent have used daily divided doses.

Doxepin (Sineguan) is another TCA that has been studied and shows promise in the management of urinary incontinence. Its efficacy has not been compared to that of imipramine, but there is some evidence that doxepin is less likely to cause orthostatic hypotention.

Although imipramine and doxepin may be useful, it is important to remember that TCAs differ significantly in their pharmacologic profile and should not be considered interchangeable in the management of urinary incontinence.

TCAs are discussed in detail in Chap. 8.

Applications

Imipramine is used in the management of detrusor instability, outlet weakness, or a combination of both.

Dosing for Imipramine and Doxepin

Initial dose: 10 mg daily.
Maximum daily dose: 75 mg in 2 or 3 divided doses; a once-daily dose may be effective.

Estrogen

Because postmenopausal urinary stress incontinence is thought to be related to estrogen deficiency, topical and oral estrogen have been a popular treatment for many years. However, most clinical studies have been short-term, poorly controlled, or confounded by the concurrent use of other treatments. Most important, these studies have tended to focus on patients under 70 years of age. These limitations notwithstanding, the present consensus is that estrogen may be effective in mild to moderate postmenopausal urinary stress incontinence, and that its efficacy is enhanced by a program of pelvic-floor exercises or concurrent use of adrenergic agents. Estrogen may also relieve a postmenopausal "urethral syndrome," which is typically characterized by dysuria, frequency, and urgency, but which may be associated with urinary incontinence in older women.

Unfortunately, long-standing urinary stress incontinence in women over 70 may be relatively resistant to estrogen.

Mechanism of Action

Estrogen acts by increasing urethral resistance in estrogen-deficient women. With estrogen replacement, histologic maturation occurs in the urethra in parallel to that occurring in the vagina. The female distal urethra is rich in estrogen receptors; estrogen receptors exist in the detrusor muscle as well but at much lower concentrations. It is perhaps for this reason that estrogen may be less effective in the management of detrusor instability than in symptoms related to the bladder neck and urethra. In older women, detrusor instability often coexists with urethral laxity, so it is difficult to know which condition is being ameliorated when patients improve.

Estrogen also increases the sensitivity of urethral tissue to endogenous and exogenous adrenergic stimulation. Estrogen and progesterone have differing effects in this regard; in the urethra, estrogen increases primarily alpha-adrenergic sensitivity while progesterone increases beta sensitivity. Beta stimulation in the urethra reduces urethral tone; thus, progesterone, which is often given in combination with estrogen, could theoretically counteract the beneficial effects of the latter in the urethra. However, this question has not been examined clinically.

Dosing and Mode of Delivery

The exact dose of estrogen for urinary dysfunction has not been determined. Estrogen should be given at the lowest possible dose to achieve a subjective response on the part of the patient. Compared to the standard oral dose given for osteoporosis (0.625 mg conjugated estrogen), lower doses are often effective in the management of postmenopausal urethral syndromes. However, in the case of urinary stress incontinence, a clinical response may not be achieved unless much higher doses are used (greater than 1.25 mg of conjugated estrogen). High doses produce greater toxicity and there is simply no published data on which to guide therapy in the geriatric patient.

The mode of estrogen delivery is also not well defined. The oral route is reliable and highly acceptable to patients, but may produce more toxicity than non-oral estrogen. Although well absorbed from atrophic tissue, systemic absorption of vaginal estrogen may be markedly reduced once maturation index has been achieved; thus, vaginal estrogen suppositories have the advantage that the delivery of estrogen is increasingly localized over time. Estrogen cream can be applied topically to the urethra using the tip of the finger. Although this method has not been adequately tested, it is conceivable that it might be more acceptable to patients than a large dose delivered intravaginally.

Transdermal estrogen has not been studied for the treatment of urinary incontinence. Transdermal preparations may be more acceptable to patients than topical creams, while just as safe, and are likely to provide sufficient estrogen stimulation in urethral syndromes. It is unknown if they have any effect in the more intractable problem of stress incontinence, however.

Recommendations

Estrogen preparations should be considered in women with postmenopausal urinary stress incontinence. Treatment should be initiated with intravaginal estrogen cream 0.3 mg of conjugated estrogen daily or its equivalent (see Chap. 20). The patient should be instructed to also apply cream directly to the urethral orifice. After 8 consecutive weeks the dose may be increased to 0.625 mg/day. Doses of 1.25 mg may be required for symptom control but higher doses should generally be avoided. If therapy is continued beyond 8 weeks in patients with intact uterus, progesterone therapy should be considered for the prevention of endometrial cancer.

Patients unwilling to use vaginal cream may take the equivalent dose of oral estrogen. The efficacy of transdermal estrogen is not known but a trial may be warranted in highly motivated patients because its toxicity is probably lower than that of oral estrogen.

For maximum benefit, a program of pelvic-floor exercises should be undertaken along with estrogen therapy. Coadministration of alpha agonists may increase the efficacy of estrogen.

Although roughly 50% of premenopausal women may experience

stress incontinence at some time, estrogen should not be used in the premenopausal period. There is no indication for estrogen in the elderly male.

A complete guide to estrogen administration is contained in Chap. 20.

Combination Treatment

It is often useful to combine agents in the treatment of urinary incontinence.

Certain agents work synergistically at the same anatomic location but few combination regimens have been studied in controlled clinical trials. Sympathomimetic agents and estrogens are a popular combination used to enhance urethral tone.

A combination agent designed for symptomatic treatment of upper respiratory infections (Ornade, others) has been used for urinary incontinence. Use of this agent was initially based on the observation that it reduced stress incontinence elicited by cold symptoms, but in fact it combines agents that act directly on the bladder. Current preparations contain chlorpheniramine, an antihistamine with anticholinergic properties, and the sympathomimetic agent phenylpropanolamine. The antihistamine reduces detrusor activity while the latter enhances urethral tone, and may be useful for people with combined bladder instability and urethral stress incontinence. This combination preparation can be purchased over the counter. However, it should not be taken by elderly patients without medical supervision because of the possibility of adverse effects from either of the two agents.

Prazosin in BPH

Prazosin is a selective alpha$_1$ adrenergic blocker that is used primarily as an antihypertensive agent. In addition to its action on the venous and arterial bed, prazosin acts at the level of the bladder outlet where it inhibits smooth muscle contraction and reduces internal urethral sphincter tone. Although this can precipitate urinary incontinence in patients with outlet weakness, prazosin may reduce symptoms of prostatism in men with BPH.

If the anatomical outlet obstruction produced by the prostate is severe, it is unlikely that pharmacologic manipulations can make an important clinical difference. However, patients theoretically stand to benefit if they have, for whatever reason, a high degree of superimposed neuromuscular tone at the outlet. Short-term clinical trials have, in fact, demonstrated symptomatic and cystometric improvement in some men. This approach is palliative, with surgery remaining the definitive treatment. Prazosin is not appropriate when surgery is urgently required. However, most patients with mild to moderate symptoms of BPH will never require surgery; for others, surgery may pose a substantial risk, and still others may be opposed to the idea of surgery or may wish to postpone it as long as possible. In these cases, a trial of prazosin may be warranted.

Long-term utility of prazosin in this setting is not known. A clear understanding of its long-term efficacy might be confounded by progression of the condition itself.

Prazosin has not been officially approved for this indication.

Recommendations

A trial of prazosin may be given to patients with mild to moderate symptoms of BPH who are unable or unwilling to undergo surgery. The drug might be particularly suitable for those patients if they required concomitant treatment of hypertension. The drug should only be given with the understanding that its efficacy is unproved, that symptoms probably will not be completely relieved, and that it may not eliminate an eventual need for surgery.

Prazosin should be used cautiously in the elderly because it may produce severe orthostatic hypotension, particularly when the drug is first initiated.

Indications and adverse effects of prazosin are discussed in detail in Chap. 12.

Dosing

Initial dose: 0.5 mg at bedtime. Dosing is initiated in the evening when the patient is supine because of the risk of orthostatic hypotension.
Dose increments: Increase total daily dose by 0.5 mg every 4 days or until clinical response is achieved. Dose should be divided.
Maximum dose: 2 mg bid.

Bethanechol (Urecholine, Others)

Bethanechol is a congenor of acetylcholine but has pure promuscarinic activity, is not inactivated by cholinesterases, and has relatively selective action at the level of the gastrointestinal and urinary tract. It stimulates bladder contraction and is used in states of detrusor underactivity to promote micturition. Its efficacy for this indication has been questioned. In the gastrointestinal tract, bethanechol increases tone and secretion.

As a muscarinic agent, bethanechol has cholinergic effects and can stimulate glandular secretion, producing **hypersalivation, sweating**, and **bronchorrhea**. Other side effects include **flushing, nausea, vomiting, diarrhea, abdominal cramps, bronchospasm**, and **bradycardia**. In high doses it can precipitate **detrusor-sphincter dyssynergy**. It is contraindicated in bowel or bladder outlet obstruction, asthma, peptic ulcer, hyperthyroidism, enterocolitis, bradyarrhythmia, Parkinson's disease, and coronary insufficiency.

Applications

Bethanechol has been recommended for use in the rehabilitation of the atonic bladder following surgery or prolonged catheterization, and for promoting micturition in chronic atonic bladder characterized by high residual urine. It has been reported to be effective in a variety of potentially reversible conditions, such as transient postoperative bladder atony, but its effectiveness in patients with preexisting disease is uncertain. Among elderly men, great caution would be required in this situation because of the frequent co-occurrence of BPH, and the possibility of underlying heart disease.

Chronic atonic bladder, which is a relatively uncommon cause of urinary retention among the elderly, may not respond at all to bethanechol. Most of the optimistic published experience with this drug has considered relatively young patients. It is possible that the doses that would be required to have a positive clinical effect (e.g., a minimum of 25–50 mg orally several times a day), would be poorly tolerated in older individuals, but there is no good clinical data to determine what the efficacy-to-toxicity ratio would be. More study is required before dosing recommendations can be made for the geriatric patient.

Patients who develop urinary retention as a side effect of another medication, most often one with anticholinergic effect, are sometimes given bethanechol. It is almost always preferable to discontinue the offending medication rather than to superimpose another potentially toxic one. In all cases, mechanical or functional outlet obstruction of the bladder must be ruled out before the drug is instituted.

NONPHARMACOLOGIC MANAGEMENT

Nonpharmacologic measures should be instituted whenever possible. Medications and other causes of acute bladder problems should be identified. The environment must be improved; there should be easy access to the toilet, commode, or urinal, and privacy should be respected.

Pelvic-floor exercises can be very effective in women with stress incontinence and have been reported to be useful in incontinent men as well. Exercises may be enhanced with biofeedback techniques. Women with bladder-urethral angle problems sometimes stay dry with the use of a vaginal pessary; this type of device must be removed and cleaned at least once a month or incarceration can develop. Credé maneuver (application of manual extrinsic pressure to the bladder) is occasionally helpful in urinary retention. Retention due to cystocele can be alleviated with manual assistance through the vagina.

Chronic indwelling catheters have little place in the management of urinary incontinence in the debilitated elderly, and, because of the inevitability of chronic bladder infection, should be adopted only in states of stubborn retention. An exception to this rule is in the presence of severe, intractable decubitus ulcers, where catheterization prevents the irritation caused by the constant urine bath. Intermittent catheterization is more benign; although self-catheterization is difficult for most geriatric patients to learn, intermittent catheterization can be taught to caregivers if they are available and willing. Condom ("Texas") catheter is useful in men with urethral incompetence and other nonretentive states, but can leak, kink, and produce infections of the bladder and skin.

Frequent toileting should be done for patients who are cognitively or physically disabled. Such patients are referred to as having "functional incontinence" because they become wet only because they are unable to toilet themselves. Frequent, scheduled toileting and bladder training should be adopted for patients with unstable bladder. In a typical bladder training program, the patient toilets every hour or less, as urinary or urgency patterns demand, until dry for 48 hours. At that point, the patient increases the interval by half an hour until dry for a second 48-hour period. This pattern is repeated until continence is maintained for 4 hours or for a realistic or acceptable time interval. The program is supplemented with strategic administration of fluid, avoidance of caffeine and alcoholic beverages, and various forms of behavioral modification. Bladder training can be effective for ambulatory as well as institutionalized patients, although the initial time intervals are not always practical and ultimate goals may differ.

Adult diapers, layered sheets, and commercially available protective garments in various sizes (Depend, Attend, others) are intended not only to keep the bed dry, but to keep the patient dry, and must be changed regularly so that skin irritation and decubitus ulcers do not result.

Surgery is the treatment of choice in severe mechanical outlet obstruction such as BPH. Surgical procedures often ameliorate certain forms of female stress incontinence. They are applied to a limited degree in the management of some forms of neurogenic bladder.

Despite a recent resurgence of research in this problem, the most effective way to manage incontinence in the elderly remains frequent toileting.

BIBLIOGRAPHY

Brown, K. H., and Hammond, C. B. Urogenital atrophy. *Obstet. Gyn. Clin. N. Amer.* 14:13–32, 1987.

Burgio, K. L., and Burgio, L. D. Behavioral therapies for urinary incontinence in the elderly, *Clin. Geriatr. Med.* 2:807–827, 1986.

Kirby, R. S., Coppinger, S. W. C., Corcoran, M. O., et al. Prazosin in the treatment of prostatic obstruction. *Brit. J. Urol.* 60:136–142, 1987.

Miodrag, A., Castleden, C. M., and Vallance, T. R. Sex hormones and the female urinary tract. *Drugs* 36:491–504, 1988.

Resnick, N. M., and Baumann, M. M. Incontinence in the nursing home patient. *Clin. Geriatr. Med.* 4:549–570, 1988.

Resnick, N. M., and Yalla, S. V. Detrusor hyperactivity with impaired contractile function. *JAMA* 257:3076–3081, 1987.

Ruffman, R. A review of flavoxate hydrochloride in the treatment of urge incontinence. *J. Int. Med. Res.* 16:317–330, 1988.

Tapp, A. J. S., and Cardozo, L. The postmenopausal bladder. *Brit. J. Hosp. Med.* 35:20–23, 1986.

Warren, J. W. Catheters and catheter care. *Clin. Geriatr. Med.* 2:857–871, 1986.

Williams, M. E. Urinary incontinence in the elderly. *Ann. Intern. Med.* 97:895–907, 1982.

24

Laxatives

CONSTIPATION IN THE ELDERLY

When a patient complains of constipation, the complaint may signify that bowel movements are too infrequent, too hard, too small, too difficult to pass, or not associated with a feeling of relief. Many people, particularly those in the current older generation, were raised to think that they have to "be regular"—that if they do not have a "good" bowel movement every day there is something wrong—so they may complain of constipation when their bowel function is actually quite normal. Since a patient's concept of constipation may refer to a variety of symptoms, it is important for the physician to focus on the new onset of a bowel complaint, complications of defecatory difficulties, patient distress, and laxative abuse.

Defecatory difficulties are not a part of normal aging but are common complaints among the elderly. Although more women than men complain of constipation in general, the female-to-male ratio decreases to unity in late life. Constipation may be chronic or may represent a change in previously normal bowel movements, and results from impaired colonic motility, or reduction of stool bulk because of lack of water in the stool, or both. Causes of constipation are listed in Tables 24–1 and 24–2. When evaluating older patients, it is important to remember that the elderly do not often consider constipation important enough to complain about to their physician, while they treat themselves with home remedies or over-the-counter preparations; that the *relief* of chronic constipation may signify the onset of a subtle medical problem such as hyperthyroidism or intestinal malabsorption; that a number of drugs may cause constipation but this problem can be ignored by patient and physician, having been attributed to the aging process.

An important cause of chronic constipation in the elderly is longstanding laxative abuse. A history of difficulty or perceived difficulty with defecation often results in daily use of potent laxatives, leading to cathartic bowel, a condition in which colonic lesions develop that resemble those seen in "burned out" ulcerative colitis. These lesions may reverse if laxatives are discontinued, but in severe cases the colon may become permanently dilated and function poorly. This damage is thought to be due to a direct toxic effect of certain laxatives on the myenteric plexus.

Dietary intake of fiber in the Western world is generally insufficient for optimal bowel function. Some elderly may curtail further fiber intake because of dental problems or because it produces flatus. In fact, a high-fiber diet can be easily maintained in edentulous patients, and flatus may gradually diminish as the intestine adapts to the new diet. Use of fiber in the management of constipation is discussed below.

Lack of physical activity can promote constipation. The most severely affected individuals are those who are bedridden or wheelchair-bound. The presence of certain neurological disease in such patients can contribute to the problem. The problem is compounded in the demented, depressed, or confused patients who do not not heed the rectal sensation to defecate, resulting in accumulation of a hard mass and constipation.

Table 24–1. Potentially Reversible Causes of Constipation

Inhospitable environment
Lack of physical activity; immobility
Hospitalization
Hypothyroidism
Depression
Tumor of colon or rectum
Benign colonic stricture
Hypercalcemia
Hemorrhoids
Hernia
Dehydration
Fecal impaction
Excessive or improper use of bulk laxatives and fiber supplements
Medications
  Antacids
  Antispasmodics
  Tricyclic antidepressants
  Antihypertensives
  Antihistamines
  Antipsychotics
  Calcium-channel blocking agents
  Colchicine
  Diuretics
  Antidiarrheal agents
  Opiates
  Cholestyramine
  Calcium carbonate
  Iron preparations

Long-standing diabetes mellitus may irreversibly affect the neurologic supply of the intestines, leading to defecatory difficulties. Constipation is much more common in such elderly diabetics than classic "diabetic diarrhea." Furthermore, although diabetic bowel may exist in 20% of type-I diabetics, most elderly diabetics have type-II diabetes and if they have bowel problems these are more likely due to causes other than diabetes.

Dehydration, which may contribute to constipation, is common in

Table 24–2. Causes of Chronic Constipation

Laxative abuse
Neurologic disease (parkinsonism, multiple sclerosis, spinal cord injury, stroke)
Chronic bed or wheelchair existence
Long-standing diabetes
Dementia

the elderly. Factors contributing to this are the aged kidney's decreased ability to concentrate urine, the use of diuretics, voluntary restriction of fluid intake because of bladder problems, and impaired thirst.

Although the most common problem associated with constipation is patient discomfort or dissatisfaction, more serious consequences may occur in geriatric patients. Excessive straining at the stool can precipitate angina or cardiac arrhythmias, and rarely, syncope. Enlargement or bleeding of hemorrhoids, anal fissure, and even rectal prolapse may occur when stool is very hard or difficult to pass. Fecal impaction is common and can result in urinary retention, or can present as paradoxical diarrhea and fecal incontinence. Diarrhea and urinary complications are often inappropriately treated while the underlying fecal impaction is ignored and worsened by the treatment.

NONPHARMACOLOGIC MANAGEMENT

Laxatives and enemas are important adjuncts to the management of constipation, but they are not innocuous and should be given only when other measures are inadequate. Treatment of constipation must include search for and remedy of underlying causes of constipation, regular physical activity, adequate hydration, and avoidance of constipating drugs. Regular toileting may be helpful in dependent patients. Diet should include adequate and appropriate intake of dietary fiber (see below). Fecal impaction should be looked for and treated promptly.

A careful history should be done to see if bowel dysfunction truly exists; if it does not, reassurance can sometimes bring about a "cure."

Fiber

Dietary fiber consists of nonstarch polysaccharides (cellulose, pectin, plant gums, and other components) and lignin. These are primarily plant components that are incompletely digested by the human small intestine, and that retain water in the colon, increasing fecal bulk and promoting defecation. Fiber may also increase stool bulk through the products of its fermentation, which include short-chain fatty acids, gases, water, and ultimately increased bacterial cell mass.

A number of claims have been made as to additional health benefits of fiber, including improved glucose tolerance in diabetes, reduction in the risk of colon cancer, and reduced risk of heart disease. While there is evidence to support some of these claims, the degree of benefit is uncertain (see Bibliography).

The term *crude fiber* refers to the amount remaining when food is subjected in vitro to chemical degradation; the actual amount of available fiber in food (*dietary fiber*) is significantly greater, gram-for-gram. Individual needs probably vary considerably, but 20 g a day of dietary fiber is considered the goal for attainment of maximum colonic function. The average American diet contains less than 10 grams. Fiber ingestion decreases with age among elderly men, and though it increases among women, it nevertheless is ingested in suboptimal amounts.

High-fiber foods, in descending order of percent fiber content, are unprocessed wheat bran, unrefined cereals, whole-grain breads, legumes, root vegetables (potatoes, carrots, parsnips), fruits, and leafy vegetables. The cooking of fruits and vegetables does not reduce fiber content, and may actually increase the amount by converting digestible starch to undigestible forms. Chopping or pureeing of food does not decrease its laxative effect to any important degree, a critical factor for the debilitated or edentulous elderly.

Unprocessed ("natural") bran is often mixed with breakfast cereal and given to constipated nursing-home patients. This may be a useful practice, but care should be taken that the bran is well mixed with moist cereal or a similar vehicle so that inhalation and aspiration of the dry material do not occur. Bran and high-fiber supplements should not be taken in excess because they may form a bulky mass, thereby *increasing* constipation and leading to fecal impaction. Excessive amounts of bran and high-fiber supplements may be harmful to bedridden patients who have a high risk of developing an obstructing mass from the fiber. Ordinary amounts of dietary fiber and fiber-enriched liquid formulas are well tolerated in such patients, however. Whenever the fiber content of a diet is increased, fluid intake should be increased as well, in order to avoid the obstructing mass effect.

Even if a high-fiber diet does not normalize bowel function, it may reduce intake of laxatives and may make the diet more interesting. Additional health benefits are probably limited, particularly if increased fiber intake begins late in life.

Recommendations

The diet should contain at least 20 g of dietary fiber per day. Fiber supplements such as unprocessed bran should be limited to an additional 5–10 g/day and should be accompanied by increased fluid intake. Fiber supplements are best avoided by nonambulatory patients with constipation, and are contraindicated in fecal impaction. Bran and other fiber supplements are often found in combination with bulk-forming laxatives such as psyllium (see below), in which case extra caution is required.

LAXATIVES

Ideally, laxatives should be prescribed for short-term use only, but in practice it is often impossible to persuade long-term users to cease or curtail laxative use. Patients often require medications that produce constipation as a side effect, and if nonpharmacologic means do not relieve the problem, laxatives may be the only alternative. Institutionalized patients with dementia, neurologic disease, or limited ambulation often fail to respond to nonpharmacologic measures and may require long-term complicated bowel regimens in order to avoid fecal impaction. In other cases, however, it may be possible to wean patients from their habit.

Laxatives, categorized by their mechanism of action, are summarized in Table 24–3. This classification is a traditional one and is presented for clarity only, since the mechanisms of action are not precisely known and may be complex. In general, all laxatives ultimately work by increasing the amount of water and electrolytes in the colon. For this reason, use of any category of laxative should be accompanied by increased fluid intake.

Innumerable preparations and combinations are available, most

Table 24–3. Laxatives

Agent (Sample Brand)	Onset of Action
Bulk-Forming Agents	12–72 hr
Psyllium (Metamucil, Fiberall, Correctol, Perdiem Plain, other)	
Methylcellulose (Citrucel)	
Polycarbophil (FiberCon, Fiberall Chewable Tablets)	
Agar	
Osmotic Agents	
Magnesium sulfate (Epsom salts)	
Magnesium hydroxide (Milk of Magnesia)	½–3 hr
Magnesium citrate	
Sodium phosphate (Fleet Phosphosoda)	
Lactulose (Chronulac)	24–48 hr
Stimulant/ Irritant Agents	6–12 hr
Cascara	
Senna (Fletcher's Castoria, Senokot)	
Aloe	
Danthron	
Casanthrol	
Bisacodyl (Dulcolax, Carter's Little Pills)	
Phenolphthalein (ExLax, Feen-a-Mint)	
Castor Oil	
Stool Softeners (Surfactants; Emollients)	24–72 hr
Dioctyl sodium sulfosuccinate/docusate sodium (Colace)	
Calcium sulfosuccinate/docusate calcium (Surfak)	
Some Combination Laxatives	
Haley's M-O (mineral oil plus magnesium hydroxide)	
Perdiem (psyllium plus senna)	
Correctol Tablets (phenolphthalein plus docusate)	
Peri-Colace (docusate sodium plus casanthranol)	
Suppositories	
Glycerin	30 minutes
Bisacodyl (Dulcolax)	
Docusate	
Enemas	minutes
Tap water	
Saline	
Sodium phosphates (Fleet Enema)	
Mineral oil (Fleet Oil Retention Enema)	
Commercial combinations	

without prescription. For a complete list, the reader is referred to the Bibliography readings (see Sewester et al.). Choice of laxative is often empiric, based on availability, cost, palatability, patient acceptance, and physician experience. The purpose of this section is to delineate the advantages and disadvantages of the types of laxatives in use.

Bulk-Forming Agents

Bulk-forming agents are preparations of natural and semisynthetic fiber, and presumably act in the same manner—by retaining water in the stool, increasing fecal bulk, and stimulating peristalsis. They are often prescribed for diarrhea due to irritable bowel syndrome since the excess water combines with the bulk forming substance, producing a gel and a formed stool. The "natural" character of these agents belies the harm that can come when they are used inappropriately. They must be taken with ample amounts of liquid or they will form a hard mass that can result in fecal impaction and even mechanical obstruction of the gastrointestinal tract. Some agents are chewable and patients may be unaware that extra liquid intake is needed. High-fiber cookies are tasty and patients ingest excessive amounts on the assumption that "more is better." A high risk of obstruction exists in immobile, dehydrated, or bedridden patients.

High-fiber diets that contain excessive amounts of phytate and other constituents have been shown to decrease the absorption of minerals, including calcium, zinc, and magnesium, under experimental conditions, but consistent development of negative mineral balance has not been demonstrated. It is unlikely that ordinary doses of bulk agents would produce clinical harm on the basis of impaired mineral balance, even if mineral intake were marginal.

Interactions with concurrently administered drugs have only infrequently been described. The calcium contained in the bulk-forming agent polycarbophil decreases the absorption of tetracycline. If there is concern about other drug interactions, it is simple to take the agents an hour or more apart.

Bulk-forming laxatives have a delayed onset of action and the effect may not be noted for 12–72 hours.

Recommendations

Bulk-forming agents are recommended for ambulatory individuals if added dietary fiber does not improve symptoms. They may be useful for weaning patients from long-term use of stimulant laxatives. They should be instituted along with increased amounts of fluid (approximately 8 oz of fluid per average dose). Because of their delayed onset of action, these agents are of limited use when rapid relief is desired. They are contraindicated in fecal impaction and should be used with great caution in nonambulatory individuals.

Osmotic Agents

Osmotic agents are poorly absorbed and act by drawing water into the intestine, increasing the bulk and water content of the stool, and promoting peristalsis by mechanical distension. Most have a rapid onset of action and are useful when rapid relief is desired. Oral agents in this group include the saline cathartics and lactulose.

Saline Cathartics

The osmotically active ions in the *saline cathartic* group are sulfate, magnesium, phosphates, and citrate, in order of decreasing potency.

Magnesium hydroxide (Milk of Magnesia) is a widely used agent that is one of the cheapest laxatives available. In addition to acting as an osmotic agent, magnesium stimulates the release of cholecystokinin, which increases intestinal secretion and stimulates peristalsis and transit. Patients who have noticed that their magnesium-containing antacids can relieve constipation sometimes use them for this purpose alone, a practice that is not advised because of the aluminum contained in them. Some patients find magnesium tablets to be more palatable than the liquid form, but these agents were designed for use as antacids and up to 8 or more tablets must be taken before a laxative effect occurs. Magnesium salts are partly absorbed into the system and excreted by the kidney; patients with renal insufficiency should avoid magnesium-containing laxatives because of the risk of hypermagnesemia.

Magnesium sulfate (Epsom salt) is the most potent of the saline cathartics. It must be mixed with water and has a bitter taste, which may account for its unpopularity. **Magnesium citrate** is considered pleasant-tasting but the dose is fairly large (10 g mixed with 8–10 oz water), and it loses its potency and palatability if it is not kept refrigerated. Oral **sodium phosphate** salts are less potent than magnesium salts. They should not be used in renal failure because of the risk of fluid retention, hyperphosphatemia, and hypocalcemia, and should be avoided by people on salt-restricted diets.

RECOMMENDATIONS. Saline cathartics are indicated when rapid, reliable relief of constipation is desired. Milk of magnesia is highly suitable for this purpose because a volume as small as 5 ml may be effective and the dose can be titrated easily. The effective dose may be given daily if necessary in the management of chronic constipation and for the prevention of fecal impaction, but diarrhea and dehydration must be avoided. The usual dose is 15–30 ml at bedtime.

Saline cathartics and other osmotic laxatives should not be used as the initial treatment of acute fecal impaction. In these cases, the mass should be cleared from below, manually or with enemas, before osmotic agents are give orally.

Magnesium-containing cathartics are contraindicated in renal failure.

Lactulose

Lactulose is a synthetic, nonabsorbable disaccharide syrup that is not degraded until it reaches the colon. Once in the colon, it promotes defecation via low-molecular-weight acids and carbon dioxide, which are its osmotically active terminal degradation products. These lower the pH of colonic contents and systemic nitrogen is trapped and excreted, making lactulose effective at higher doses for the treatment of hepatic encephalopathy. At lower doses than those used for hepatic encephalopathy, lactulose remains a potent laxative. It contains small amounts of absorbable disaccharides but is felt to be safe for most diabetics, and may be used safely in patients with renal failure. It may cause **belching, flatulence,** and **abdominal cramping** and **distension,** but these symptoms sometimes subside with time. The sweet taste of lactulose is perceived as pleasant to some, and impalatable to others; for the latter, it may be mixed with water, milk, or juice.

Lactulose is probably no more effective than other osmotic agents, and has a slower onset of action of 24–48 hours after dosing is initiated. The onset of action is partly dependent on colonic transit time. Since colonic transit time may be prolonged with age, lactulose could have an even slower onset in the elderly. The impatient individual desiring rapid relief could ingest excessive amounts and develop severe diarrhea if not properly instructed on correct use of this agent.

The major drawback of lactulose, however, is its cost. It is marketed as a laxative (Chronulac) and for use in hepatic encephalopathy (Cephulac), the latter being somewhat less expensive. The hepatic dose is much higher than the laxative dose, however, and the patient who wishes to purchase the less expensive brand should be cautioned not to follow the package instructions, but to take only the prescribed cathartic dose, or severe diarrhea and electrolyte imbalance may result.

RECOMMENDATIONS. Lactulose is a suitable alternative to magnesium-containing agents for patients with renal failure, but relief may not be as rapid as with saline cathartics. As with saline cathartics, lactulose is suitable for chronic use.

The initial dose of lactulose is 15–30 cc/day. The dose may be increased by 15–30 cc every 24–48 hours until effect is achieved, to a recommended maximum dose of 60 cc. Patients should be closely instructed as to its use and its delayed onset of action so that they do not self-administer increasing doses to the point of diarrhea.

Although lactulose is unlikely to produce hyperglycemia in diabetics, it is prudent to monitor blood sugar periodically in such patients. Electrolytes, including serum bicarbonate, should be monitored in patients using lactulose for prolonged periods.

Polyethylene Glycol-Electrolyte Solution (PG-ES; Brands: Golytely, Colyte)

PG-ES is an osmotic agent intended for bowel preparations. It has been used successfully as adjunctive treatment in the management of fecal impaction (see Puxty & Fox), but it has not been specifically compared to high doses of other osmotic agents. It is probably effective in the management of chronic constipation but the volume required may be impractical or annoying to the patient.

The onset of action is from 30 to 60 minutes. PG-ES is not absorbed and is not associated with significant loss of electrolytes into the colon, but it may produce **nausea, vomiting,** and **abdominal cramps.** If the jug is **refrigerated,** the patient may experience **chills.**

RECOMMENDATIONS. PG-ES should generally be reserved for use as a bowel prep, where the dose is 3–6 liters (average, 1 gallon) given as an 8-oz glass every 10–15 minutes. Patients who are unable or unwilling to ingest such large amounts may be given smaller doses over a 2-day period.

PG-ES may be given as adjunctive treatment of fecal impaction without complete obstruction at a dose of 2 liters (½ gal) for 2 days, in addition to conventional methods such as manual disimpaction and enemas. It is not known if this method is superior to those using conventional, more convenient laxatives.

As an ordinary laxative, the dose is 8–16 oz/day, but this may be less acceptable to patients than other osmotic agents, which are given in much smaller volumes.

PG-ES is suitable for installation into the stomach via enteral tube.

Stimulant/ Irritant Laxatives

The traditional notion regarding the stimulant laxatives is that they act directly on the myenteric plexus and stimulate colonic peristalsis, but their mechanisms may be diverse and more complex. They are potent laxatives and are the agents most often implicated in the cathartic bowel syndrome. Since they are available without prescription, most in convenient tablet form, they have a high abuse potential.

The anthraquinone irritant laxatives (**senna, cascara, aloe, casanthrol,** and **danthron**) may be partly absorbed, producing a falsely positive urine test for urobilinogen, but systemic toxicity does not occur. However, danthron has been associated with hepatotoxicity when taken with surfactant laxatives, which increase its absorption.

The diphenylmethane **phenolphthalein** is partly absorbed and undergoes enterohepatic circulation, so that the cathartic effect may be very prolonged, and **excessive purgation** is a risk if this agent is not used cautiously. It has also been implicated in **skin rashes** and more serious dermatopathology, as well as **malabsorption** and even osteomalacia. If the urine is alkaline, phenolphthalein will turn the urine a pink or red color, and may produce a red-colored stool if a soapsuds enema is given. These effects are harmless but can cause consternation to the uninformed. **Bisacodyl** is chemically related to phenolphthalein but is minimally absorbed and has not been reported to cause systemic toxicity. It is potent, however, and has been abused. Bisacodyl is enteric-coated and should not be given with antacids since raising gastric pH can disrupt the coating and lead to gastrointestinal symptoms. Both diphenylmethane compounds are ineffective in the presence of biliary obstruction or diversion. **Prune juice** and prunes contain a phenolphthalein derivative and do indeed have a cathartic action. It is not known if chronic ingestion is harmful.

Recommendations

Irritant laxatives may be used when rapid relief of constipation is desired, but are recommended for short-term use only. They should not be used in fecal impaction, which should be first cleared from below, manually or with the use of enemas.

Stool Softeners (Surfactants; Emollients)

Stool softeners (docusate sodium, docusate calcium) have a detergent action that reduces surface tension and promotes the admixture of water and fat allowing their penetration into feces and softening the stool. They may also act directly on the intestine and it has been suggested that long-term use of these agents could alter intestinal morphology. Although surfactants are not absorbed themselves, their detergent action enhances the absorption of danthron, mineral oil, and possibly other laxatives, increasing their systemic toxicity. However, in general, these agents are considered quite safe.

It is possible that their safety record is related to the fact that they have a mild action and are not often abused.

Recommendations

Stool softeners may be used as adjunctive treatment of hemorrhoids and other anal pathology, or in other situations when it is desirable to avoid straining during defecation. As with true laxatives, fluid intake should be increased. There are no known contraindications.

Other Laxatives

Mineral Oil

Mineral oil is in a category by itself. It acts as a lubricant, coating the intestine and its contents, preventing the absorption of water, and easing the passage of stool. It is a powerful cathartic and an old remedy still used by many elderly patients. Unfortunately, mineral oil can be **inadvertently aspirated**, particularly when it is taken at night, and **lipid pneumonia** can result. Chronic use can interfere with the absorption of fat-soluble vitamins. Systemic absorption of mineral oil can occur if it is taken with surfactant laxatives, and foreign-body reactions in lymphoid tissue have been described.

RECOMMENDATIONS. Mineral oil should be avoided by geriatric patients because they are at increased risk of aspiration, and this agent has no advantages over other potent laxatives. It is contraindicated in patients with an impaired gag reflex.

Castor Oil

Castor oil has been traditionally grouped with the irritant cathartics, but it acts partly in the small intestine, reducing smooth muscle contractility and speeding the passage of feces to the large intestine. It may also increase salt and water content of feces. It must first be hydrolyzed to its active form, ricinoleic acid, a substance that increases intestinal secretion and has been found to disrupt intestinal villi and promote **malabsorption**. Castor oil is unpalatable, potent, and sometimes acts very quickly. Although castor oil is a time-worn home remedy, it has no apparent advantages over other potent laxatives.

Suppositories

When patients are unable to take medication by mouth, suppositories can be given, and are preferred to more irritating enemas. **Bisacodyl** and **docusate** are available in suppository form. **Glycerin** is an osmotic agent that is absorbed when given orally and therefore is effective only when given by suppository. Its only side effect with ordinary use is occasional rectal irritation.

Enemas

Tap water, saline, sodium phosphates, mineral oil, and soapsuds, in order of increasing peril, have all been used as cathartic enemas. Combinations and liquid forms of bisacodyl are also available commercially. All can be **locally irritating**. However, **soapsuds enemas are particularly irritating**; they frequently cause cramping and distention and may produce hypovolemia and mucorrhea with potassium depletion. Although rare, **anaphylaxis, rectal gangrene,** and **hemorrhagic colitis** have been reported. The constituents of **sodium phosphate (Fleet) enemas** can be absorbed systemically and, if used injudiciously, they have the potential of enhancing **fluid retention** or **hyperphosphatemia** in high-risk patients.

RECOMMENDATIONS. In the management of constipation, enemas should be reserved for adjunctive treatment of acute fecal impaction. Prevention of recurrent impaction is best managed with oral agents or suppositories, with enemas being reserved for the occasional patient who is refractory to other methods.

Oil enemas should be reserved for intractable cases of fecal impaction. Soapsuds enemas should generally be avoided.

BIBLIOGRAPHY

Alessi, C. A., and Henderson, C. T. Constipation and fecal impaction in the long-term care patient. *Clin. Geriatr. Med.* 4:571–588, 1988.

American College of Gastroenterology Committee on FDA-Related Matters. Laxative use in constipation. *Amer. J. Gastroenterol.* 80:303–309, 1985.

Brandt. L. J. *Gastrointestinal Disorders in the Elderly.* New York: Raven Press, 1984. Pp. 261–275.

Lanza, E., and Butrum, R. A critical review of food fiber analysis and data. *J. Amer. Diet. Assoc.* 86:732–743, 1986.

Pietrusko, R.G. Use and abuse of laxatives. *Am. J. Hosp. Pharm.* 34:291–300, 1977.

Pike, B. F., and Phillippi, P. J. Soap colitis. *N. Engl. J. Med.* 285:217–218, 1971.

Puxty, J. A. H., and Fox, R. A. Golytely: a new approach to faecal impaction in old age. *Age Ageing* 15:122–124, 1986.

Sewester, C. S., Olin, B. R., Hebel, S. K., et al. *Facts and comparisons.* St. Louis: Lippincott, 1990. Pp. 316–323.

Wrenn, K. Fecal impaction. *N. Engl. J. Med.* 321:658–662, 1989.

Liquid Enteral Formulas and Tube Feeding

An important use of liquid formulas in geriatric practice is in enteral-tube feeding of debilitated patients. Tube feeding is given when a patient cannot or will not take in enough nutrition through the mouth to satisfy nutritional needs, but when gastrointestinal function does not mandate parenteral feeding. Specific uses of tube feeding include physical or neurologic impairment preventing oral intake or swallowing, anorexia secondary to medication or psychiatric disease, refusal to eat, and increased nutritional or metabolic demands that cannot be met orally (e.g., in the setting of trauma, burns, severe wasting disease, and decubitus ulcers). Patients with advanced Alzheimer's disease frequently lose the ability to swallow or may fail to take in sufficient food to satisfy nutritional requirements. It has recently been noted that calorie requirements may be higher than normal in Alzheimer's disease, an observation that requires further study.

Liquid formulas designed for tube feeding can be given orally. If oral intake is possible, flavored formulas are preferred because they are more palatable. Liquid feeds can be used as the sole source of nutrition in individuals who cannot swallow solid or semisolid food, or they may be used as nutritional supplements in patients whose normal intake is not sufficient to satisfy nutritional or caloric requirements.

SELECTION OF FORMULA

Standard

A standard formula is one that satisfies 100% of the U.S. Recommended Daily Allowance (RDA) of vitamins and minerals while providing adequate caloric intake, and can be used as a sole source of nutrition. Supplementary nutrients and additional liquid may be added in specific circumstances. In tube-fed patients, the liquid (water or fruit juice) that is often added during periodic flushing of the tube may also serve to satisfy requirements that might otherwise not be met.

RDA levels are intended to reflect the needs of healthy individuals, so that actual nutrient requirements may vary depending on the presence or absence of disease or drug use. Controversy exists as to the RDA of certain nutrients in the elderly. However, for the nursing home patient who receives long-term tube feeding, such considerations may be academic; in these patients, adequate nitrogen balance, prevention of overt deficiency disease, and the provision of physical and psychological comfort are of paramount importance.

The gastrointestinal tract acts to maintain its osmolality at the same level as that of normal body fluids (roughly 300 mOsm/kg water). Since standard formulas are somewhat hyperosmolar (400–600 mOsm/kg water), they may produce net secretion of water into the gut, resulting in diarrhea. Osmotic effects may be particularly pronounced in patients with feeding tubes placed in the jejunum.

Patients who are able to tolerate a standard commercial formula may also be given diluted pureed food ("home-brew"), although as a practical matter this is seldom used for tube-fed patients in institutions today. Pureed food is, of course, suitable for patients who are able to feed orally. Likewise, powdered breakfast products mixed with milk (Instant Breakfast) may be substituted for standard-formula liquid feeds and may be less expensive.

Isotonic

Isotonic (isosmotic) feeds are highly suitable for tube-fed patients because their osmolarity is roughly 300 mOsm/kg water, approximating that of normal body fluids. For this reason, such feeds are less likely to produce diarrhea. The lower osmolality of these feeds is achieved through the use of glucose polymers instead of simple sugars as the carbohydrate source, and by reducing sodium content. Low sodium content makes these feeds additionally useful when salt restriction is desirable, although salt restriction should by no means be assumed to be a requirement in all geriatric patients. High molecular carbohydrates are theoretically beneficial to the poorly controlled diabetic, but the clinical significance of this is not known.

Fiber-Containing Formulas

Fiber-containing formulas are designed for patients with constipation and chronic impaction, and would appear to be ideal for nursing-home patients, but clinical advantage over standard formulas has yet to be scientifically demonstrated. The addition of dietary fiber has other theoretical benefits, such as improved glucose tolerance, but further study is required.

Fiber formula provides 3.4 g of dietary fiber per 8-oz can, so that if used as a total source of nutrients it would provide the amount comparable to the average American diet. The disadvantage of these preparations is that they are more viscous and may flow through a small-bore tube sluggishly.

High-Calorie (Calorie-Dense)

High-calorie formulas contain 1½–2 times the calories per unit volume of standard formulas and are designed for patients who require additional energy support because of a hypermetabolic state, trauma, or a wasting disease such as cancer. In chronically tube-fed elderly, calorie-dense formulas may be useful when fluid restriction is desired, as in the case of refractory congestive heart failure or hyponatremia. These highly concentrated supplements do, however, have high osmolality (600 mOsm/kg water or more) and should be instituted carefully so that diarrhea, electrolyte disturbances, and dehydration do not occur. Because of high carbohydrate content, these formulas should be used with extra caution in diabetics or those with stress- or illness-induced insulin resistance.

Calorie-dense formulas are not intended for routine use and should be instituted only when a specific indication exists.

Specialized Formulas

The following preparations are rarely used in geriatric practice and should be reserved only for situations for which they were designed.

Elemental (hydrolyzed, predigested) feeds are designed for patients with protein or fat malabsorption or maldigestion. Elemental formulas may have oligopeptides or free amino acids rather than whole proteins as their protein source, or medium chain triglycerides as a portion of their fat source. Although useful in patients with pancreatic insufficiency, inflammatory bowel disease, or short bowel syndrome, predigested feeds are expensive and unlikely to alleviate formula-related diarrhea in the chronically tube-fed geriatric patient with presumably normal gastrointestinal function (see Gastrointestinal Complications below).

High-nitrogen formulas are designed for patients with severe burns, multiple trauma, and protein depletion. Although occasionally used in the cachectic cancer patient, they are not intended for the typical nursing-home patient.

Formulas with a nitrogen source consisting of high levels of **branched-chain amino acids** have been shown to be superior to those high in aromatic amino acids for patients with hepatic encephalopathy, in that branched-chain formulas are capable of maintaining positive nitrogen balance while inducing a lower rate of cognitive impairment. However, they do not consistently improve hepatic encephalopathy. These formulas have also been promoted for use in states of high physiologic stress, but their efficacy in improving nitrogen balance in such situations is controversial.

Individuals with severe pulmonary disease may fare better with a **decreased carbohydrate-to-nitrogen ratio** and a formula exists for this purpose.

Other Considerations

Most prepared formulas today are completely or nearly lactose-free. This probably has come about for commercial reasons more than scientific considerations, since the link between lactose and formula-related gastrointestinal symptoms has not been proved. Of course, powdered formulas prepared with milk may worsen symptoms in lactose-intolerant patients. All commercially prepared formulas are gluten free.

The number and complexity of commercially prepared formulas is proliferating, in an effort to provide the "ideal" formula for each specific patient. A summary of formulations most commonly used in geriatric practice is found in Table 25–1.

SELECTION OF TUBE

Large-bore tubes (roughly 12 French or greater) are less likely than small-bore tubes to become clogged and are therefore practical when feeds with high viscosity are used. However, large-bore tubes are stiff and extremely uncomfortable, and are associated with a wide spectrum of mechanical complications, including nasal erosions, hoarseness, impaired cough, esophagitis, and erosions or ulcers of the esophageal and gastric mucosa. Although acceptable for gastrostomy feeding, they should rarely if ever be used for long-term nasogastric feeding. Because of their extreme discomfort, they should be strictly avoided in patients who are conscious.

Small-bore tubes (roughly smaller than 10 French) produce less discomfort and trauma than large-bore tubes. Although they are less likely to reduce the competency of the lower esophageal sphincter, they are unlikely to reduce the risk of aspiration in high-risk patients (see Complications below). The softness and small diameter of small-bore tubes make it possible for certain patients to swallow so that tube feeding can be supplemented by oral feeding, a patient-

Table 25-1.   Commonly Used Enteral Formulas

Type	Brand	Osmolarity (mOsm/kg H_2O)	Kcal/ml
Standard	Sustacal	625	1.0
	Ensure	470	1.06
	Meritene[a]	505	0.96
	Instant Breakfast[a]	677–715[c]	1.06
	Compleat Regular[b]	405	1.07
Isotonic	Isocal	300	1.06
	Osmolite	300	1.06
	Compleat Modified	300	1.07
Fiber-Added	Enrich	480	1.1
	Jevity	310	1.06
Calorie-Dense	Sustacal HC	650	1.5
	Ensure Plus	690	1.5
	Magnacal	590	2.0

[a]Milk-based.
[b]Meat-based.
[c]Prepared with 8 oz whole milk per packet.

assisted maneuver that gives sensory gratification and psychological benefit.

Small-bore tubes have a tendency to become clogged. The frequent flushing needed to ensure tube patency may increase nursing time, a problem that is sometimes overcome by changing to a soft tube with a slightly larger diameter, by diluting a viscous feed, or by using an infusion pump. Small-bore tubes have a tendency to collapse under negative pressure, making it difficult to evaluate gastric residual by aspirating gastric contents. They may become knotted, tend to coil up in the oropharynx during installation, and, because they are more likely to become displaced, have been known to end up in the bronchial tree, sometimes with disastrous consequences. Nonetheless, purely from the point of view of patient comfort, they are preferable to the large-bore tube if the nasogastric route is used for feeding.

Small-bore tubes are made out of soft Silastic or polyurethane material and may require special techniques for insertion. Many are now available with a removable stylet to facilitate insertion.

COMPLICATIONS OF TUBE FEEDING

Aspiration

Tubes that cross the esophagogastric junction reduce the competency of the lower esophageal sphincter, increasing the risk of regurgitation and aspiration. At greatest risk are patients who are neurologically impaired, mechanically ventilated, severely debilitated, or moribund, those with impaired gag reflex, and those who are restrained. Aspiration is certain if the tube rides up into the esophagus or is inadvertently inserted into the trachea when it is first placed. Unfortunately, aspiration may not be immediately apparent in the very patients who are at highest risk.

Feed instilled below the gastroesophageal junction, as with gastrostomy, does not prevent aspiration pneumonia in most chronically tube-fed patients. Regurgitation of food may occur regardless of feeding route, and recent evidence suggests that even jejunostomy feedings can be regurgitated. In addition, it is important to emphasize that neurologically impaired patients with impaired deglutition continually aspirate oropharyngeal secretions and are likely to develop aspiration pneumonia on that account. Finally, since tube feeding is a passive process, the patient cannot reduce food intake when there is anorexia, satiety, or gastrointestinal disease, and may thus lose a natural protection against regurgitation. Thus, patient factors are at least as important as, if not more important than, feeding method in determining the risk of aspiration.

Gastrointestinal Complications

Distension, cramping, and diarrhea occur commonly, especially when the feed is first instituted. Although these symptoms can be due to bacterial contamination of the feed or to gastrointestinal disease such as malabsorption and maldigestion, most often they are due to the high osmotic load delivered to the upper small intestine as a function of the osmolarity of the feed itself and of the speed with which the osmotic load is delivered. Osmolarity of the feed can be reduced by diluting with water or by changing to a feed of reduced osmolality. The feeding rate can be reduced by giving smaller bolus feeds more frequently, or by reducing the rate of a continuous feed, or by using a mechanical infusion pump to precisely regulate the rate of infusion. Switching to an elemental feed containing hydrolyzed protein or medium-chain triglycerides is generally not helpful for patients who do not have malabsorption or maldigestion, and can be expensive.

Diarrhea and cramping have also been attributed to the use of cold feed or to concurrent antibiotics. Immobilized patients who are chronically tube-fed could also have fecal impaction with secondary diarrhea. Symptoms should be attributed to lactose intolerance only if commercial formulas are prepared with added milk.

If secondary factors are ruled out, and if adjusting the content and speed of the feed fails to eliminate the problem of diarrhea, antidiarrheal agents such as loperamide or diphenoxylate are often effective.

Metabolic Complications

Hypernatremia or hyponatremia occurs commonly in debilitated elderly and may develop with the use of enteral nutrition as well. Hypernatremia is most likely to occur in calorie-dense feeds, in the presence of diarrhea, or in the presence of medical conditions predisposing to dehydration, such as infection or hyperglycemia. Geriatric patients are prone to hypernatremia because of the kidney's age-related decrease in urinary concentrating ability. There is also an age-associated lack of thirst in response to dehydration, which could be exacerbated in the passively tube-fed patient who is unable to request hydration. Hypernatremia can be avoided if adequate free water is given and if electrolytes are monitored in the event of illness.

The occurrence of hyponatremia is related to the fact that many aged individuals have impaired free-water clearance. If hyponatremia develops in tube-fed patients, the tube should be flushed with fruit juice rather than free water, and calorie-dense formulas should be carefully instituted until hyponatremia is corrected.

Hypokalemia and **hyperkalemia** can occur when the potassium content of the feed does not match the needs of the patient. If *hyper*kalemia develops, a formula that is low in potassium can be substituted. If a formula change does not correct *hypo*kalemia, potassium supplements can be added to the feed; in such cases, care should be taken if the tube lies in the jejunum, since potassium supplements are extremely hyperosmolar.

Hyperglycemia sometimes occurs in tube-fed patients and is theoretically preventable in high-risk patients if feeds using complex carbohydrates rather than simple sugars are used as a carbohydrate source. However, feed that has sat out too long may be deficient in glucose. Fortunately these problems are uncommonly linked to enteral feeds and are rarely serious.

Nutrient-drug interactions occur in tube feeding just as they do when food and medications are taken orally. Such interactions are potentially avoidable when bolus feeds are given, but the tube must be thoroughly flushed before and after medication is administered. Continuous feeds should be stopped for instillation of certain medications. Important interactions have been described for theophylline, warfarin, and phenytoin. In these cases nutrients may bind to the drug, reducing its absorption. Since these drugs have a narrow therapeutic-to-toxic ratio, caution must be observed when there is a change in the drug or feeding regimen. The drug should be administered at least 2 hours prior to instillation of the feed. If this is impractical, the drug should at the very least be given at a constant interval in relation to the feed.

It is also important to remember that drug absorption may be altered if the feed and drug are instilled below the pylorus, as with jejunostomy feeding.

Liquid forms of medications should be used when available. Enteric-coated drugs should not be crushed and may sometimes have to be substituted by alternative medication. Timed-release preparations should be avoided.

ETHICAL CONSIDERATIONS

Patients have the right to refuse artificial feeding as they are able to refuse any medical treatment. If they are incompetent, they may do so through a surrogate decision-maker or advance directive such as a living will. This right has been upheld in the courts and is supported by respected professional organizations. Patients or their decision-makers need to be completely informed about the benefits and burdens of tube feeding for the patient in question.

In general, patients should be fed orally as long as possible, not only because it is more physiologic, but because it is pleasurable. Artificial feeding lacks a sensory component and sometimes can only be effected if restraints are used, which may produce discomfort, intense anxiety, and agitation in the patient who does not understand what is going on. Physicians and family members may become concerned when patients do not take in enough calories to maintain their ideal body weight, but it is important to remember that the imposition of nutrients in response to strictly calculated nutritional requirements does not necessarily improve patient comfort. In fact, this practice may pose an undue burden on patients who are unable to express the fact that they are satiated or that they are feeling unwell.

There is no evidence that withholding artificial feeding from neurologically impaired or dying patients is painful. For further discussion of this issue, the reader is referred to the Bibliography readings (see Ahronheim & Gasner; Steinbrook & Lo).

BIBLIOGRAPHY

Ahronheim, J. C., and Gasner, M. R. The sloganism of starvation. *Lancet* 1:278–279, 1990.

Ciocon, J. O., Silverstone, F. A., Graver, M., et al. Tube feeding in elderly patients. Indications, benefits, and complications. *Arch. Intern. Med.* 148:429–433, 1988.

Eisenberg, P. Enteral nutrition. Indications, formulas, and delivery techniques. *Nurs. Clin. North. Am.* 24(2):315–338, 1989.

Kahn, S., Hunter, W., and Thomas, E. Gastroesophageal reflux in patients with percutaneous endoscopic gastrostomy or percutaneous endoscopic jejunostomy. *Gastroenterology* 96:A245, 1989 (abstract).

Rombeau, J. L., and Caldwell, M. D. *Enteral and Tube Feeding.* Philadelphia: Saunders, 1984.

Silk, D. B. A. Topics and controversies in enteral nutrition. *Gut* 27 (Suppl. 1):1–122, 1986.

Steinbrook, R., and Lo, B. Artificial feeding—solid ground, not a slippery slope. *N. Engl. J. Med.* 318:286–290, 1988.

Drugs for Peptic Ulcer and Gastritis

Although both duodenal and gastric ulcer are common in late life, the proportion of gastric disorders increases with age. By the age of 75, gastric lesions, notably ulcer and gastritis, are probably twice as common as duodenal ulcer. The age-related predilection for the stomach is probably related to the high incidence of underlying atrophic gastritis and gastric atrophy, which is associated with loss of secretory cells and thinning of the mucosa, increasing the vulnerability to disruption from a variety of insults. Although these age changes are by no means universal, hypo- or achlorhydria is present in at least 20% of people 65 and older, and this proportion continues to increase in the later decades of life.

Gastropathy from nonsteroidal anti-inflammatory agents (NSAID gastropathy) is most common in the elderly population. This is related both to age changes in the stomach and to the fact that older individuals are the chief consumers of NSAIDs. NSAIDs indirectly contribute to duodenal pathology, and exacerbation of duodenal ulcer disease may occur.

Ulcers and gastritis may present atypically in the elderly. Epigastric pain is frequently modest or absent, with occult or even massive bleeding not uncommonly the first sign. In the case of NSAID gastropathy, this presentation may be partly related to the fact that the cause of the problem is an analgesic. "Painless" and subtle presentations in elderly patients may also have to do with factors such as altered pain perception or the presence of dementia or other neurological impairments. This is likely to lead to delayed diagnosis, missed diagnosis, and increased morbidity. Major complications such as perforation increase dramatically after the age of 75, resulting in a much higher need for emergency surgery.

Heliobacter (Campylobacter) pylori infection has been increasingly invoked in the pathogenesis of peptic ulcer and gastritis. A direct cause-and-effect relationship has not been established, but the association is under intensive study. The incidence of colonization with *H. pylori* increases with age, so the role of this bacterium in the geriatric age group is even less well defined. Until the meaning of *H. pylori* colonization is better understood, standard antiulcer treatment should be given, as described below. Gastroenterologists often direct treatment at the organism by prescribing agents with activity against the organism itself, including bismuth and metronidazole. Although this practice has been discouraged by others, who recommend that such treatment be reserved for refractory cases, there is evidence that eradication of *H. pylori* reduces recurrence rate of ulcer treated with standard therapy.

Therapy of peptic ulcer, gastritis, and dyspepsia in the elderly is based on the same pathophysiologic principles as in younger groups. However, doses of certain agents may differ, and selection of agent may have to be based on practical principles such as compliance, drug regimen, and side-effect profile.

SPECIFIC AGENTS

Antacids

Antacids, the mainstay of ulcer therapy for many years, have lost popularity to a newer generation of agents. The reasons for this are manifold. Compliance with long-term antacid therapy is poor. Many patients find an antacid regimen to be unpalatable and inconvenient. Although there is evidence that low-dose therapy is just as effective as high doses, multiple daily doses are still viewed as obligatory to effect healing. Antacids may impair absorption of a number of medications; the requirement that they must be taken at least 1 hour away from these agents can seriously complicate a patient's drug regimen. Although antacids are available without prescription, the total dose taken can make the regimen as costly as other agents. Finally, although toxicity is generally not serious, there is a high incidence of side effects, notably alteration in bowel function, which may damage compliance or which may ultimately produce systemic symptoms.

Despite these pitfalls, antacids still have an important place in the management of gastroduodenal disease.

Pharmacologic Considerations

MECHANISM OF ACTION. Antacids are believed to act by buffering gastric contents and increasing the pH. Standard antacids contain magnesium or aluminum hydroxide. These compounds react with hydrochloric acid to form a salt and water, raising the pH of gastric juices that remain in the stomach or that are delivered to the duodenum. If pH approaches 4, the proteolytic action of gastric enzymes is reduced. Recent evidence indicates that antacids act by other mechanisms as well, conferring "cytoprotection," perhaps by enhancing secretion of protective prostaglandin. This would explain the fact that antacid regimens with very low buffering capacity may be as effective as high-dose regimens. It would also explain the apparent paradox that antacids may work in patients with gastric hypoacidity.

Antacids are at least as effective for the management of stress ulcer as other antiulcer agents when given in a controlled setting where frequent (hourly) dosing can be assured. They are widely used in the management of nonulcer dyspepsia because of their convenience and probably because of the reluctance of physicians to prescribe systemic therapy when no ulcer is demonstrable. The efficacy of antacids in the prevention and management of NSAID gastropathy is not known because controlled studies are lacking.

Calcium carbonate is an effective antacid but it is less commonly used today than in the past because of the widely held notion that calcium, by stimulating the parietal cell, produces "acid rebound" and counterproductive hypersecretion. Sodium bicarbonate, once a popular antacid, is infrequently used because of its sodium load and tendency to produce alkalosis.

PHARMACOKINETICS. In the fasting state, the pH-increasing effect of antacids lasts for approximately 30 minutes; after meals, this effect may last for as long as 3–5 hours. Both the magnitude and duration of effect are highly variable, depending on buffering capacity of the agent used and on patient characteristics such as gastric acidity and gastric emptying time.

Sodium bicarbonate that is not converted to salt and acid is well absorbed, while calcium and magnesium are less well, and aluminum minimally absorbed. Calcium, magnesium, and aluminum are converted to compounds in the intestine that are largely insoluble and poorly absorbed.

OTHER CONSTITUENTS. **Alginic acid** combined with antacid produces a foaming gel that floats on top of gastric contents and reduces symptoms of acid reflux. Alginic acid itself has no intrinsic antiulcer properties but is available in combination with antacid (Gaviscon). It delivers the antacid directly to the irritated mucosa at the gastroesophageal junction and reduces the antacid requirement.

Combination agents often contain **simethicone** (Mylecon, others), a surfactant that reduces the surface tension of bubbles, making them coalesce into larger bubbles that are easier to expel, or that dissipate. Simethicone may help to reduce symptoms of belching or bloating in a variety of clinical states, but has no known ability to enhance ulcer healing.

Adverse Effects

Short-term antacid use rarely produces serious harm, but in at least 50% of cases, **alterations in bowel function** occur.

Magnesium-containing antacids frequently produce **diarrhea**, which may be severe, resulting in **dehydration** and **electrolyte imbalance**. Magnesium is thought to exert its cathartic effect by producing insoluble salts in the intestine or by stimulating the secretion of cholecystokinin, increasing water in the gut. Most magnesium-containing antacids also contain aluminum to counterbalance the cathartic effect. The cathartic effect of these antacids is often perceived as beneficial by the chronically constipated patient. This encourages some patients to use antacids inappropriately.

In renal failure, the limited degree to which magnesium is absorbed is offset by reduced excretion; **hypermagnesemia** may result.

Aluminum-containing antacids may produce **constipation** and **fecal impaction**, a problem that is probably limited to agents that contain no magnesium. Constipation is thought to be related to the ability of aluminum to bind bile acids, hampering their digestive and laxative effect. By binding intestinal phosphate, aluminum may also produce **hypophosphatemia**, and long-term, high-dose use can produce **osteomalacia**. The risk of osteomalacia increases in patients with hyperparathyroid bone disease or chronic renal failure, when accumulation of aluminum itself can impair bone mineralization. Increased aluminum burden from antacids and dialysate has also been implicated in "dialysis dementia" of chronic renal failure. However, there is no convincing evidence that elevated brain aluminum produces Alzheimer's disease or other forms of dementia.

Calcium-containing antacids may also produce **constipation, flatulence**, and, in susceptible individuals, **hypercalcemia** and **hypercalciuria**. A full blown "**milk-alkali**" **syndrome** with hypercalcemia, renal stones, and metabolic alkalosis may result when doses are high. This syndrome, also described with high milk intake and sodium bicarbonate antacid, is rarely seen today. It has not become a problem with the recent wide use of calcium carbonate in the management of osteoporosis, probably because calcium is poorly absorbed in late life.

All antacids may produce various degrees of **systemic alkalosis,** but significant alkalosis is unlikely except with long-term use of sodium bicarbonate or calcium carbonate. **Sodium bicarbonate** may also cause clinically significant **fluid retention** in susceptible individuals.

If recent evidence is borne out that low-dose regimens are as effective as traditional high-dose regimens, these side effects should diminish in importance.

Important Drug Interactions

These interactions are critically reviewed in the Bibliography readings (see D'Arcy & McElnay) and summarized in Table 26–1. Antacids may bind to or chelate agents, or may change the pH of the stomach and upper small intestine, altering dissolution properties and absorption of concurrently administered medications. Consequently, they may impair or delay the absorption of a wide variety of drugs and nutrients, but the clinical importance of this is probably limited to a few. Much depends on the type of antacid and the formulation of the drug administered, and inter-individual differences in gastric emptying time and pH will determine the time interval required between antacid and drug ingestion. As a general rule, the antacid should be given at least 1 hour away from other medications. Two hours or more should transpire before giving agents with a narrow therapeutic-to-toxic ratio, such as digoxin and phenytoin.

Antacids are commonly administered as a protective maneuver with an anti-inflammatory agent, and in most cases will delay but not impair overall absorption. Antacids should not be administered concurrently with enteric-coated agents, including aspirin, because the resultant increase in gastric pH may speed dissolution of the pill's protective coating. This could potentially enhance rather than lower gastric toxicity.

Contraindications and Precautions

Magnesium-containing antacids are contraindicated in renal failure. Calcium-containing antacids are contraindicated in hypercalcemic states, and in patients with urinary tract stones, particularly those

Table 26–1. Agents Whose Bioavailability Is Reduced by Antacids

Iron (due to increased gastric pH)
Tetracycline (due to increased gastric pH)
Phenothiazines
Certain NSAIDs
Digoxin
Isoniazid
Prednisolone
Ranitidine
Cimetidine?
Phenytoin

associated with abnormalities in calcium metabolism. Sodium bicarbonate should be avoided in fluid-retaining states and in poorly controlled hypertension.

If an aluminum-only antacid is required in a patient with a history of fecal impaction, the need for a laxative should be assessed early on in therapy.

Patients who self-administer magnesium-aluminum combination antacids for purposes of "bowel regularity" should be discouraged from using antacids in this way.

Choice of Agent

Combination magnesium-aluminum antacids are the most widely used antacids today. These antacids are the formulation of choice except in renal failure, where hypermagnesemia is a risk. Aluminum-only antacids are generally used in that setting and can be used in other patients as well if combination antacids produce diarrhea.

Patients who wish to increase their intake of calcium for dietary reasons sometimes inquire about the use of calcium carbonate as an antacid (TUMS, others). Although calcium carbonate may be appropriate for occasional use in the management of nonulcer dyspepsia, it should not be relied upon for ulcer healing.

Sodium bicarbonate has no important advantages over other antacids and should generally be avoided.

Agents differ in their acid-neutralizing capacity (see Sewester et al.). On the whole, liquid preparations have higher acid-neutralizing capacity than tablet forms, and have traditionally been considered more effective. Some investigators feel that tablets may be as effective as liquid antacids, however, and patients who are physically and socially active may wish to use the tablet form at various times during the day for the sake of portability and convenience.

Palatability of a particular formulation or brand may differ, and is a matter of personal taste. Since palatability will affect compliance, the patient should be told that preparations and brands differ in flavor and consistency.

Indications

Antacids are indicated in short-term treatment of nonulcer dyspepsia and as adjunctive treatment in peptic ulcer. Although their efficacy in the prophylaxis of NSAID-related peptic disease is not known, they are probably suitable for patients who take occasional doses of NSAIDs.

Antacids are indicated for the treatment of peptic ulcer and gastritis if more convenient agents cannot be given. They are also indicated for the prevention or treatment of stress ulcer, given alone or in combination with intravenous histamine$_2$ antagonists (see below).

Dosing (Magnesium- or Aluminum-Containing Agents)

Peptic ulcer: 15–30 cc 1–3 hours after meals and at bedtime. Dosage may be given more frequently if symptoms break through. Full-dose therapy should be continued for 8–12 weeks.

Note: Low-dose regimens of 15–30 cc qid may be equally effective.

Stress ulcer: 30–60 cc up to once an hour. If administration is by nasogastric tube, the dose can be titrated to keep gastric pH at 5 or greater.

Histamine$_2$ (H$_2$) Blockers

Pharmacologic Considerations

MECHANISM OF ACTION. H$_2$ blockers act by competitively inhibiting the histamine$_2$ receptor in gastric parietal cells. Binding of histamine at these sites promotes gastric acid secretion. By blunting histamine action, H$_2$ blockers inhibit basal and stimulated gastric acid secretion, speed the healing of peptic ulcers, relieve pain, and, when taken chronically, prevent ulcer recurrence. Cimetidine has proven to be as effective in elderly patients as in younger adults and it is anticipated that the same will be true for all agents of this class. However, while highly effective in the treatment of duodenal ulcer, H$_2$ blockers like most other antiulcer medication have variable effects on the healing of benign gastric ulcer.

H$_2$ blockers have no effect on histamine$_1$ receptors and do not share activities with traditional antihistamines (H$_1$ blockers). Also, while H$_2$ receptors do exist outside the stomach, pharmacologic blockade of these receptors by H$_2$ blockers appears to have limited clinical applicability.

There are some chemical differences among the four H$_2$ blockers that are now available. Although they are approximately equal in efficacy, they have a somewhat different profile of adverse effects and drug interactions.

Cimetidine (Tagamet)

The first H$_2$ blocker in use, cimetidine has a track record of efficacy and relative safety in elderly patients. However, it has a number of disadvantages that make it less preferable than other H$_2$ blockers.

ACTIONS NOT RELATED TO GASTRIC SECRETION. Cimetidine binds to cytochrome P-450, decreasing the activity of hepatic microsomal enzymes. It is thought to reduce hepatic blood flow, but this effect is controversial.

Cimetidine has antiandrogenic effects; it binds to androgenic receptors and reduces hepatic degradation of estradiol, the most potent form of endogenous estrogen. In addition, cimetidine increases the secretion of prolactin.

Cimetidine binds to peripheral lymphocytes and increases their responsiveness to mitogens. While attempts have been made to harness this immunostimulatory action in disorders such as cutaneous herpes zoster, there are at present no recognized clinical applications.

PHARMACOKINETICS. Cimetidine is well absorbed from the upper small intestine with peak plasma levels being achieved in 1–2 hours. It undergoes first-pass metabolism but 70% is excreted unchanged by the kidney. Although half-life is brief at 2 hours, gastric acid secretion is suppressed for 5–7 hours after a 300-mg dose. Serum half-life tends to be prolonged in elderly patients, but it is not known if biologic action in the stomach is altered.

Cimetidine and the other H$_2$ blockers are not highly bound to serum proteins.

ADVERSE EFFECTS. Cimetidine can produce a variety of **central nervous system (CNS) symptoms,** including confusion, lethargy, dizziness, agitation, and hallucinations. Elderly patients with overt or subclinical CNS impairments are probably more susceptible to these effects than other groups of patients. These effects appear to be dose-related and the predilection for the elderly may also be due to diminished renal excretion of the drug. Intravenous is more likely than oral cimetidine to produce these problems.

The antiandrogen actions of cimetidine may result in **gynecomastia**. Baseline gynecomastia is not unusual in elderly men and should be noted before cimetidine is instituted so that it should not be incorrectly attributed to the drug. **Impotence** has also been reported with cimetidine. It is not known if the estrogenic actions of cimetidine have clinical effects in women.

By binding to cardiac H_2 receptors, large doses of rapidly administered **intravenous** cimetidine have been reported to produce **bradycardia, arrhythmias,** and **hypotension**. These effects are rare. Concurrent use of other drugs and coexistent cardiac disease in ill elderly patients would tend to confound the clinical picture in such cases. However, as a precaution, intravenous H_2 blockers should be administered very slowly.

Other reported side effects include nausea, pruritus, skin rash, and transient elevation in serum transaminases. Increase in intraocular pressure has been reported with cimetidine and ranitidine in a patient with chronic open angle glaucoma; this association has not been explained.

Cimetidine reduces creatinine excretion by a competitive inhibition of tubular secretion. As a result, serum creatinine levels may become elevated; however, this is not an indication of renal dysfunction.

Long-term use of H_2 blockers is thought to be generally safe, but concern has been raised over the **potential consequences of prolonged gastric acid suppression**. This is of particular concern in older patients who often have gastric hypoacidity at baseline. Both cimetidine and ranitidine have been found to reduce the absorption of vitamin B_{12}, which is dependent on acid-mediated release from binding sites in dietary protein. Although there are no reports of clinical deficiency due to these drugs, vitamin B_{12} deficiency resulting from gastric hypoacidity is probably far more prevalent in the geriatric age group than previously recognized and should be watched for in all older patients on long-term H_2 blockers. Chronic gastric acid suppression may also result in bacterial overgrowth, which could increase the risk of aspiration pneumonia. Another potential risk would be the development of phytobezoars, rare lesions that result from faulty digestive processes in the stomach. The exact prevalence of these problems has not been determined.

IMPORTANT DRUG INTERACTIONS. By reducing the activity of the hepatic cytochrome P-450 enzyme system, cimetidine decreases the metabolism of certain drugs, increasing their potency. Important drugs affected by cimetidine in this way include warfarin, theophylline, phenytoin, and a number of other agents. Some of these drug interactions have been explained by cimetidine's action in reducing hepatic blood flow, but this mechanism has been disputed. In the presence of hepatic insufficiency and congestive heart failure, hepatic-mediated drug interactions may be accentuated.

The metabolism of cimetidine is enhanced by coadministration of enzyme-inducing agents such as phenobarbital, which would reduce the efficacy of the former.

Cimetidine is largely excreted by the kidney. Other drugs may compete with cimetidine for tubular secretion sites and their clearance may be reduced. Important interactions have been reported for procainamide, triamterene, and flecainide. This property is shared by ranitidine and possibly by the newer H_2 blockers as well.

Suppression of gastric acid may reduce the absorption of certain drugs including ketoconazole, indomethacin, and chlorpromazine. Such an effect should be assumed to occur with the other H_2 blockers until other evidence exists to the contrary.

Concurrent administration of antacid reduces the systemic absorption of cimetidine. It is not known if this impairs antiulcer efficacy, since the antacid itself would be expected to exert a therapeutic effect.

Drugs whose activity can be enhanced by cimetidine are summarized in Table 26-2.

INDICATIONS. H_2 blockers are indicated in the management of peptic ulcer, duodenitis, and gastritis. Gastric lesions due to NSAIDs appear to respond better to misoprostol (see below), which is presently the only agent officially approved for this indication.

DOSING. Doses of H_2 blockers are summarized in Table 26-3. Doses listed on the table are derived from data on nongeriatric adults. These doses should be initiated in patients with active gastroduodenal disease who have normal serum creatinine. In the elderly, a normal creatinine may mask diminished ability of the kidneys to clear these drugs. If dose-related adverse effects such as confusion occur, downward dose adjustment may maintain clinical

Table 26-2. Some Drugs Whose Activity May Be Enhanced by Cimetidine

Antiarrhythmic agents
   Quinidine*
   Procainamide*
   Lidocaine
   Encainide
   Flecainide
Anticonvulsants
   Phenytoin*
   Carbamazepine
   Valproic acid
Benzodiazepines (long-acting)
Beta adrenergic blockers*
Calcium channel blocking agents*
Digitoxin
Metronidazole
Oral hypoglycemic agents
Salicylates
Theophylline*
Triamterene
Tricyclic antidepressants
Warfarin* (variable)

*Drug or member of group may also interact with ranitidine according to scattered case reports.

Table 26–3. Dosing of H_2 Blockers (mg)

Agent (Brand)	Initial Oral	Intravenous[a]	Maintenance
Cimetidine (Tagamet)	400 bid or 800 hs	300 q6–8 h	400 hs
Ranitidine (Zantac)	150 bid or 300 hs	50 q8–12 h	150 hs
Famotidine (Pepcid)	40 hs	[b]	20 hs
Nizatidine (Axid)	150 hs	—	150 daily or on alternate days

Doses based on data in nongeratric adults. Dosage given for nizatidine is adjusted for adult with moderate renal impairment.
[a]May be given by continuous infusion.
[b]Insufficient information to recommend to geriatric patients.

efficacy in some cases, but this cannot be predicted with certainty. Among the H_2 blockers this is particularly important with cimetidine, which may not only cause mental confusion but can increase serum creatinine without altering renal function. Given the ever-expanding choice of agents, it is advisable in these circumstances to switch to another H_2 blocker or to an agent from another class.

In benign peptic ulcer disease, full doses of H_2 blockers should be given until the ulcer heals. In younger patients, the disappearance of symptoms generally correlates well with healing and takes about 4–6 weeks. It is not known if healing is delayed in older individuals. However, because disease is more often silent and since initial and recurrent ulcer is associated with greater morbidity and mortality, full ulcer treatment should probably be given for at least 8 weeks. In gastric ulcer, healing may take up to 12 weeks and should be demonstrated objectively with radiographic or endoscopic evaluation. It is usually not necessary to document healing of duodenal ulcer, but if there is any reason to suspect delayed healing or in the presence of other serious medical problems, maintenance doses should be instituted.

Ranitidine (Zantac)

PHARMACOLOGIC CONSIDERATIONS

Actions. Ranitidine resembles cimetidine and other H_2 blockers in its antiulcer action. However, ranitidine binds to cytochrome P-450 much less avidly than cimetidine. Consequently, while it has the potential of participating in related drug interactions, these have been reported less frequently.

Ranitidine has less antiandrogenic effect than cimetidine and does not bind to lymphocytes.

Pharmacokinetics. Ranitidine is well absorbed with peak plasma levels being achieved in 1–3 hours. It undergoes first-pass metabolism in the liver, but at least 50% is excreted unchanged by the kidney. The serum half-life of 2–3 hours may be prolonged in some elderly. Inhibition of gastric acid secretion lasts for 8–12 hours, somewhat longer than for cimetidine.

ADVERSE EFFECTS. Ranitidine appears to be capable of producing the same spectrum of CNS effects as cimetidine, despite earlier claims that its relatively lower penetration of the blood-brain barrier would eliminate this risk. Ranitidine appears to be more likely than cimetidine to produce **headache.** All in all, however, CNS effects are uncommon. Unlike cimetidine, ranitidine does not bind to androgen receptors and has no effect on prolactin secretion, but gynecomastia has been reported. The drug has rarely been reported to produce bradycardia.

Potential long-term consequences of gastric acid suppression are discussed above.

IMPORTANT DRUG INTERACTIONS. Ranitidine has the potential to participate in the same drug interactions as cimetidine. Although hepatically mediated interactions are less likely with ranitidine because of its weaker inhibition of microsomal enzymes, cimetidinelike interactions have been reported. In addition, conclusions regarding the lack of interactions from ranitidine have often been based on experimental data derived from healthy subjects, and interactions based on competition for renal excretion may still occur. Because of occult reductions in renal function often seen in older patients, levels of ranitidine could be higher than expected, and perhaps high enough to produce an important drug interaction in an aged patient. It is prudent to anticipate a cimetidinelike drug interaction when ranitidine is given with drugs that have a narrow therapeutic index. However, it is generally safer to give ranitidine than cimetidine under those circumstances.

Famotidine (Pepcid)

Famotidine differs from cimetidine and ranitidine in several ways. It has a longer half-life and duration of antisecretory activity and is marketed as a once-a-day drug, but current evidence indicates that other H_2 blockers may be just as effective when the entire dose is taken once a day. Famotidine is metabolized and only about 20%–30% of oral drug is excreted unchanged by the kidney; however, elimination may be delayed in elderly patients.

Famotidine is at least as well tolerated as other H_2 blockers. However, it has been reported to produce **negative inotropic effects under experimental conditions** in healthy volunteers. This effect has been attributed to antagonism of histamine-mediated enhancement of cardiac contractility, but it has not been observed to date with other H_2 antagonists. Famotidine does not possess antiandrogenic effects, but it has been reported to cause confusion. It reduces prolactin levels, but the consequences of this are not known. One potential advantage of famotidine for the geriatric patient is that it does not appear to interfere with hepatic metabolism of other drugs and may not participate in drug interactions on that basis. It is not yet known if drug interactions occur on some other basis, and it is probably premature to assume that famotidine is completely safe to use with other drugs.

Nizatidine (Axid)

This H_2 blocker is the most recently introduced and it is expected to be well tolerated and participate in fewer drug interactions than cimetidine. It is too early to know whether these properties will make the drug more applicable for use in the geriatric patient than the other H_2 blockers.

As with other H_2 blockers, excretion may be delayed in aged patients. This could ultimately be problematic in the elderly because oral nizatidine is even more dependent than other H_2 blockers on renal function for its elimination.

Which H_2 Blocker for the Elderly?

Presently, there is little reason to prescribe cimetidine to geriatric patients. Although famotidine and nizatidine have a theoretical advantage over ranitidine in that they may prove to participate in fewer drug interactions, ranitidine has a proven track record of relative safety. Therefore, until there is firm evidence that other H_2 blockers are safer, ranitidine should be considered the H_2 blocker of choice for the elderly.

Sucralfate (Carafate)

Pharmacologic Considerations

MECHANISM OF ACTION. Sucralfate is structurally unrelated to other agents used in peptic ulcer and does not act by reducing gastric acid secretion. It is an aluminum salt of sucrose sulfate that is transformed in acid pH to a sticky gel. This substance acts locally in the stomach and duodenum, binding to ulcerated mucosa and forming a protective coating. Sucralfate may also stimulate local synthesis and release of protective prostaglandin. Aluminum itself may stimulate prostaglandin secretion, a property shared by certain other ions.

Sucralfate speeds the healing of duodenal ulcer. It is less effective in the healing of gastric ulcer, but does not differ in this regard from most other antiulcer drugs.

PHARMACOKINETICS. Sucralfate is minimally absorbed by the gastrointestinal tract. The amount of aluminum that is absorbed is of no significance, except perhaps in renal failure when blood levels may be increased.

Adverse Effects

Because of its lack of absorption, sucralfate is virtually devoid of systemic side effects under ordinary circumstances. **Constipation,** the most commonly described effect, occurs in only about 2% of patients, and is probably related to its ability to adsorb bile acids. In renal failure, however, plasma aluminum levels may rise, as they do when aluminum-containing antacids are given. Sucralfate also binds intestinal phosphate and may lead to **phosphate depletion.**

Important Drug Interactions

Because of its binding characteristics, sucralfate has the potential of altering the absorption of concurrently administered drugs. Such an interaction has been reported with warfarin, but the importance of this has been disputed. Drug interactions are probably rare, but caution should be observed in patients taking any drug with a narrow therapeutic-to-toxic ratio when sucralfate is added and withdrawn from the regimen.

Indications

Sucralfate is indicated for short-term treatment of duodenal ulcer, for which it has been approved. It is also indicated for the prevention of ulcer recurrence, but once-nightly dosing may not be effective. Contrary to earlier expectations, sucralfate may be less effective than other agents in the management of gastric lesions due to

NSAIDs. It appears to be useful in treating the resulting duodenal lesions, however.

Dosing

Initial dose: 1 g tid and at bedtime. The drug should be administered on an empty stomach, 1 hr before or 2 hr after meals.
Note: There is some evidence that 2 g bid may be as effective as the qid regimen in duodenal ulcer, but this is not an approved dosage regimen.
Maintenance dose: 1 g bid.

Special Considerations

Sucralfate is a large pill and its size may be a disincentive. The pill can be broken in half. Some gastroenterologists administer sucralfate as a "slurry," by crushing the pill and dissolving it in warm water. Although this liquid preparation has not been widely tested, it may prove to be an important option for patients with swallowing difficulties and may be very effective in reflux esophagitis. The slurry has also been used with success as mouthwash in the treatment of aphthous ulcers.

Anticholinergic Agents

Once widely used for the treatment of peptic ulcer because of their ability to inhibit gastric acid secretion, anticholinergic agents are hardly if ever used for this indication today, although their use as adjunctive treatment in Zollinger-Ellison syndrome is being explored. Anticholinergic agents have not been compared to contemporary antiulcer therapy but indirect evidence suggests that they would not stand up to the newer agents. Adverse effects of anticholinergic agents are particularly common in the elderly. They are mentioned here because geriatric patients are occasionally found to be taking drugs that were prescribed in the distant past.

Anticholinergic agents are discussed in Chap. 10 in connection with Parkinson's disease.

Misoprostol (Cytotec)

A synthetic analogue of prostaglandin E_1, misoprostol was developed to mimic the protective properties of that substance on gastric mucosal integrity. Misoprostol has antisecretory and cytoprotective actions. It binds to receptor sites on parietal cells and inhibits acid secretion. Its cytoprotective effects are thought to be achieved in a number of ways: by neutralizing gastric pH via the stimulation of bicarbonate secretion, by potentiating the production of protective mucus, by increasing mucosal blood flow, and by preventing mast cell destruction that occurs from a variety of insults and contributes to ulcer formation. These cytoprotective actions may be particularly important in the management of patients who are prone to gastric toxicity of NSAIDs, which exert their adverse effects by inhibiting protective prostaglandin. To date, misoprostol appears to be more effective than both H_2 blockers and sucralfate in such patients. However, it appears to be no more effective in the treatment of peptic ulcer not associated with NSAIDs.

Pharmacokinetics

Misoprostol is rapidly converted in the liver to active and inactive metabolites, many of which are renally excreted. The active metabolite may be primarily responsible for the biologic action of misoprostol. The drug disappears rapidly from serum, owing to its rapid distribution within the gastrointestinal system, but the terminal half-life of active drug may be as long as several days. The pharmacokinetics of this drug have not been defined in the elderly.

Adverse Reactions

The most common adverse effect of misoprostol is **diarrhea.** This is due to prostaglandin-mediated stimulation of intestinal secretion. Diarrhea may subside with time or with reduction of dosage but is sometimes severe and may be accompanied by **abdominal pain.** It is not known if older patients have increased or reduced susceptibility to this effect, for it could manifest as "normalization" of bowel habits in a chronically constipated patient. It is important to remember that NSAIDs themselves occasionally cause diarrhea by inhibiting the cytoprotective effects of prostaglandin. **Other nonspecific gastrointestinal complaints** are offered, but less commonly. Some, such as nausea and dyspepsia, may be difficult to distinguish from the discomforts of gastroduodenal disease itself.

Nongastrointestinal symptoms have not been generally reported. However, the long-term effects of misoprostol are not known. Indirect evidence suggests that misoprostol has immunosuppressant properties. T-cell function is inhibited physiologically by endogenous prostaglandins of the E series, an effect that increases with age. To date, clinical adverse effects of misoprostol have not been noted on the basis of immunosuppressant activity.

Indications

At present, the only approved indication for misoprostol is the prevention of gastropathy related to NSAIDs, including aspirin. In general, it should be reserved for patients on long-term NSAID therapy and not for those using NSAIDs casually.

Dosing

Usual dose: 200 μg qid. If not tolerated, 100 μg qid may be given.

Omeprazole (Prilosec [formerly Losec])

Recently released, omeprazole is chemically unrelated to other antiulcer agents. The drug irreversibly blocks hydrogen-potassium adenosinetriphosphatase (HK-ATPase), the enzyme responsible for activating the "proton pump," which is the final common pathway of gastric acid secretion regardless of stimulus. Thus, omeprazole differs from other agents, which are more specific in their effect; for example, H_2 blockers inhibit histaminelike stimuli, but fail to prevent cholinergic or gastrinlike stimuli from producing gastric secretion.

Omeprazole disappears rapidly from serum but its effect on gastric secretion far outlasts its presence in serum. This has been attributed to preferential distribution of the drug to gastric tissue and its irreversible effect on HK-ATPase. Omeprazole appears to be equal to or more effective than other agents in the management of gastroduodenal peptic disease and gastroesophageal reflux. It is currently approved for use only in severe reflux esophagitis and Zollinger-Ellison syndrome.

Limited study of omeprazole in the elderly indicates reduced elimination rate and increased bioavailability. It is not known if the pharmacodynamic effects of this agent differ in the aged gastric mucosa.

Omeprazole inhibits hepatic microsomal enzymes and may reduce the metabolism of drugs such as warfarin and phenytoin. Caution is advised when omeprazole is given together with drugs metabolized by this system.

At this time, the drug appears to be quite safe and highly effective. Although it is not known if the commendable benefits of its prolonged biologic effect could be outweighed by adverse effects in the long term, theoretical concerns about carcinogenesis (e.g., gastric carcinoid) might be of diminished importance in late life when life span is limited.

Dosing
In severe reflux esophagitis: 20 mg daily.

NONPHARMACOLOGIC MANAGEMENT
Whether or not drug treatment is used in managing patients with ulcers and related disorders, nonpharmacologic approaches are essential. The use of potent anti-inflammatory agents should be limited. It should be recognized that they do not necessarily offer therapeutic advantages over less toxic agents, such as acetaminophen or nonacetylated salicylates, for the majority of elderly patients with osteoarthritis. Cigarette smoking has been strongly linked to peptic ulcer recurrence and should be discontinued. Use of alcoholic beverages should be curtailed. Attention should be given to the avoidance of psychological and physiological stress and to the correction of other medical conditions. There is no specific dietary modification that has been shown to improve ulcer healing, but patients should avoid foods and beverages that they feel worsen their symptoms.

BIBLIOGRAPHY
Berstad, A., and Weberg, R. Antacids in the treatment of gastroduodenal ulcer. *Scand. J. Gastroenterol.* 21:385–391, 1986.

Brandt, L. J. *Gastrointestinal Disorders of the Elderly.* New York: Raven Press, 1984. Pp. 101–249.

D'Arcy, P. F., and McElnay, J. C. Drug-antacid interactions: assessment of clinical importance. *Drug. Intell. Clin. Pharm.* 21:607–617, 1987.

Gilinsky, N. Peptic ulcer disease in the elderly. *Gastroenterol. Clin. N. Amer.* 19:255–291, 1990.

Graham, D. Y. Prevention of gastroduodenal injury induced by chronic nonsteroidal anti-inflammatory drug therapy. *Gastroenterol.* 96 (2, Part 2):675–681, 1989.

Jones, J. B., and Bailey, R. T. Misoprostol: a prostaglandin E_1 analog with antisecretory and cytoprotective properties. *Drug Intell. Clin. Pharm.* 23:276–282, 1989.

Kirch, W., Hoensch, H., and Janisch, H. D. Interactions and non-interactions with ranitidine. *Clin. Pharmacokin.* 9:493–510, 1984.

Lanza, F. L., and Sibley, C. M. Role of antacids in the management of disorders of the upper gastrointestinal tract. Review of clinical experience 1975–1985. *Am. J. Gastroenterol.* 82:1223–1241, 1987.

Maton, P. N. Omeprazole. *N. Engl. J. Med.* 324:965–975, 1991.

Sewester, C. S., Olin, B. R., Hebel, S. K., et al. *Facts and comparisons.* St. Louis: Lippincott, 1990. Pp. 293–297a.

Somogyi, A., and Muirhead, M. Pharmacokinetic interactions of cimetidine 1987. *Clin. Pharmacokin.* 12:321–366, 1987.

Metoclopramide

PHARMACOLOGIC CONSIDERATIONS

Mechanism of Action

Metoclopramide is structurally related to procainamide but does not share its local anesthetic and antiarrhythmic properties. Rather, metoclopramide possesses a number of pharmacologic actions that affect the gastrointestinal system. It antagonizes dopamine in the central nervous system, and blocks dopamine receptors in the chemoreceptor trigger zone. It enhances the action of acetylcholine at peripheral muscarinic sites, and acts directly or indirectly on smooth muscle, enhancing contractility. Used therapeutically, metoclopramide increases lower esophageal sphincter tone and increases gastric peristalsis. As such, it reduces symptoms of gastroesophageal reflux such as heartburn and regurgitation, and may promote the healing of related esophagitis. It reduces postprandial bloating, nausea, and belching in patients with diabetic gastroparesis, and, by increasing gastric emptying, reduces nausea. The drug also has a general antiemetic effect, reducing nausea in a variety of other clinical situations. There is some evidence that the antiemetic effect is enhanced in the elderly, possibly because of loss of central dopaminergic neurons and a decreased sensitivity to emetogenic insults. In addition to enhancing gastric emptying, metoclopramide decreases small-intestinal transit time, but it does not appear to enhance distal small intestinal and colonic motility.

The dopamine blocking action of metoclopramide produces a number of effects on endocrine systems, the best known of which is enhanced prolactin secretion. Dopamine blockade is also responsible for important extrapyramidal toxicity.

Pharmacokinetics

Metoclopramide is well absorbed orally with peak plasma levels being attained within 1 hour. It is extensively metabolized in the liver to inactive conjugates, with roughly 20% being excreted unchanged in the urine. Apparent extensive first-pass metabolism reduces the bioavailability of absorbed metoclopramide. This reduced bioavailability occurs with significant interindividual variation, a fact that may partly account for individual susceptibilities to adverse effects. It is not highly protein-bound.

Ordinarily, elimination half-life ranges from 3 to 6 hours. Direct and indirect evidence indicates that elimination may be decreased in elderly patients, leading to higher levels for any given dose.

ADVERSE EFFECTS

Troublesome neurologic side effects may occur with metoclopramide. A variety of dystonic reactions have been reported in young patients but are less likely to occur in the elderly with ordinary oral use. However, **parkinsonian symptoms**, including rigidity, tremor, akathesia, and dyskinesia, are adverse effects that occur almost exclusively in the elderly. Although this may in part reflect prescribing patterns, the age-related predilection may be due to underlying alterations in dopamine receptors or, in other cases, an unmasking of subclinical idiopathic Parkinson's disease. There may also be an increased risk in patients with family history of movement disorders. Metoclopramide-induced movement disorders generally subside when the drug is discontinued, but in some patients the symptoms persist for months and tardive dyskinesia has been reported. Extrapyramidal effects may be dose-related and gastrointestinal symptoms can sometimes be controlled on lower doses without full reappearance of adverse effects in selected patients. However, continuation of the drug in this manner may not reduce the risk of tardive dyskinesia, to which older patients are particularly prone. As with other agents possessing antidopaminergic action, tardive dyskinesia is thought to occur when prolonged dopamine antagonism produces hypersensitivity of dopamine receptors. Tardive dyskinesia is sometimes held in abeyance when the responsible agent is resumed or the dose increased. Thus, the development of tardive dyskinesia may be masked by metoclopramide. Interestingly, low-dose metoclopramide does not necessarily worsen parkinsonian symptoms in patients who already have the disease.

Other reported neurologic effects include sedation, lassitude, and confusion. The **neuroleptic malignant syndrome** has been associated with the use of metoclopramide on rare occasions. Drug-induced parkinsonism and the neuroleptic malignant syndrome are discussed further in Chap. 6.

Metoclopramide stimulates the secretion of prolactin. Although the theoretical side effects in geriatric patients might include gynecomastia, impotence, and stimulation of existing breast tumors, the exact clinical implications are not known. Metoclopramide also increases the secretion of catecholamines and has been reported to produce **hypertensive crisis in patients with pheochromocytoma.**

High-dose parenteral metoclopramide often produces **diarrhea** and is the route most often associated with acute dystonic reactions.

IMPORTANT DRUG INTERACTIONS

By decreasing small-intestinal transit time metoclopramide may reduce the absorption of some digoxin preparations. Increased absorption of other agents has been reported, including acetaminophen, aspirin, beta blockers, lithium, and certain sedatives. The actual occurrence and importance of such interactions are not known, but in general metoclopramide should be instituted cautiously with any agent that has a narrow therapeutic-to-toxic ratio.

Metoclopramide may increase systemic absorption of levodopa; while this may have a beneficial effect in the treatment of Parkinson's disease, toxicity of levodopa could be enhanced. Conversely, parkinsonian symptoms could be enhanced by metoclopramide. The combination of levodopa and metoclopramide is illogical; metoclopramide should be avoided in Parkinson's disease if possible. The risk of parkinsonian activity, including tardive dyskinesias, may be increased when metoclopramide is used in conjunction with other agents possessing antidopaminergic activity, such as phenothiazines and haloperidol, so that concurrent use is discouraged.

Metoclopramide may produce an additive effect when used with central nervous system depressants and should be used cautiously in conjunction with them. If used with monoamine oxidase inhibitors (MAOIs) a hypertensive crisis may occur.

The efficacy of metoclopramide may be reduced by concurrent administration of anticholinergic agents, which counteract cholinomimetic effects of metoclopramide.

CONTRAINDICATIONS AND PRECAUTIONS

Metoclopramide should not be used in gastrointestinal obstruction, perforation, or hemorrhage. Because of its ability to release catecholamines, metoclopramide is contraindicated in patients with pheochromocytoma, those with poorly controlled hypertension, and patients taking MAOIs.

Idiopathic Parkinson's disease is not an absolute contraindication to the use of metoclopramide, although the drug must be used very cautiously in this setting and the indications must be strong.

INDICATIONS AND NONINDICATIONS

Because of the risk of troublesome neurologic effects in the elderly, metoclopramide should only be used when safer agents are ineffective. It is therefore indicated for short-term use in the treatment of gastroesophageal reflux that does not respond to antacids or other agents used for nonulcer dyspepsia (see Chap. 26). Metoclopramide is highly effective in the treatment of diabetic gastroparesis. However, diabetic and nondiabetic patients with nonspecific symptoms of postprandial bloating and belching may respond to dietary manipulations or to agents containing simethicone. If the symptoms are mild to moderate, these approaches should be instituted before metoclopramide is prescribed.

Metoclopramide is not the first-line treatment for the management of nausea. However, in the case of nausea associated with cancer chemotherapy, intravenous metoclopramide is indicated if other agents are ineffective or poorly tolerated.

Although preoperative metoclopramide has been used with some success in reducing the incidence of aspiration pneumonia in surgical patients, this drug should not be used to prevent aspiration pneumonia in nonsurgical patients because the risks and benefits are not known. Neurologically impaired elderly who develop recurrent aspiration pneumonia have difficulty swallowing oropharyngeal secretions as well as gastric contents and would not be expected to respond to maneuvers that hasten gastric emptying.

Metoclopramide is not useful in the treatment of constipation.

DOSING

Oral Use

Initial dose: 5 mg once daily 30 min prior to the most troublesome meal. If well tolerated and if symptoms require, dose may be increased after 2 or 3 days to 5 mg bid or tid. In general, dosage should be keyed to the time of day when symptoms actually occur.

Intravenous Use in Nausea of Chemotherapy

Initial dose: 1 mg/kg 30 min before chemotherapy. The dose should be given as an intravenous drip over approximately 15 min.
Note: Downward dose adjustments may be required in renal impairment and higher doses may be needed in some patients.

BIBLIOGRAPHY

Albibi, R., and McCallum, R. W. Metoclopramide: pharmacology and clinical application. *Ann. Intern. Med.* 98:86–95, 1983.

Grimes, J. D., Hassan, M. N., and Preston, D. N. Adverse neurologic effects of metoclopramide. *Can. Med. Assoc. J.* 126:23–24, 1982.

Miller, L. C., and Jankovic, J. Metoclopramide-induced movement disorders. Clinical findings with a review of the literature. *Arch. Intern Med.* 149:2486–2492, 1989.

Shaughnessy, A. F. Potential uses for metoclopramide. *Drug Intell. Clin. Pharm.* 19:723–728, 1985.

Medical Treatment of Gallstones: Ursodiol and Chenodiol

GALLBLADDER DISEASE IN THE ELDERLY

The likelihood of developing gallstones increases with age so that by the age of 80 between 30% and 80% of people have gallstones, the highest prevalence being in native Americans. In most cases, these gallstones are silent, and are discovered incidentally during testing for other disease, or at autopsy. In fact, because of the common co-existence of gallstones, a number of other conditions are frequently misdiagnosed as being due to gallbladder disease, notably gastroesophageal pathology, peptic ulcer, coronary artery disease, and right lower lobe pneumonia.

The male-to-female ratio of patients with gallstones increases with age, approaching unity by late life. The actual number of affected women is still greater simply because more women survive to old age.

Assuming that the diagnosis is correct, elective surgery is the treatment of choice for symptomatic gallstone disease and is tolerated well by healthy elderly. In contrast, morbidity and mortality are unacceptably high in emergency surgery. However, the natural history of silent gallstones does not justify prophylactic surgery. Although there is some evidence to suggest that the presence of gallstones increases the risk of gallbladder cancer, a disease primarily seen in the elderly, this lesion is too uncommon for the risk to justify routine cholecystectomy.

Unfortunately, many older patients have medical conditions that increase the risk of this surgery. Notable among them are unstable coronary artery disease, heart failure, cerebrovascular disease, and obstructive lung disease. This problem is compounded by the fact that it is often extremely difficult to know whether gallbladderlike symptoms are truly related to gallbladder disease in a population with such a high prevalence of silent gallstones. Alternatives to abdominal surgery would seem highly appropriate for selected patients.

Ursodiol and chenodiol, which are naturally occurring bile acids, may dissolve gallstones when given over a period of several months, and may be alternatives for some. Of the two, ursodiol is far better tolerated than chenodiol, and since its introduction in 1988 has offered the medical option to increasing numbers of patients.

WHO IS A CANDIDATE FOR GALLSTONE DISSOLUTION?

Before embarking on a prolonged trial of medical treatment, it is important to identify patients who are most likely to achieve benefit. The treatment regimen may last for a year or more, is costly, and does not preclude recurrences, which approach a rate of 50% within 5 years. If recurrent gallstones become symptomatic, retreatment may be required.

Currently, treatment with gallstone-solubilizing agents is recommended in patients with moderate to severe symptoms who are not candidates for or refuse surgical treatment, and who do not respond to appropriate dietary maneuvers. Sol bilizing agents cannot be used in patients with unstable symptoms, biliary obstruction, ascending cholangitis, or liver disease.

Gallstone composition determines the outcome of dissolution therapy. Only cholesterol gallstones will respond, whereas those composed of salts of bilirubin (pigment stones) or calcium will not. Genetic factors and other variables determine gallstone composition, but age alone may play an important role. Compared to younger patients, who usually have cholesterol stones, elderly patients at cholecystectomy are more likely to have calcified pigment stones, which will not respond to medical therapy. Statistics based on patients coming to cholecystectomy leave open the question of whether pigment stones form later in life or merely remain quiescent longer. In fact, many older patients do have stones that make them candidates for dissolution therapy.

Although the chemical composition of a stone cannot be ascertained without removing and analyzing it, radiographic clues are predictive in the majority of cases.

Radiographic criteria should strongly suggest cholesterol gallstones. On plain film, stones should be radiolucent. The plain film should be done prior to a dye study, since dye can coat stones and make them appear radio-opaque. On oral cholecystogram, stones should float; floating stones tend to be high in cholesterol content, low in calcium content, and small in size. In general, stones should not be larger than 1.5–2.0 cm in diameter. However, large stones do not preclude medical treatment as long as they are pure cholesterol stones. These will probably eventually dissolve, although treatment may take longer.

Radiographic criteria are not exact. One third of stones with small amounts of visible calcification may still consist primarily of cholesterol, although densely calcified stones probably will not dissolve. Conversely, about one third of radiolucent stones contain significant amounts of calcium and pigment. Floating stones consist primarily of cholesterol.

URSODIOL (ACTIGALL)

Pharmacologic Considerations

Mechanism of Action

Ursodiol (ursodeoxycholic acid) is a naturally occurring bile acid. When ingested, ursodiol enters the liver where it acts to decrease the secretion of hepatic cholesterol, possibly through an effect on hepatic enzymes involved in the metabolism and synthesis of cholesterol. Ursodiol also increases the solubility of cholesterol by sequestering it in micelles and perhaps by altering its physicochemical properties in other ways. These actions reduce the ratio of cholesterol to bile acid in the bile, reducing its lithogenicity. The reduction in cholesterol concentration of bile ultimately results in stone dissolution.

Only gallstones that are predominantly cholesterol stones will be dissolved. Pigment gallstones and those that contain substantial amounts of calcium are not subject to dissolution by bile acids.

Pharmacokinetics

Ursodiol is well absorbed and is heavily extracted by the liver where most is conjugated. Conjugates enter the bile and undergo enterohepatic circulation. In the intestine, they are partly reconverted to ursodiol, reentering the bile, and partly degraded by intestinal bacteria to lithocholic acid. Lithocholic acid is a compound that has been held responsible for the hepatotoxicity seen with chenodiol, the other agent used for gallstone dissolution (see below). The extent to which bacterial degradation occurs depends greatly on the individual's gut flora. However, bacteria appear to produce far less of this putative hepatotoxin from ursodiol than from chenodiol. This small concentration of lithocholic acid is absorbed and rapidly inactivated or is excreted in the feces. Ursodiol conjugates eventually become part of the circulating bile pool and have a half-life of several days.

Certain patients may interconvert ursodiol and chenodiol in the gut, depending on the nature of gut flora.

The disposition and action of bile acids have not been studied specifically in the elderly. There does not appear to be any particular rationale for adjusting the dose for age, since efficacy depends on the concentration in bile, and toxicity appears to depend on the presence of undeactivated lithocholic acid. Presently, ursodiol appears to be rather nontoxic. The most important factor to consider in older patients is whether they satisfy eligibility criteria for a full course of treatment or a treatment trial.

Adverse Effects

Ursodiol is far better tolerated than chenodiol (see below). It is less likely to produce diarrhea and it does not elevate serum levels of low-density lipoprotein cholesterol.

Important Drug Interactions

Absorption of ursodiol may be inhibited by cholestyramine and colestipol, and by aluminum-containing antacids. Agents that increase the lithogenicity of bile, such as estrogens, may counteract the therapeutic effect of bile acids.

Contraindications

Gallstone dissolution therapy is contraindicated in acute cholecystitis, biliary obstruction, and ascending cholangitis.

Indications

Gallstone dissolution therapy is indicated in patients with mild to moderate symptoms clearly related to the presence of gallstones, but who are not candidates for surgical procedures and whose symptoms do not respond to dietary maneuvers. Radiologic criteria predicting dissolution should be satisfied.

In robust patients, surgery is generally preferable to medical treatment because the latter has a high failure rate, shows a significant recurrence rate, and may actually be more expensive for the patient when in-hospital insurance coverage is considered.

Dissolution therapy is also given to symptomatic patients about to embark on a major weight loss, which can mobilize cholesterol and increase its concentration in bile and worsen symptoms.

Dosing

Daily dosage: 8–10 mg/kg in 2 to 3 divided doses. Therapy should continue for a minimum of 9 months, or until dissolution occurs. The progress of gallstone dissolution should be followed by baseline and periodic ultrasound. If there is no evidence of partial dissolution at 6–9 months, treatment should be discontinued.

CHENODIOL (CHENIX)

Chenodiol (chenodeoxycholic acid) is similar in its mechanism of action to ursodiol, but is associated with a high incidence of **diarrhea**, and may produce **elevations in liver enzymes** and **serum levels** of **LDL cholesterol**. Diarrhea is a particularly troublesome side effect for patients and a frequent cause of noncompliance. Although certain older patients would be less likely to develop disabling diarrhea from chenodiol, it is far less effective than ursodiol.

Although the efficacy-toxicity ratio of chenodiol is unfavorable when used alone, this agent is presently less expensive than ursodiol, a factor of considerable importance in view of the protracted treatment course required. This has led to combined use of the two agents, which may be more effective in dissolving gallstones but just as safe as treatment with ursodiol alone. Safety of combined use may be related to the fact that a lower dose of chenodiol is used or that ursodiol may have a protective effect, specifically at the level of the liver cell membrane. However, more study is needed before specific recommendations can be made. Presently ursodiol should be regarded as the drug of choice.

NONPHARMACOLOGIC TREATMENT

Dietary manipulations may improve symptoms in many patients. The traditionally recommended diet is low in fat and moderate in protein, since fat and to a lesser extent protein stimulate gallbladder contraction. If between-meal snacks cannot be avoided, food taken at those times should be limited to small amounts of carbohydrates, which do not stimulate gallbladder contraction. Meals should generally be taken 3 times a day with calories evenly distributed throughout the day. Large "banquet" meals should be avoided.

Obesity is a risk factor for gallstone formation, so avoidance of obesity is desirable. However, fasting and calorie restriction resulting in rapid weight loss may increase the formation of gallstones. It is not known what type of weight reduction diet is the most desirable in these patients, but in general rapid weight loss is strongly discouraged.

Elective surgery is an acceptable treatment for most patients with symptomatic disease provided they are otherwise in good health. Laparoscopic cholecystectomy is a new approach that is being offered with increasing frequency.

BIBLIOGRAPHY

Broomfield, P. H., Chopra, R., Sheinbaum, R., et al. Effects of ursodeoxycholic acid and aspirin on the formation of lithogenic bile and gallstones during loss of weight. *N. Engl. J. Med.* 319:1567–1572, 1988.

Croker, J. R. Biliary tract disease in the elderly. *Clin. Gastroenterol.* 14:773–809, 1985.

Hyams, D. E., and Fox, R. A. The gastrointestinal system—the liver and biliary system. In J. C. Brockelhurst (ed.), *Textbook of Geriatric Medicine and Gerontology.* Edinburgh: Churchill Livingstone, 1985. Pp. 576–580.

Liddle, R. A., Goldstein, R. B., and Saxton, J. Gallstone formation during weight-reduction dieting. *Arch. Intern. Med.* 149:1750–1753, 1989.

Podda, M., Zuin, M., Battezzati, P. M., et al. Efficacy and safety of a combination of chenodeoxycholic acid and ursodeoxycholic acid for gallstone dissolution: a comparison with ursodeoxycholic acid alone. *Gastroenterol.* 96:222–229, 1989.

Rosenbaum, C. L., and Cluxton, R. J. Ursodiol: a cholesterol gallstone solubilizing agent. *Drug Intell. Clin. Pharm.* 22:941–945, 1988.

Tint, G. S., Salen, G., and Shefer, S. Effect of ursodeoxycholic acid and chenodeoxycholic acid on cholesterol and bile acid metabolism. *Gastroenterol.* 91:1007–1018, 1986.

Bronchodilators

WHEEZING IN THE ELDERLY

The management of wheezing in the elderly is subject to the same principles as treatment in younger adults, but the differential diagnosis of bronchospasm is more complex. Wheezing can be due to chronic obstructive pulmonary disease (COPD), allergic bronchitis, or bronchial asthma, as in young or middle-aged adults, but other, less frequent causes of wheezing, such as left ventricular failure, aspiration, and pulmonary embolus, may also be seen. Bronchial asthma itself can be a continuation of a lifelong affliction, or can actually begin late in life. Late-onset asthma is clinically indistinguishable from other forms of asthma, but is only infrequently associated with overt allergic or atopic symptoms. Because of long-held views that asthma is a disease that is "outgrown," the physician may approach this entity with disbelief.

In the geriatric patient, the physician must also more frequently give consideration to the contribution of drugs, such as beta blockers, aspirin, or nonsteroidal anti-inflammatory agents, or those that contain the yellow dye tartrazine, all of which may produce bronchospasm in susceptible individuals. If bronchospasm first develops late in life, a careful drug history should be done and should include queries about the use of over-the-counter medications and eyedrops. Ocular beta blockers, including "selective" betaxolol, are quite capable of producing bronchospasm in highly sensitive patients (see Chap. 34) but are often not part of a drug history.

Whatever the cause of wheezing, bronchodilators are generally part of the treatment regimen. Even cardiac asthma in some instances is managed more smoothly if a bronchodilator is cautiously added to the regimen. According to traditional teaching, wheezing in the setting of pulmonary edema is due to narrowing of the airways by fluid, and the hallmark of treatment is the relief of pulmonary congestion with diuretics. However, recent evidence suggests that there is a true bronchospastic component to this clinical entity. Although bronchodilators do not relieve airways obstruction in all of these patients, added to a regimen of diuretics they may be useful in many. It should be emphasized that the use of bronchodilators in cardiac asthma is controversial since this disorder generally occurs in conjunction with ischemic heart disease. Moreover, theophylline is eliminated very slowly in congestive heart failure and toxicity is likely to occur if the dosing is not adequately adjusted.

THEOPHYLLINE PREPARATIONS

Although not as well tolerated as inhaled beta$_2$-adrenergic bronchodilators (see below), oral theophylline is often an important part of treatment in the elderly, many of whom are unable to master the use of the metered-dose inhaler, even when auxiliary devices are used. In these cases, oral agents are often the only effective way of managing the patient, and, compared to *oral* beta-adrenergic agents, the therapeutic index of theophylline tends to be more favorable. Despite this, theophylline must be used judiciously and cautiously

in the elderly. It is far from nontoxic for older individuals and participates in a number of drug-drug interactions.

Pharmacologic Considerations
Mechanism of Action
Theophylline is a methylxanthine, structurally and chemically related to caffeine and theobromine, but with greater bronchodilating
properties than these and other members of this class of drugs. The
precise mechanism of action of theophylline is not known, traditional explanations that it is a phosphodiesterase inhibitor having
been disputed. It relaxes bronchial smooth muscle, promoting bronchodilation, and has wide-ranging pharmacodynamic effects on
other organ systems. Most important among these effects are central nervous system excitation, inotropic and chronotropic effects
on the heart, and irritation of the gastrointestinal tract. Theophylline also has a diuretic effect, which may be related to a direct action
on the renal tubule.

Pharmacokinetics
The disposition of theophylline is subject to complex factors. This
complexity contributes to the unpredictability of dose and response.
   All forms of theophylline are well absorbed, but absorption may be
considerably delayed by food, and formulations differ widely in the
timing of absorption in relation to meals. Theophylline is only 60%
bound to serum proteins so that large changes in serum protein levels would have to occur before a significant increase in the free fraction had an impact on drug effect. Debilitated elderly, who are often
severely hypoproteinemic, generally require downward dose adjustments in any case, because of illness and reduced body mass.
   The rate at which theophylline is initially cleared from the serum
depends on urine flow rate, which increases in response to fluid intake and to the diuretic properties of the drug itself. At steady state,
the clearance rate is dependent on metabolism by hepatic microsomal enzymes, but this is a saturable process, so that with increasing dosages of the drug less enzyme is available for metabolism.
Thus, therapeutic index narrows further at the high end of the dose
range. The metabolic enzyme system itself can be turned on or inhibited by a number of factors (see below). Congestive heart failure,
which is associated with decreased hepatic blood flow, and liver disease greatly impair theophylline metabolism, and in these settings
the half-life may be markedly prolonged. Age-related reduction in
the activity of this enzyme system probably prolongs the metabolism of theophylline somewhat, but the exact contribution of age
cannot be quantified, owing to the multiplicity of other modifying
factors. The average serum half-life of theophylline is 8 hours, but
there is wide variation. It is generally agreed that clearance is reduced by roughly 30%, on the average, in elderly patients.
   Diurnal variations in pharmacokinetics occur. Younger patients
may attain higher blood levels in the morning than in the evening,
but there is some evidence that the reverse is true in elderly patients.
These age differences are difficult to explain and are subject to great
variability.
   Other factors that affect the pharmacokinetics of theophylline in-

clude genetic variations in metabolic enzymes, cigarette smoking, disease, and concurrent drug use (see Table 29–1).

Oral Preparations Available

Oral theophylline is available in rapid- and slow-release tablets and elixir. Individual differences in pharmacokinetics and patient response exist among and within these groups.

Table 29–1. Important Theophylline Interactions

Drugs/Factors That Increase Theophylline Levels

Drugs
    Erythromycin
    Ciprofloxacin
    Cimetidine
    Ranitidine (inconstant)
    Propranolol
    Allopurinol
    Calcium channel blockers?
    Postmenopausal hormone replacement?
    Influenza vaccine (live virus only)

Disease states
    Left ventricular heart failure
    Liver disease
    Severe hypoproteinemia
    Hypoxemia
    Viral illness
    Severe acute illness or chronic debility

Drugs/Factors That Decrease Theophylline Levels

    Barbiturates
    Phenytoin
    Rifampin
    Cigarette smoking
    High-protein diet
    Hyperthyroidism?

Other Interactions

    Diuretics—Increased diuretic effect
    Sympathomimetic agents—Increased cardiac and central stimulation
    Antacids—Altered absorption
    Food—Altered absorption
    Tube feeding—Decreased absorption

Drug Effects Decreased by Theophylline

Phenytoin—Decreased phenytoin levels
Lithium—Decreased lithium levels
Carbamazepine—Decreased carbamazepine effect

Rapid-release tablets and elixirs of theophylline tend to have a speedy onset (less than 1 hour) and short duration of action (average 8 hours). They are generally recommended for patients who require occasional, immediate relief, but who are unable to use inhaled bronchodilators. However, in individual patients, their efficacy in this regard may not be greater than certain slow-release preparations. Furthermore, while their serum half-life is probably somewhat prolonged in older individuals, the frequency of administration may still be impractical for the majority of patients whose condition requires constant blood levels in order to avert wheezing.

Aminophylline and oxtriphylline (Choledyl) are short-acting agents that contain approximately 80% and 65% theophylline, respectively, the remainder consisting of a base, which is designed to enhance solubility and absorption. These compounds have not been found to increase the absorption of oral theophylline and have no therapeutic advantage. It is important to point out that the dosage of aminophylline and oxtriphylline is not comparable to plain theophylline, an underrecognized fact that occasionally leads to inappropriate prescribing. Aminophylline is the most widely used form of parenteral theophylliine.

Slow-release preparations are designed for twice-daily (Theo-Dur, Slo-bid, others) or once-daily (Uniphyl) dosing.

There are many twice-daily forms available; each brand has unique physicochemical properties that contribute to the slow-release effect, and hence they differ in their rate of absorption and duration of action. Some brands may not be completely absorbed for several hours, and, when taken regularly, the duration of action for nonelderly adults ranges from 3 to 16 hours. Thus, many patients will require dosing more frequently than every 12 hours to be free of wheezing, while patients with mild symptoms often are satisfied with only occasional doses. If patients switch from one brand to another, there may be significant differences in the pattern and degree to which symptoms are controlled, and toxicity may develop unexpectedly, even if the dose is held constant.

Limited study of a once-daily preparation (Uniphyl) indicates that it is as well tolerated as twice-daily preparations. However, time to peak blood levels and perhaps clinical effect may be less predictable.

It is important to point out that most studies of these preparations have been conducted on nonelderly patients. Although interindividual variability is most likely as great or greater among older patients, initial dosing choices should be made with the assumption that the half-life of any preparation is prolonged, until the patient's clinical response is known.

Adverse Effects

Theophylline may produce **cardiac arrhythmias,** sometimes when therapeutic levels have not been exceeded. Geriatric patients are particularly susceptible to this effect and are probably more likely than younger adults to develop arrhythmias despite a subtoxic blood level. This situation is confounded by the fact that arrhythmias in wheezing patients are often due to the respiratory condition itself and not the bronchodilator. Differential diagnosis is still more complicated in elderly patients, who frequently have unrelated cardiac arrhythmias.

CNS excitation may result in restlessness and sleeplessness. Confusional states are generally considered a symptom of overdose; however, indirect evidence from cerebral blood flow studies and from observations in children suggest that elderly patients might be at risk of developing confusion earlier on.

Tremor is an effect seen often in older patients, but this occurs less often than with beta-adrenergic agents. **Seizures** may occur, although age per se does not increase the risk.

Gastrointestinal symptoms are not uncommon and may consist of nonspecific dyspepsia, anorexia, cramps, nausea, or vomiting. Although this may be a result of direct gastrointestinal irritation, these side effects may also be related to a dose-dependent effect on the CNS. Tolerance to gastrointestinal symptoms may occur over time.

Theophylline has a mild diuretic action at the doses used for the treatment of wheezing. Frank incontinence is probably uncommon, but any drug with diuretic effect has the potential of causing bladder complaints in the predisposed elderly patient.

The **ethylenediamine portion of aminophylline** is sensitizing and may produce **rash** or other allergic symptoms in certain individuals.

Serious theophylline toxicity may not be preceded by warning signs in the form of milder adverse effects. This may be because premonitory signs are unrecognized or mistaken for disease in other organ systems, or because one end organ may be unduly sensitive to the effects of the drug.

Important Drug and Nutrient Interactions

Theophylline participates in a number of interactions. The most important interactions occur when the drug is given with agents that impair or stimulate hepatic microsomal enzymes. The most consistent interactions are listed in Table 29-1. The interaction with influenza vaccine is inconstant; earlier reports of an interaction are probably explained by the fact that it is mediated by interferon, which is present only in vaccines containing live and attenuated virus. Viral interferon impairs hepatic microsomal enzymes and is the means by which viral disease itself increases theophylline levels. Recent vaccines have been primarily produced from killed virus, with which a theophylline interaction has not been reported.

Other interactions with theophylline may exist but are less well documented. For example, oral contraceptives have been reported to decrease the metabolism of theophylline preparations, increasing their effect. Thus, the potential exists for an interaction between theophylline and postmenopausal hormone regimens. Certain calcium channel blockers have been reported to increase theophylline levels, but an interaction has not been proved and a mechanism has not been established. Despite lack of consistency in these reports, it is wise to exercise precaution whenever new drugs are added to a regimen that contains theophylline. The physician should also be on the lookout for both increased and decreased theophylline effect.

As mentioned earlier, food unpredictably delays the absorption of various theophylline preparations; continuous enteral tube feeding with artificial nutrients has also been reported to do this.

Theophylline may also alter levels of other drugs. This is particularly important for drugs with a narrow therapeutic window (see

Table 29–1). For a detailed discussion of theophylline interactions, the reader is referred to the Bibliography readings (see Jonkman).

Use of Serum Levels

Determination of serum levels is an important part of theophylline therapy, since the therapeutic-to-toxic ratio of this drug is narrow, and it is difficult to predict clinical response from dose. In general, the therapeutic range of theophylline concentrations is considered to be 10–20 $\mu g/ml$. However, in sensitive patients, toxic symptoms may occur when blood levels are in the subtoxic range. Thus, serum levels must always be viewed critically in conjunction with the clinical response. This is very important in elderly patients who may be unduly sensitive to low tissue levels of theophylline, particularly in the cardiovascular system.

Because of variability among patients and products, it is difficult to predict the optimum time of sample collection. Despite evidence that elderly patients may exhibit altered diurnal variations in blood levels, it is generally recommended that the sample be collected approximately 4 hours after the morning dose of a slow-release preparation in order to detect the highest level attained. If the patient has breakthrough or toxic symptoms at particular times of the day, it may be helpful to sample at those times if possible. Serum levels should be determined if toxicity is suspected, even if no dose change has been made, since so many factors may alter absorption or disposition. Serum levels can also be determined when another drug that might interfere with the disposition of theophylline is added to a regimen or if poor compliance is suspected.

Once-daily preparations tend to produce peak blood levels 8–12 hours after ingestion, but this is highly variable, with wide fluctuations occurring in relation to meals. Clinical monitoring becomes very important in these situations, both in the timing of the blood sample and in making decisions about dose changes.

Contraindications

In active peptic ulcer, other bronchodilators should be considered before theophylline. Like other bronchodilators, theophylline should be used with extreme caution in unstable cardiac disease. Aminophylline should be avoided in patients known to be allergic to the ethylenediamene component; other theophylline preparations can be used in these circumstances.

Precautions

Marked variations among theophylline formulations, even within subgroups, have been mentioned above. A change in brand may lead to enhanced, diminished, or altered clinical response. It is important for patients to be informed of this because brands may be changed at the drugstore if the prescription provides for generic substitution. If there is any doubt as to the patient's capability to understand this factor and to report brand changes to the physician, as is often the case in geriatric practice, the prescription should be written by brand name.

Continuous tube feeding should be interrupted for at least 1 hour before and after enteral theophylline is administered, or, if the feed-

theophylline regimen is changed, the patient should be observed for alterations in clinical response.

Indications

Theophylline is indicated in patients with wheezing who are unable to use inhaled beta$_2$-adrenergic agents. Theophylline is also indicated as adjunctive treatment to these agents. It may also be used for the treatment of nocturnal and early morning wheezing that cannot be conveniently prevented by inhaled bronchodilators.

Parenteral theophylline, generally given as aminophylline, is indicated in the management of acute asthma in patients unable to take or responding incompletely to other rapidly acting agents.

Dosing

Oral Preparations

Initial dose: 100–200 mg every 6–12 hr. Alternatively, a loading dose of 6 mg/kg theophylline may be given, followed by 2 mg/kg every 6 hr for 2 doses, then every 8 hr. Total dose should not exceed 12 mg/kg in the first 24 hours.

Note: 100 mg theophylline is equivalent to 127 mg aminophylline and 156 mg oxtriphylline.

Maintenance dose: 6 mg/kg/24 hr in 2 to 3 divided doses.

Maximum dose: Dose should not exceed that which will produce toxicity. Toxicity is most likely to occur when serum levels of theophylline approach or exceed 20 μg/ml, but may occur at lower-than-expected levels in older patients.

Parenteral Theophylline (as Aminophylline)

Loading dose: 6 mg/kg IV given at a maximum rate of 25 mg/min. This should be followed by 0.6 mg/kg/hr for the first 12 hours and 0.3 mg/kg/hr thereafter.

In congestive heart failure: Loading dose should not be adjusted. It should be followed by 0.5 mg/kg/hr for 12 hr and 0.1–0.2 mg/kg/hr thereafter.

Note: These doses are intended for patients who have not been taking oral theophylline just prior to intravenous administration. Total daily dose may be given as a continuous infusion or in 4 divided doses. Theophylline levels should be monitored in all cases.

BETA-ADRENERGIC DRUGS

Mechanism of Action

Beta-adrenergic agents are sympathomimetic catecholamine derivatives, which act by stimulating beta$_2$ receptors in bronchial smooth muscle, producing relaxation and bronchodilation. Ephedrine, which has no direct beta$_2$ action, acts by releasing endogenous catecholamines from nerve terminals. Additional effects of these drugs include a reduction in certain chemical mediators of allergy and local inflammation, but these actions are not as important as their effect on the bronchial smooth musculature itself.

Sympathomimetic agents used for the treatment of bronchospasm have varying degrees of alpha-, beta$_1$-, and beta$_2$-adrenergic properties. Important alpha-adrenergic properties include smooth muscle contraction, resulting in vasoconstriction, elevations of blood pressure, and constriction of smooth muscle in the gastrointestinal and urinary tracts; beta$_1$ properties include positive inotropic and chronotropic effects on the heart, and lipolysis; and beta$_2$ properties include relaxation of smooth muscle of the vasculature, bronchi, and gastrointestinal and urinary tracts. Adrenergic stimulation also takes place in the brain, producing excitation, and in sweat glands, producing secretion.

When high blood or tissue levels of active drug are achieved, adrenergic agents exhibit less selectivity, producing effects mediated by beta$_1$, beta$_2$, and alpha receptors. Clinically, this may be manifested as a wider range of toxicity than predicted by receptor selectivity. Receptor selectivity of these agents is summarized in Table 29-2.

The amount of drug reaching the systemic circulation depends on the route of administration. The intravenous and subcutaneous routes produce the highest levels; orally administered agents, which are subject to extensive metabolism, produces lower levels. Inhaled bronchodilators act predominantly on the lung, with only small amounts being systemically absorbed through the lung and gastrointestinal tract. Although as much as 90% of drug delivered by the inhaler is actually swallowed, of that portion, a substantial amount is degraded in the liver and intestinal wall. In some cases, however, enough can reach the systemic circulation to produce side effects. Patients who are unable to coordinate administration and inhalation well retain even more in the mouth. Less active substance reaches the preferred site of action, more is absorbed through the gastrointestinal tract, and less via the pulmonary vessels.

Beta$_2$-Selective Agents

Metaproterenol (Alupent, Metaprel), **albuterol** (Proventil, Ventolin), and **terbutaline** (Brethine, Bricanyl; Brethaire) have predominantly beta$_2$-selective activity, with less prominent beta$_1$ activity than the agents discussed above, and virtually no alpha-adrenergic properties. This selectivity makes them the best suited to the treatment of bronchospasm. Although they are available for oral use, and terbutaline for injection, these agents are primarily administered by inhalation. When inhaled, their duration of action is longer than that of isoproterenol and epinephrine, an additional advantage.

Isoetharine (Bronkometer, Bronkosol), another adrenergic agent that is administered by inhalation, has less beta$_2$ selectivity and a shorter duration of action than agents such as albuterol and metaproterenol. **Pirbuterol** (Maxair) and **Bitolterol** (Tornalate), which are beta$_2$-selective, probably have no specific advantages over albuterol and metaproterenol but may be preferred by some patients.

When inhaled bronchodilators are indicated, beta$_2$-selective agents are the first choice.

Pharmacokinetics

When administered properly, approximately 10% of aerosolized drug reaches the respiratory tract. Of the portion that remains in the mouth, much is swallowed and degraded by the liver. Little active drug reaches the systemic circulation. The standard dosage of 2 puffs delivers microgram doses, which are extremely active topically, producing bronchodilation, but minimally active systemically.

The orally administered forms are substantially degraded in the liver. Their bioavailability varies, the percentage of ultimate absorption ranging from less than 30% for terbutaline to 60%–80% for al-

Table 29-2. Adrenergic Agents

Agent (Brand)	Receptor Activity	Suggested Route	Onset of Action (min)	Duration of Action[a]	Maximum Dose
First Line					
Albuterol[b] (Proventil, Ventolin)	$\beta_1 < \beta_2$	MDI[c]	≤ 15	Intermediate	2 puffs qid
		NEB[d]			
Bitolterol (Tornalate)	$\beta_1 < \beta_2$	MDI	≤ 5	Intermediate	2 puffs qid
Metaproterenol[b] (Alupent, Metaprel)	$\beta_1 < \beta_2$	MDI	≤ 5	Intermediate	2 puffs qid
		NEB			
Pirbuterol (Maxair)	$\beta_1 < \beta_2$	MDI	≤ 5	Intermediate	2 puffs qid
Terbutaline (Brethaire)	$\beta_1 < \beta_2^{\text{e}}$	MDI	≤ 30	Intermediate	2 puffs qid
Other					
Isoetharine (Bronkometer)	$\beta_1 < \beta_2$	MDI	≤ 5	Short	2 puffs qid
Isoproterenol (Isuprel)	β_1, β_2	MDI	≤ 5	Short	N.R.[f]
Epinephrine	α, β_1, β_2	MDI	< 5	Short	N.R.
		SQ	5–15	Short	0.3 mg
Ephedrine	α, β_1, β_2	Oral	15–60	Intermediate	N.R.

[a] Short = < 3 hours; intermediate = 3–6 hours (may last up to 8); derived from data in nongeriatric adults.
[b] Available as solution for nebulization.
[c] Metered-dose inhaler.
[d] Solution for nebulization; dosage depends on concentration.
[e] When administered by inhalation.
[f] Not recommended.
Adapted from Sewester, C. S., Olin, B. R., Hebek, S. K., et al. *Facts and Comparison.* St. Louis: Lippincott, 1988. Pp. 173a–177a.

buterol. The extent of bronchodilation depends on blood levels achieved, which must be substantially higher for oral drug than aerosolized drug. Consequently, oral drug produces adverse effects much more often than inhaled drug.

There is little pharmacokinetic data on these drugs in elderly patients. Drug profiles summarized in Table 29–2 are derived from observations on the average nonelderly adult.

Adverse Effects of Inhaled Beta$_2$ Agonists

Adverse effects are said to be uncommon when these agents are administered by inhalation, since the amount of drug reaching systemic circulation is very small. However, the published safety profile has been determined from observations on nonelderly asthmatics who are in relatively good health, and who use the agents properly. Adverse effects are more likely to occur when beta$_2$ agonists are used concurrently with theophylline preparations, when inappropriately high doses are administered, or when patients are frail, elderly, chronically ill, or medically unstable. Adverse effects in the elderly are probably limited by the fact that so many are unable to use the metered dose inhalers correctly.

Tremor is the most common side effect of beta$_2$ agonists and is more common in older than in younger patients. It may occur de novo, or may present as an accentuation of an existing tremor, such as essential tremor and tremor due to Parkinson's disease. Tremor is thought to result from stimulation of peripheral beta$_2$ receptors in muscle spindles, rather than from a central mechanism.

Tachyarrhythmias are a potential side effect but are uncommon when the drugs are given by inhalation. The incidence of this effect in older patients is not known. It is unclear if tachycardia, when it occurs, is reflex in origin—a response to beta$_2$ vasodilation—or due to a direct nonselective effect on the heart. In general, elderly patients are somewhat less likely to experience reflex tachycardia from any cause because of impaired baroreceptor function.

Because these drugs penetrate the blood-brain barrier poorly, centrally mediated effects are uncommon.

All adverse effects are far more likely to occur when the drug is administered by routes other than direct inhalation. In the case of terbutaline, which can be administered subcutaneously, beta$_2$ selectivity seems to be eradicated when this route is used. Thus, injected terbutaline seems to have few advantages over epinephrine in the emergency room setting.

Oral Versus Aerosolized Beta$_2$ Agonists

The main advantage of aerosolized agents is that most active drug remains at the site of action, namely, in the lung, while only a small proportion reaches the systemic circulation. This minimizes the likelihood of side effects, in contrast to oral agents, which not uncommonly produce side effects at therapeutic doses. This may be an important limiting factor in the older patient. An additional advantage of aerosolized agents is their rapid onset of action, which allows most patients to achieve some relief within a few minutes. Oral agents may not begin to act for at least half an hour.

There are nonetheless disadvantages of aerosolized agents. Many patients do not use them properly, a common, often insurmountable problem in geriatric practice. Patients often fail to develop the necessary hand-breath coordination and some simply lack the manual dexterity to operate the canister. Repeated instruction may fail to overcome these handicaps and some patients may not even benefit from additional appliances, such as spacers (see below). Patients with dementia and other neurological impairments generally are unable to use any inhaler properly. Another disadvantage of inhalers is that some patients may be embarrassed to use them in public. Finally, the duration of action may be too short to control symptoms adequately, particularly through the night.

There is little rationale for using oral adrenergic agents today. If an inhaler cannot be used or produces insufficient abatement of symptoms, elderly patients should generally use a theophylline preparation rather than an *oral* adrenergic agent, since cardiac toxicity and tremor are less common with the former. In addition, theophylline serum levels can readily be obtained in most communities. Adrenergic agents may be better tolerated in certain patients, however, and they are subject to a different spectrum of drug interactions, so an occasional patient may benefit.

Dosing

Recommended dosages are summarized in Table 29–2.

Spacers and Other Auxiliary Devices for Inhalers

Patients with poor hand-breath coordination often benefit from the use of a *spacer*. This device is a valved holding-chamber that is attached to the commercial inhaler. The spacer retains the aerosolized spray emitted from the metered-dose inhaler and allows the patient to breathe in the medication using ordinary tidal volume without having to coordinate inspiration with manual operation of the canister. By increasing delivery of small-diameter aerosolized particles, spacers may increase the actual amount delivered to the lung over what would have occurred with the metered-dose inhaler alone. This theoretically increases the effective dose delivered by the commercial inhaler.

Patients with poor manual dexterity due to paralysis, arthritis, or other factors may benefit from another auxiliary device (Vent-ease), which requires a less forceful motion for canister activation.

A new delivery system is available for albuterol (Rotahaler with Ventolin rotacaps). A capsule containing 200 μg of albuterol is inserted into an opening in the dispenser, which is then twisted, releasing the medication into the dispenser as a powder. The device is held between the lips like a cigarette and the medication is inhaled directly. This device eliminates the need for strict hand-breath coordination, but the powdered preparation occasionally produces cough. Only 1 capsule should be used per dose and the patient should be strictly instructed not to take the capsule orally.

Hand-bulb (also called "handheld") nebulizers (Devilbis Pulmoaid, others) are used for the administration of adrenergic agents, most commonly the beta$_2$-selective variety. This type of device delivers bronchodilator by mouthpiece or face mask and is inhaled at tidal volume; it is thus helpful to the patient who is unable to produce adequate inspiratory flow because of respiratory compromise or because of failure to comprehend the method. Although generally used in severe acute exacerbations of bronchospastic disease, either at home or in the hospital, there may be a place for the hand-bulb nebulizer in the less severely ill patient who cannot use other delivery systems. However, it is essential that this type of device be used or monitored by someone who fully understands its use. A fixed amount of bronchodilator solution is mixed with saline and is available for inhalation for approximately 15 minutes. The usual amount of drug in a 1-unit vial is far in excess of the amount delivered by metered-dose inhaler (e.g., a total of 15 mg metaproterenol in nebulized solution versus 0.65 mg per metered puff). While only a small proportion of this is actually inhaled by the patient, the total amount delivered in 1 treatment cannot be measured and toxicity can occur. This, of course, can be more severe in a geriatric patient.

Important Drug Interactions

The central and cardiovascular effects of concurrently administered theophylline preparations may be potentiated by beta-adrenergic agents; however, the combination may also provide additive bronchodilating effects and is often therapeutically useful.

Adrenergic agents with alpha-stimulating properties should not be used in conjunction with monoamine oxidase inhibitors, because hypertensive crisis may occur. Adrenergic agents in general may produce hypertension when used in conjunction with tricyclic antidepressants and ganglionic blockers; this interaction is unlikely with inhaled $beta_2$ bronchodilators but caution should be observed.

Precautions

While the inability to use a metered-dose inhaler limits the adverse effects of bronchodilators, it obviously limits the therapeutic effects. If an appliance such as a nebulizer is then utilized and the patient is finally able to use the system correctly, adverse effects may only then manifest themselves. Careful monitoring should be undertaken when these accessories are first instituted.

OTHER ADRENERGIC AGENTS

Epinephrine

Like endogenous catecholamines, exogenously administered epinephrine is rapidly degraded by enzymes that not only are concentrated in the liver, but are ubiquitous. Epinephrine is not orally active since its rapid degradation begins in the gastrointestinal tract, and in the treatment of bronchospasm it is administered parenterally or by inhaler. Epinephrine has alpha-, $beta_1$-, and $beta_2$-stimulating properties and can produce a wide range of side effects. Its short duration of action limits the duration of adverse effects, but elderly patients are extremely sensitive to systemic effects and dose adjustments are required.

Epinephrine products are available without prescription as respiratory inhalers, as well as nasal and ocular decongestants. Toxicity may occur if these over-the-counter preparations are used injudiciously.

The most common adverse effects are **tachycardia, elevations in blood pressure, tremor,** and **sweating. Symptoms of myocardial ischemia** may occur in patients with heart disease. Beta-adrenergic effects on the liver and pancreas may result in **transient hyperglycemia.**

Contraindications

Parenteral epinephrine should not be given to elderly asthmatics with ischemic heart disease or cardiac arrhythmias.

Indications

Epinephrine administered subcutaneously is indicated for severe, acute asthma that cannot be managed with other bronchodilators. Although parenteral epinephrine has been used successfully for years, its use has always been discouraged in the elderly and the availability of inhaled bronchodilator beta$_2$-selective agonists has all but supplanted its use in asthma.

Parenteral epinephrine is indicated in the treatment of anaphylaxis.

Inhaled epinephrine is not recommended for elderly patients, since better-tolerated inhaled agents are available.

Precautions

Aerosolized epinephrine is available without prescription. Elderly patients should be instructed to avoid this agent or to use it only under the physician's care.

Dosing

Acute asthma: 0.3 cc (0.3 mg) SQ.

Ephedrine

Ephedrine has both alpha- and beta-adrenergic properties, but acts primarily by releasing endogenous catecholamines. It is less potent than epinephrine, but it has a longer duration of action and penetrates the CNS to a greater degree. The duration of action of ephedrine is up to 5 hours in nonelderly adults, and although there is little information regarding this drug in the elderly, it is largely eliminated by the kidney and probably has a longer duration of action in this age group.

Because of significant alpha-adrenergic activity, ephedrine may stimulate contraction of the internal urethral sphincter. This is generally seen as a positive effect in older women with urethral incompetence or unstable bladder, and the drug has been used therapeutically in this setting (see Chap. 23). However, urinary dysfunction could be worsened in those with urinary retention syndromes, such as prostatic outlet obstruction.

Adverse effects are similar to those produced by epinephrine, but may be milder or longer lasting. Because ephedrine readily penetrates the CNS, effects such as dizziness, insomnia, and headache may be prominent. Confusional states are a potential risk in geriatric patients.

Although ephedrine is available without prescription, it is not recommended for the treatment of bronchospasm in elderly patients because there are more effective, better-tolerated agents.

Precautions

Oral ephedrine is available without prescription. Elderly patients should be instructed to avoid this agent or to use it only under the care of the physician.

Isoproterenol (Isuprel)

Like epinephrine, isoproterenol is potent and short-acting, but unlike epinephrine, it has little or no alpha-adrenergic activity. It is a nonselective beta agonist and is primarily used in aerosolized form for the management of acute asthma and exacerbations of emphysema. The most common adverse effects are tachyarrhythmias, tremor, dizziness, and flushing.

Isoproterenol should generally be avoided by elderly patients because of the prominent cardiac effects that may occur at therapeutic doses. Inhaled beta$_2$-selective agents are excellent alternatives.

IPRATROPIUM (ATROVENT)

Mechanism of Action

Ipratropium is the chief anticholinergic (atropinelike) aerosol agent used in the treatment of bronchospasm. Like other anticholinergic agents, ipratropium acts by competitively inhibiting acetylcholine at muscarinic receptor sites. Physiologically, tonic endogenous cholinergic stimulation in the tracheobronchial tree enhances bronchial tone, but patients with asthma and other forms of bronchospasm have hyperresponsiveness to cholinergic stimulation. This response can be prevented or reversed by atropine, although the response to ipratropium varies greatly on a clinical level. Cholinergic stimulation also increases the production of secretions by submucosal glands in the tracheobronchial tree, and, although systemic anticholinergic agents inhibit production and clearance of these secretions, inhaled ipratropium does not appear to have a drying effect that is harmful in the usual clinical situation. Cholinergic mechanisms in wheezing are thought to increase in importance with age, perhaps because of reductions in the sensitivity of the parallel beta-adrenergic system. This does not presently appear to have importance in clinical management of the elderly asthmatic, however.

Ipratropium is chemically related to atropine, but possesses a quaternary ammonium structure so that it neither passes through the blood-brain barrier nor is absorbed through the gastrointestinal tract. Like other aerosols inhaled through the mouth, substantial amounts are swallowed, but unlike inhaled adrenergic agents, only negligible amounts of ipratropium enter the systemic circulation through the lung and gut, and the drug does not enter the CNS. Swallowed drug is excreted in the feces and the small amount that appears systemically is metabolized to inactive substances by the liver. Systemic effects at recommended doses are close to nil, making it potentially one of the best-tolerated agents.

Compared to inhaled sympathomimetic agents, ipratropium has a slower onset of action. Thus, it has limited utility in the management of acute asthma. In addition, it has no known effect on noncholinergic mediators of bronchospasm, such as histamine, and fewer asthmatics achieve substantial clinical benefit from ipratropium than from adrenergic agents. However, ipratropium may be equally as or more effective than adrenergic agents and theophylline in the treatment of COPD, although the benefit derived in COPD is less than in asthma, regardless of the intervention. In both conditions, one cannot predict which patients will benefit from ipratropium without a therapeutic trial.

As expected, the utility of ipratropium is limited by the fact that many patients are unable to use the metered-dose inhaler correctly.

Adverse Effects

Patients may complain that ipratropium has a **bitter taste** and many complain of **dry mouth**.

Because very little drug reaches the systemic circulation, reports of systemic anticholinergic effects are rare. There is a paucity of data on its specific use in patients over 75 years of age, who are notoriously more sensitive to small doses of anticholinergic medication. However, older individuals may have a diminished cardiac response to atropine. In any case, it is probably safe to say that this agent is even less likely to produce cardiac effects than inhaled sympathomimetic agents, and it does not produce tremor. Confusional states are unlikely to occur. Toxicity of anticholinergic medication is discussed elsewhere in this book (see Chap. 10).

The main disadvantage of ipratropium is that it is not as effective as adrenergic agents in as wide a range of clinical settings.

Contraindications and Precautions

Unlike systemic anticholinergic agents, ipratropium has no absolute contraindications. However, the spray can be inadvertently instilled into the eyes, in which case the potential exists for the drug to precipitate acute angle closure glaucoma. Susceptible patients should be advised to use caution.

Indications

Ipratropium is indicated as adjunctive treatment in patients with bronchospasm who are unable to tolerate or who do not fully respond to treatment with other agents. It may be used for the prevention of bronchospasm as a first-line agent in patients, particularly those with COPD, who demonstrate a good therapeutic response following a therapeutic trial. It may be used alone or in combination with inhaled sympathomimetic agents or theophylline.

Dosing

Dosage: 1–2 puffs qid.

PROPHYLACTIC AGENT: CROMOLYN SODIUM (INTAL)

Cromolyn sodium is thought to act by preventing the release of endogenous mediators of allergy and inflammation in response to exposure to allergens. It is not chemically related to bronchodilators or histamine$_1$ blockers (antihistamines). It is used to prevent rather than treat bronchospasm that results from various stimuli and probably has no acute bronchodilating effects when used clinically. It may be less effective than theophylline in preventing exacerbations in chronic asthma. However, the anti-inflammatory nature of cromolyn gives it an important role in the management of chronic asthma and it may reduce the need for bronchodilators.

Cromolyn has been used most widely in treating children, but it is effective in adults as well. There is no specific information as to its efficacy in elderly asthmatics, but there is no reason to discount its potential usefulness. The advantages of cromolyn are that it does not produce cardiac side effects, tremor, or CNS excitation, and does not possess anticholinergic effects seen with the first-generation antihistamines.

Aside from its lack of acute benefit, the chief disadvantage of cromolyn is that it must be inhaled and is subject to the same practical problems that other inhalers pose for geriatric patients. Two types of inhalers are available, a metered-dose inhaler and the Spinhaler turboinhaler, which activates a capsule that must first be placed in the device. The latter may require slightly less hand-breath coordination but perhaps more manual dexterity.

Adverse Effects

Cromolyn may produce **irritation and dryness of the oral mucosa. Cough** may occur and is probably more common with the inhaled powder (Spinhaler turboinhaler) than with the more recently developed metered-dose inhaler. Some patients may develop wheezing after inhalation. While paradoxical wheezing has been reported with other inhalers, **hypersensitivity reactions,** including laryngeal edema, have been reported with cromolyn. These effects are rare.

It should be emphasized that cromolyn is a prophylactic agent and that its beneficial effects in some patients might not be apparent until it has been used for many weeks.

Indications

Cromolyn is indicated for the prevention of wheezing in patients with chronic or seasonal asthma. It may be used in conjunction with bronchodilators. It is not indicated in COPD.

Dosing

Metered dose inhaler: 2 puffs qid.
Spinhaler: 1 capsule activated by turboinhaler qid.

After 1–2 months, or until symptoms are controlled, the dose may be reduced to tid or bid. In seasonal asthma, therapy should begin at least 2 weeks before symptoms are expected.

CORTICOSTEROIDS

Systemic Use

It is increasingly being recognized that asthma is a chronic inflammatory disease and that corticosteroids may be underutilized in patients, such as the average elderly asthmatic, who do not have severe, classic steroid-dependent asthma. Although the side effects of corticosteroids are exaggerated in aged individuals, fear of adverse effects should not deter the physician from prescribing them in a timely albeit judicious fashion. A major advantage for certain frail elderly patients is that, unlike bronchodilators, corticosteroids are devoid of cardiac toxicity. Side effects and other aspects of corticosteroids are discussed in Chap. 3.

The smallest effective dose should be used. Elderly patients with bronchospasm sometimes achieve dramatic resolution of bronchodilator-resistant symptoms with small doses of oral corticosteroids (as low as 10–20 mg of prednisone) and rarely require high doses for prolonged periods.

Indications

Systemic corticosteroids are indicated in bronchospasm that does not respond to bronchodilators.

Dosing

Doses of corticosteroids must be individualized. Knowledge of a patient's response can assist the physician in tailoring the dose to a particular patient. In general, the elderly asthmatic has less severe disease than the classic steroid-dependent younger asthmatic and when systemic corticosteroids are required to break an attack small doses are sometimes very effective. High doses of intravenous corti-costeroids are rarely required but may be used if necessary.

In moderate bronchospasm: 30–40 mg by mouth, tapered rapidly over 1 week.

Note: Some patients may respond to initial doses as small as 10–20 mg. Those who have shown a satisfactory response to higher doses may be tried on a lower-dose regimen at a later date if the clinical situation allows.

In severe disease: 40–60 mg prednisolone every 6 hr given by IV drip until symptoms resolve.

Note: Higher doses may be used if needed, but these clinical situations are unlikely to be encountered in geriatric practice.

Maintenance oral therapy should be determined by patient response and can be given on alternate days.

Inhaled Use

As in all age groups, inhaled corticosteroids are better tolerated than systemic corticosteroids by elderly patients, who should be switched to the former as quickly as tapering and symptoms allow. As with other agents delivered by metered-dose inhaler, inhaled corticosteroids may be difficult for the aged patient to use. A spacer is particularly important for the patient inhaling corticosteroids, since it will reduce the risk of developing steroid-associated oropharyngeal candidiasis.

Adverse Effects

Oropharyngeal and esophageal candidiasis may occur. **Sore throat** is common. These side effects can be minimized if the mouth is rinsed with water after each use and if a spacer or other auxiliary device is used. Inhaled corticosteroids may produce candidiasis of the upper airways, but this is quite unusual. **Dysphonia** may occur from candida or from the agent itself. **Mild suppression of the pituitary-adrenal axis** may occur with prolonged use.

Precautions

Because of the potential for pituitary-adrenal axis suppression, patients who use these agents on a long-term basis must be instructed carefully on their use. A problem frequently encountered in geriatric practice is that, even with repeated explanations, many patients fail to understand that inhaled corticosteroids are used as prophylaxis and not as bronchodilators. They often fail to distinguish corticosteroid inhalers from inhaled bronchodilators, and use them interchangeably. Instructions should be repeated at each visit until it is certain that the patient and caregiver understand this concept. Inhalers should be clearly marked with instructions if necessary.

Indications

Inhaled corticosteroids are indicated in steroid-responsive asthmatics who are being successfully weaned from systemic corticosteroids. They may occasionally be useful as adjunctive treatment in patients not on oral corticosteroids but who fail to respond fully to other bronchodilators.

Available Agents

Three agents are available in the United States (see Table 29–3). Differences in potency among these agents are circumvented as fixed

Table 29-3. Inhaled Corticosteroids

Agent	Brand	Usual Dose
Beclomethasone	Beclovent, Vanceril	2 puffs bid-qid
Triamcinolone	Azmacort	2 puffs bid-qid
Flunisolide	AeroBid	2 puffs bid

amounts are delivered by the metered-dose inhaler. Beclomethasone has been in use the longest and is said to have the most favorable topical-to-systemic potency of the three. Although it is difficult to detect a different clinical response among the available agents, it should be emphasized that flunisolide is much more potent on a per-weight basis and should be taken no more than twice daily.

Dosing
Doses are summarized in Table 29-3.

BIBLIOGRAPHY
Barnes, P. J. A new approach to the treatment of asthma. *N. Engl. J. Med.* 321:1517–1527, 1989.

Braman, S. S., and Davis, S. M. Wheezing in the elderly. Asthma and other causes. *Clin. Geriatr. Med.* 2:269–283, 1986.

Fanta, C. H. Asthma in the elderly. *J. Asthma* 26:87–97, 1989.

Fishman, A. P. Cardiac asthma—a fresh look at an old wheeze. *N. Engl. J. Med.* 320:1346–1348, 1989.

Gal, P., and Layson, R. Interference with oral theophylline absorption by continuous nasogastric feedings. *Ther. Drug Monitor.* 8:421–423, 1986.

Gross, N. J. Ipratropium bromide. *N. Engl. J. Med.* 319:486–494, 1988.

Hendeles, L., and Weinberger, M. Selection of a slow-release theophylline product. *J. Allerg. Clin. Immunol.* 78:743–751, 1986.

Jenne, J. W. Effect of disease states on theophylline elimination. *J. Allerg. Clin. Immunol.* 28:727–735, 1986.

Johnson, C. E. Aerosol corticosteroids for the treatment of asthma. *Drug Intell. Clin. Pharm.* 21:784–790, 1987.

Jonkman, J. H. Therapeutic consequences of drug interactions with theophylline pharmacokinetics. *J. Allergy Clin. Immunol.* 78:736–742, 1986.

Petty, T. L., Rollins, D. R., Christopher, K., et al. Cromolyn sodium is effective in adult chronic asthmatics. *Am. Rev. Resp. Dis.* 139:694–701, 1989.

Weinberger, M., Hendeles, L., and Bighley, L. The relation of product formulation to absorption of oral theophylline. *N. Engl. J. Med.* 299:852–857, 1978.

Ziment, I., and Au, J. P. Anticholinergic agents. *Clin. Chest Med.* 7:355–366, 1986.

Antihistamines

Antihistamines (histamine$_1$ [H$_1$] blockers) are structurally related to histamine and reversibly bind to H$_1$ receptor sites, competitively blocking the action of histamine. When histamine is released from mast cell granules in response to provocation by specific antigens, it binds to cell receptors, producing a variety of effects, including vasodilation, smooth muscle contraction, stimulation of peripheral nerve endings, and gastric secretion. Among the H$_1$-receptor effects blocked by antihistamines are vasodilation, vascular permeability, and bronchial smooth muscle constriction. Antihistamines do not prevent the actual release of histamine, but do block its action, and while they may prevent the occurrence and worsening of a range of allergic phenomena, they do not reverse the effects of histamine once they have become established. Furthermore, many allergic phenomena are mediated by factors other than histamine, a fact that probably accounts for the incomplete efficacy of H$_1$ blockers in preventing these symptoms.

H$_1$ antagonists are structurally dissimilar from histamine$_2$ (H$_2$) antagonists, such as cimetidine and ranitidine, and do not block the effects of histamine at H$_2$ receptors. Therefore, they have no ability to inhibit H$_2$-mediated effects such as gastric secretion. H$_1$ blockers are referred to as *antihistamines,* their traditional appellation, in this chapter.

The side-chains of antihistamines determine pharmacokinetics and side effects. First-generation antihistamines, such as diphenhydramine and chlorpheniramine, are highly lipid-soluble and cross the blood-brain barrier readily. H$_1$ receptors are present in the brain, and competitive blockage of histamine binding at these sites is thought to be responsible for the common side effect of sedation. This sedation often limits daytime usefulness of antihistamines but is an effect that has been harnessed in the treatment of insomnia.

Antihistamines also exert varying degrees of anticholinergic, antiserotonin, and anti-alpha-adrenergic effects, characteristics that may produce side effects that are often troublesome in geriatric patients.

These drawbacks paved the way for the development of a second generation of antihistamines. The new agents do not readily enter the brain and produce sedation far less often than first-generation antihistamines. They are furthermore virtually devoid of anticholinergic activity and thus do not produce urinary retention, constipation, blurred vision, or acute angle closure glaucoma. These characteristics increase the safety with which allergic phenomena can be treated in the geriatric patient.

FIRST-GENERATION ANTIHISTAMINES

Pharmacokinetics

There is a paucity of pharmacokinetic data on the older antihistamines, because accurate assays were lacking when these agents were developed. Data that exists is confusing because of methodologic differences and variability in outcome of trials. In general, the duration of action may be in the range of 24 hours or more for many of these agents. Thus, both efficacy and side effects can be prolonged.

Adverse Effects

Sedation is the most common side effect of antihistamines and occurs to some degree with all of the first-generation agents. Tolerance develops to this sedation within days or a few weeks when the drug is used chronically.

Anticholinergic effects such as dry mouth, urinary retention, and constipation, blurred vision, and acute angle closure glaucoma, may occur. **Confusion** may be precipitated in susceptible patients.

Long-term use of antihistamines has been reported to produce **tardive dyskinesia,** but this side effect is very rare.

Skin reactions to antihistamines are rare, and when they do occur they are generally acute in onset because they are probably mediated by acute release of histamine from the receptor rather than due to a typical allergic reaction.

Characteristic chemical profiles for commonly used agents are summarized in Table 30–1.

Drug Interactions

Antihistamines participate in few if any pharmacokinetic interactions. Sedation and the anticholinergic effects of antihistamines may be enhanced by other agents possessing these properties, and concurrent use should be avoided if possible.

Table 30–1. Actions of Commonly Used Antihistamines

Agent (Brand)	Sedative	Anticholinergic	Chief Use
First Generation			
Diphenhydramine (Benadryl)	3+	3+	Allergy; sleep
Brompheniramine (Dimetane)	1+	2+	Allergy
Chlorpheniramine (Chlor-Trimeton	1+	2+	Allergy
Hydroxyzine (Atarax, Vistaril)	3+	2+	Pruritus; anxiety
Cyproheptadine (Periactin)	1+	2+	Urticaria
Meclizine (Antivert)	2+	2+	Vertigo; motion sickness
Promethazine (Phenergan)	3+	3+	Nausea
Second Generation			
Terfenadine (Seldane)	<1	0	Allergy
Astemizole (Hismanal)	<1	0	Allergy

0 = absent
<1 = negligible
1+ = mild
2+ = moderate
3+ = strong

Indications

Antihistamines are indicated in the treatment of seasonal and perennial allergy, relieving symptoms such as sneezing, runny nose, and watery and itchy eyes. Allergic conjunctivitis may respond well to systemic antihistamines, and ocular preparations are available. Antihistamines are indicated in the treatment of urticaria, angioedema, and pruritus that is related to allergic phenomena.

Other Uses

Owing to unique chemical properties, some antihistamines are particularly useful in the treatment of vertigo, motion sickness, and nausea (see Meclizine, below).

Antihistamines are commonly prescribed in the management of pruritus, regardless of etiology, but their efficacy in most settings is probably slight. The extent to which histamine mediates itch in the absence of a wheal and flare reaction is not known. It is likely that the sedating property of antihistamines may be one of the more important factors in their efficacy, and the placebo effect may play a role as well. Antihistamines probably have little effect in pruritus associated with cholestasis or Hodgkin's disease, although the sedative effect may play an adjunctive role here. Idiopathic pruritus in the elderly is thought to be related to dryness of the skin and antihistamines are unlikely to play a central role. In that condition, the physician should first prescribe nonpharmacologic treatment, including the elimination of prolonged bathing, drying soaps, and other irritants, and the use of emollients. Regardless of etiology, however, a trial of antihistamines should be considered in the treatment of refractory pruritus.

The use of antihistamines in asthma is under investigation. Traditionally, antihistamines were contraindicated in acute asthma because the drying effect was thought to produce inspissated secretions with possible disastrous consequences. There is some evidence that this may not be the case, and it is clear that antihistamines taken prophylactically may reduce the frequency and severity of attacks in certain asthmatics, and may actually have a small bronchodilating effect. Until more is known, antihistamines should be reserved for asthmatics who have shown clear benefit in the past. Otherwise, they should generally not be a part of routine treatment once an asthma attack has become established.

The use of antihistamines in the common cold is also a matter of some controversy. Antihistamines are found in a number of cold preparations that also contain adrenergic agents, but there is conflicting data on the efficacy of antihistamines alone in the treatment of cold symptoms, such as nasal obstruction and secretions. Claims of efficacy have been made even for antihistamines not possessing the anticholinergic effects thought to be responsible for drying the nasal mucosa, prompting some investigators to suggest that many symptoms produced in the common cold are actually mediated by histamine. The controversy notwithstanding, antihistamines probably do have a place in palliation of cold symptoms and would be suitable alternatives to adrenergic agents in patients with cardiac disease or hypertension. Certainly for the patient with cardiac disease or hypertension, it is wiser to prescribe a mild antihistamine for a cold, rather than a combination pill containing an adrenergic agent.

The use of antihistamines for sleep and anxiety is discussed in Chaps. 6 and 7.

Specific Agents

A large number of antihistamines are available in the United States. Many antihistamines offer no particular advantage over other ones. The antihistamines that are discussed here are those that are particularly applicable to geriatric practice. For further discussion of antihistamines, the reader is referred to the Bibliography readings (see Douglas).

The pharmacokinetic aspects of first-generation agents have not been well studied and little or no pharmacokinetic data on elderly patients exists.

Brompheniramine (Dimetane, Others)

This drug has an elimination half-life of at least 24 hours in healthy adults, but the pharmacokinetics after chronic ingestion have not been well studied. It is extensively metabolized in the liver. The sedating effects of brompheniramine may correlate well with serum levels and are greatest 3–4 hours after administration. The antihistaminic and perhaps other effects greatly outlast peak serum levels. Traditional recommendations that the drug be taken up to 4 times a day may be inconsistent with more recent understanding of the drug's pharmacokinetics.

Compared to other first-generation antihistamines, brompheniramine is relatively nonsedating, but it should be used cautiously in patients with confusional states and should not be taken in conjunction with other drugs having a sedating effect.

DOSING

Initial dose: 4 mg once daily.

Maximum dose: 4 mg qid.

Note: Response to once-daily therapy should be observed for several days before dose increases are made.

Chlorpheniramine (Chlor-Trimeton, Others)

Chlorpheniramine is chemically related to brompheniramine and shares its pharmacologic profile. It has been better studied than other agents in use.

Chlorpheniramine is absorbed slowly, with peak levels and maximum effect occurring within 2–6 hours, but with highly variable onset of action, which may be as soon as 15 minutes. Absorption as well as bioavailability may vary widely among the many preparations and brands on the market. The drug is extensively metabolized in the liver, with variable amounts being excreted unchanged in the urine. The elimination half-life may be as long as 24 hours in healthy adults. Although no specific pharmacokinetic data are available in older patients, its pharmacologic profile suggests that elimination would tend to be prolonged in older patients.

As with most other antihistamines, antihistaminic activity may outlast "therapeutic" serum concentrations. Like brompheniramine, traditional dose recommendations may be inconsistent with the actual pharmacokinetics of chlorpheniramine.

DOSING

Initial dose: 4 mg once daily.

Maximum dose: 4 mg qid.

Note: Response to once-daily therapy should be observed for several days before dose increases are made.

Diphenhydramine (Benadryl, Others)

Except for the phenothiazines, diphenhydramine is one of the most sedating antihistamines. For this reason, it is commonly used in the treatment of insomnia (see Chap. 7), and is available over the counter in many preparations. Although the tendency to produce sedation may reduce its daytime usefulness, diphenhydramine seems to have a shorter elimination half-life than chlorpheniramine and brompheniramine, with a closer correlation between plasma levels and both antihistaminic activity and sedation.

DOSING
Initial dose: 10–25 mg daily to tid.
Maximum dose: 50 mg tid.

Hydroxyzine (Atarax, Vistaril)

Hydroxyzine is more effective than most other antihistamines in suppressing the itch associated with experimental histamine-induced wheal and flare. Limited clinical study suggests that it may be more effective in reducing itch produced by a variety of causes. The potent sedating effect of hydroxyzine may be in part responsible for this purported antipruritic efficacy.

After oral dose, peak plasma levels occur within 2 hours, and elimination half-life of a single dose in nonelderly adults averages 20 hours. One renally excreted metabolite is pharmacologically active and itself has a half-life of 24 hours. There is some evidence that the half-life is further prolonged in older patients. This has been attributed to an increased volume of distribution. The antihistaminic effect in the skin apparently outlasts peak serum levels by many hours.

Hydroxyzine hydrochloride (Atarax) and hydroxyzine pamoate (Vistaril) are essentially equivalent. Only the former is available in the small 10-mg dosage form.

INDICATIONS. Hydroxyzine is commonly used in the management of pruritus. However, the efficacy of antihistamines in pruritus is controversial (see Other Uses, above). It is suitable for use in allergy but may be more sedating than other agents.

This agent is also used occasionally for the management of anxiety and insomnia (see Chaps. 6 and 7).

DOSING
Initial dose: 10 mg once daily.
Maximum dose: 25 mg qid.

Meclizine (Antivert)

Meclizine has a slow onset of action but is useful in suppressing symptoms of vertigo and nausea associated with disease of the central and peripheral vestibular system. It is probably overprescribed in geriatric practice, where it is sometimes given inappropriately for nonspecific complaints of dizziness.

Although meclizine is probably less effective for vestibular symptoms than the phenothiazines and their derivatives, such as promethazine, it is also less sedating and less likely to produce extrapyramidal symptoms.

RECOMMENDATIONS. Meclizine is indicated for nausea and vomiting due to vertigo, Meniere's disease, and other labyrinthine syndromes. It is often effective when vertigo is due to central lesions as well.

Meclizine should not be given routinely for nonspecific complaints of dizziness. Such symptoms should be thoroughly evaluated in all elderly patients before such prescribing decisions are made.

DOSING

Usual dose: 12.5–25.0 mg as needed up to 3 times daily. Symptoms are often controlled with a once-daily dose.

Cyproheptadine (Periactin, Others)

Cyproheptadine is a member of the piperidine family of antihistamines, and is structurally more similar to phenothiazinelike antihistamines than other groups. In addition to its antihistaminic activity, cyproheptadine possesses antiserotonin effect, which is not thought to be directly useful in the treatment of allergies but which may responsible for its unique side-effect profile. In addition to its general antiallergy properties, cyproheptadine is thought to be particularly useful in the treatment of pruritus and cold urticaria. The theoretical basis for this application is that serotonin serves to moderate itch in some cases. However, limited clinical study suggests that hydroxyzine is more effective in this regard than cyproheptadine.

Cyproheptadine is absorbed slowly and is extensively metabolized. Elimination half-life is about 16 hours in nonelderly adults.

The antiserotonin activity of cyproheptadine is thought to be responsible for the increased appetite and modest weight gain experienced by some patients. Although it produces sedation in some patients, it can cause stimulation in others.

Compared to most other first-generation antihistamines, cyproheptadine has relatively mild anticholinergic effects.

ADVERSE EFFECTS. **Weight gain** and **increased appetite** are seen as a disadvantage in most patients who use this agent for its antihistaminic properties. However, when weight gain does occur, it is quite mild.

Less likely than other first-generation antihistamines to produce sedation, cyproheptadine is more likely to produce **stimulation, agitation,** or even **psychosis.** Fortunately, these effects are rare.

Despite its relatively **mild anticholinergic properties,** side effects may occur.

RECOMMENDATIONS. Cyproheptadine is indicated in the management of cold urticaria. Although its efficacy in pruritus is probably minimal, it can be offered as an alternative to hydroxyzine if the latter is too sedating.

Cyproheptadine should not be used to stimulate the appetite in the elderly because there is no evidence that it is particularly useful in that regard. Patients with anorexia require a careful medical and psychological evaluation.

DOSING

Usual dose: 4 mg daily to bid.

SECOND-GENERATION ANTIHISTAMINES

The second-generation antihistamines differ from first-generation antihistamines in their markedly reduced tendency to produce sedation, and their virtual lack of anticholinergic activity.

Terfenadine (Seldane)

Although controlled studies generally demonstrate that terfenadine is comparable in its efficacy to standard antihistamines in the treatment of allergic rhinitis and urticaria, many clinicians disagree, claiming that this agent is of limited value. Nonetheless, many patients attain sufficient relief of symptoms and are pleased with the lack of sedation that occurs. Of all the antihistamines considered in this chapter, terfenadine probably has the best safety profile, and, if cost is not a factor, it can be considered the drug of choice in the treatment of allergy in geriatrics.

Currently terfenadine is considerably more expensive than older, sedating antihistamines.

Pharmacologic Considerations

MECHANISM OF ACTION. Like other antihistamines, terfenadine selectively binds to H_1 receptors and antagonizes typical responses of histamine in various organ systems. It does not appreciably cross the blood-brain barrier and therefore does not antagonize histamine-mediated arousal mechanisms. It does not possess significant anticholinergic effects and does not block H_2 receptors.

PHARMACOKINETICS. Terfenadine is extensively metabolized to one inactive and one partly active metabolite. The terminal half-life is approximately 20 hours. The duration of action is only about 12 hours, however, a discrepancy that has not been fully explained. Terfenadine kinetics have not been well studied in older patients, but the pharmacologic profile suggests that excretion should be somewhat prolonged in late life.

Adverse Effects

Although central nervous system effects such as **sedation** have been reported by a minority of patients, double-blind studies have shown that the incidence of these complaints is no more than that produced by placebo and is significantly less than that produced by first-generation antihistamines. Likewise, terfenadine does not appear to produce anticholinergic effects, such as dry mouth, urinary retention, constipation, and visual reactions. **Dermatologic hypersensitivity** reactions have been reported rarely. **Ventricular arrhythmias** have been reported **in overdose.**

Important Drug Interactions

Although terfenadine is highly protein-bound, no important drug interactions have been reported to date. Terfenadine does not appear to enhance central nervous system depressant effects produced by other CNS depressants.

Indications

Terfenadine is indicated in the treatment of allergic phenomena when antihistamine use is desired. Although it lacks sedative effect, some relief of pruritus from a variety of causes may be achieved with this drug.

If cost is not a factor, terfenadine is the antihistamine of first choice in elderly patients. It is particularly suitable for patients who cannot tolerate the sedative or anticholinergic effects of first-generation antihistamines. However, patients who have been satisfactorily treated with older agents and who have experienced no untoward effects do not need to switch to terfenadine.

Dosing
Usual dose: 60 mg once or twice daily.

Astemizole (Hismanal)
Astemizole is a nonsedating antihistamine, which has equal or greater antihistaminic efficacy than terfenadine.

Pharmacologic Considerations
MECHANISM OF ACTION. Astemizole is structurally unrelated to histamine and to antihistamines currently in use. Like terfenadine, astemizole does not penetrate the blood-brain barrier significantly, and is devoid of anticholinergic and antiadrenergic effect. There is some evidence that its antihistaminic effect is somewhat greater than those of terfenadine. However, it has been suggested that superior clinical efficacy can be due to compliance factors.

PHARMACOKINETICS. Astemizole is well absorbed orally, but antihistaminic effect may be delayed for 2 or more *days*. It undergoes extensive first-pass metabolism in the liver to a number of active and inactive metabolites, and substantial enterohepatic circulation of metabolites occurs. Some metabolites are excreted in the urine, but their relative inactivity and shorter half-life reduce their contribution to biologic effect. Despite significant hepatic extraction, astemizole does not affect hepatic microsomal enzymes.

The overall elimination half-life of astemizole (including active metabolites) is time-dependent, at 9–13 days after 1 dose but as high as 18–20 days after 2 or more months of daily administration. There are no specific pharmacokinetic studies in elderly patients, but the pattern of metabolism suggests that half-life could well be even more prolonged in elderly patients, and substantial drug accumulation could occur over time.

The antihistaminic effect of astemizole not only appears later, but lasts for much longer, than serum levels would predict. Thus, antihistaminic effect may persist for up to a few weeks after the drug has been discontinued, depending on how long the drug has been taken. This discrepancy may be due to its intense binding to tissue receptors and the potential that this drug has for accumulation. Since elimination is most likely further delayed in older individuals, this delay could well be enhanced.

Astemizole is found in tissues at far greater concentration than in plasma. Likewise, it is highly protein-bound.

Adverse Effects
Although some patients report that they experience **sedation** with astemizole, controlled studies generally have shown that sedation occurs no more commonly than with placebo, and less frequently than with other antihistamines, with the possible exception of terfenadine. Like cyproheptadine, astemizole may **increase appetite,** and has been associated with **modest weight gain** in some patients. This effect has been attributed to an antiserotonin effect, but this explanation conflicts with the observation that astemizole exhibits antiserotonin activity only at high doses. It is not known if drug accumulation plays a role here.

Prolongation of QT interval and **ventricular tachycardia** have been reported **with overdose.** The mechanism is thought to be related to blockage of cardiac H_1 receptors, although the significance of these receptors is unclear.

Important Drug Interactions

No important drug-drug interactions have been reported to date.

Recommendations

There are no contraindications to the short-term use of astemizole in the older patient. However, long-term experience with this drug in the elderly is limited. Ventricular tachycardia has been reported in overdose. Reported cases involved healthy young people with one-time ingestion of 20 times the recommended dose. Although limited study of healthy young adults indicates no effect on electrocardiographic parameters after 2 weeks, this drug has not been well studied in well or ill elderly. Since the potential for significant drug accumulation exists, and is greater in the older individual, it would seem prudent to exercise caution when prescribing this drug until more is known abut its long-term effects.

Like other antihistamines, astemizole is indicated in the treatment of allergy. However, it has a delayed onset of action and may not be useful if immediate relief is desired. If symptoms are not relieved rapidly enough, a shorter-acting antihistamine can be added for the first few days, until clinical activity of astemizole sets in.

Dosing

The usual recommended dose is 10 mg daily. After 3 successive days, a once-weekly dosage of 10 mg may be effective in some patients. Although the weekly dosage schedule has not been well studied, it should be attempted in preference to daily dosing in geriatric patients. Loading doses as high as 30 mg for 3 days have been given in studies involving younger patients.

BIBLIOGRAPHY

Carter, C. A., Wojciechowski, N. J., Hayes, J. M., Skoutakis, V. A., and Rickman, L. A. Terfenadine, a nonsedating antihistamine. *Drug Intell. Clin. Pharm.* 19:812–817, 1985.

Cohen, B., and Vianney deJong, J. M. B. Meclizine and placebo in treating vertigo of vestigular origin. *Arch. Neurol.* 27:129–137, 1972.

Douglas, W. W. Histamine and 5-hydroxytryptamine (serotonin) and their antagonists. In A. G. Gilman, L. L. Goodman, T. W. Rall, et al. (eds.), *The Pharmacological Basis of Therapeutics.* New York: Macmillan, 1985. Pp. 605–638.

Henauer, S. A., and Gluck, U. Efficacy of terfenadine in the treatment of common cold. A double-blind comparison with placebo. *Eur. J. Clin. Pharmacol.* 34:35–40, 1988.

Olzem, R., Zeisner, M., and Amery, W. K. Astemizole (R 43 512) in the treatment of hay fever. An international double-blind study comparing a weekly treatment (10 mg and 25 mg) with a placebo. *Curr. Ther. Res.* 29:24–35, 1981.

Popa, V. The classic antihistamines (H_1 blockers) in respiratory medicine. *Clin. Chest Med.* 7:367–382, 1986.

Use of Antibiotics

INFECTIONS IN THE ELDERLY

Although the selection of antimicrobial agents depends largely on the susceptibility of the etiologic organism, there are particular aspects of infections in late life that merit discussion and clarification.

There is an increased susceptibility to certain infections with age because of alterations in host defense and host environment. Unfortunately, the diagnosis of infection is not always apparent, because infections often present atypically. For example, fever may be absent; infections frequently present with altered states of consciousness, even though the organism lies outside the central nervous system; abdominal catastrophes may present with a minimum of symptoms; cough may be absent in pneumonia; tuberculosis often presents atypically and is misdiagnosed.

Bacteremia occurs more commonly in older infected patients than in younger ones with similar infections. Not only does this affect prognosis but it means that the blood is often a more reliable if not more easily accessible source of specimen for culture than the primary site. Gram-negative infections increase in incidence with age, a fact that should be taken into account when antibiotic selection is made.

With a few important exceptions, which are discussed below, antibiotics tend to have a wide therapeutic index. Thus, age-related dose adjustments are infrequently required. In geriatrics, when and how to prescribe the antibiotic are as important principles as which agent to prescribe and at what dose. This section deals with key infections encountered in geriatric practice, and provides some practical tips that modify antibiotic treatment in these situations.

URINARY TRACT INFECTIONS

Asymptomatic Bacteriuria: To Treat or Not to Treat?

The incidence of asymptomatic bacteriuria rises dramatically after midlife in men and is 10 times as common in men over 80 than in those between the ages of 65 and 70. As many as 50% of older women have chronic asymptomatic bacteriuria, with or without pyuria, and antibiotic treatment frequently fails to eradicate the organisms. The stubborn persistence of bacteriuria may be due to age-related factors, such as changes in the genital mucosa and changes in urinary osmolality and pH. How aggressively, then, should this be treated?

Although there is some evidence that individuals with chronic, asymptomatic bacteriuria have a higher mortality than those without bacteriuria, it has never been made clear whether this has to do with disease or physical impairments that encourage the development of bacteriuria or whether the bacteriuria itself leads to higher mortality. One reason that this dilemma remains unresolved is that infection soon recurs after antibiotic therapy is concluded.

Recurrent antibiotic treatment has the potential risk of producing resistant strains without clear-cut benefit for the asymptomatic host.

Recommendations

A course of antibiotics should be given to the patient who is found to have bacteriuria. Recurrent asymptomatic bacteriuria in the absence of an overt urinary tract lesion should be treated expectantly. In the symptomatic patient, causes other than infection should also be sought. If there is no other explanation for the symptoms, antibiotics directed at the urinary pathogen should be given. It is important to emphasize that symptoms may be subtle or may suggest disease outside the urinary tract.

Single-dose antibiotic therapy, which has been successful in younger women, is usually not effective in asymptomatic "cystitis" of older women.

Bacteriuria in the Catheterized Patient

Bacteriuria associated with a chronic indwelling catheter is an important management problem in nursing homes. After 3 days of catheterization, the incidence of colonization increases logarithmically and is virtually 100% after 1 week. Bacteriuria cannot be eradicated unless the catheter is removed. Maneuvers such as bladder irrigation, urinary acidification, increasing or decreasing catheter changes, use of highly sterile technique when inserting the catheter and when emptying and changing bags, and intravesical installation of antimicrobial agents or antiseptics have not been shown to reduce the overall incidence or chronicity of this type of infection although they may delay the onset. Chronic suppression with systemic antibiotics is inadvisable, since this approach may attenuate the growth of some organisms but encourages the development of resistant strains.

Indwelling catheters are overused. There are several alternatives to indwelling catheters in the management of urinary incontinence. These are discussed in detail in Chap. 23 and should be employed if possible.

In cases where the indwelling catheter is unavoidable, how does the physician approach the problem of chronic bacteriuria?

The incidence of infection is not reduced by sterile technique; however, infection can be passed from patient to patient if staff does not wash and change gloves before and after treating colonized patients. Although colonization per se may not lead to systemic illness, it is conceivable that patients living comfortably with certain strains of organisms may become ill if confronted with a new pathogen. Thus, the staff should be instructed to wash and change gloves before and after treating a catheterized patient, in order to prevent interpatient transmission of pathogens.

It is not known how frequently the catheter should be changed. Many nursing homes adopt the policy of changing the catheter monthly on a routine basis, or more often if crusting or blockage occurs. The exact timing is an arbitrary decision, there being little or no data calling for a particular time interval.

Recommendations

Antibiotics should not be instituted for urinary tract infections in chronically catherized patients unless symptoms occur. It must be emphasized that catheterized patients are frequently debilitated or neurologically impaired and either do not manifest or do not complain of symptoms. Symptoms are replaced by signs, and tend to consist of somnolence, restlessness, agitation, altered mental status, metastatic infection, or fever alone.

Chronically catheterized bladders are colonized with several species of organisms at a time. If symptoms occur and an antibiotic is indicated, a culture of the urine in the bladder (not the bag) should be done, but with the awareness that the organism causing the symptoms is not necessarily the one that will grow out on culture. Concurrent cultures of blood and other sites, if indicated, may yield the etiologic organism. It is a useless exercise to "routinely" culture the bladder contents while the patient is asymptomatic because the organism that grows out in culture may not be one to succeed on a subsequent culture.

Because specimen for culture is readily accessible and can be reliable, empiric treatment should be avoided except in urgent situations. If empiric treatment is necessary, as in possible urosepsis, broad-spectrum coverage should be given with ampicillin or a cephalosporin plus an aminoglycoside. Local institutional susceptibility patterns should also be considered in selecting the antibiotic. It is important to remember that the presence of the catheter does not exclude the possibility that the origin of the sepsis may be outside the urinary tract.

DECUBITUS ULCERS (PRESSURE SORES)

Decubitus ulcers commonly become infected. The likelihood of infection and the need for antibiotic intervention depends on the depth of the decubitus ulcer and the presence or absence of associated signs and symptoms.

The hallmark of treating decubitus ulcers is the removal of pressure and irritation. The treatment of skin ulcers and their four-stage classification is covered in Chap. 33.

Topical Antibiotic Ointments: Use or Avoid?

Physicians as well as nurses disagree on the utility of topical antibiotics in skin ulcers. The ulcer exists in a polymicrobial environment and is likely to become contaminated by organisms from the skin, gut, urinary tract, and the environment. The topical antibiotic sets up a sort of barrier against extrinsic infection and reduces local bacterial counts. While this may be of aesthetic value when wounds are purulent or foul smelling, there is no convincing evidence that topical antibiotics contribute to ulcer healing or patient comfort above and beyond other strict forms of wound care.

Routine use of topical antibiotics has the potential of producing resistant strains of organisms. This is an important consideration in closed communities such as nursing homes, where long-term infection control is so important.

Topical antibiotics may produce contact dermatitis. Less commonly, systemic allergy may occur. Allergic reactions are more likely to occur in patients with repeated exposure to these agents.

Recommendations

Topical antibiotics should be employed for short-term use in individual cases rather than as part of a routine regimen or institutionwide skin ulcer policy.

Specific Topical Antibiotics

Bacitracin is an antibiotic produced by *Bacillus subtilis* and is unrelated to other major groups of antibiotics. It is predominantly active against gram-positive organisms, including some anaerobes, but gram-negative enteric organisms are generally resistant. It is available alone or in combination with polymyxin B (Polysporin) or neomycin and polymyxin (Neosporin), providing a broader spectrum of coverage. Systemic bacitracin commonly produced nephrotoxicity and is no longer in use, but topical bacitracin is benign in this regard.

Contact dermatitis, urticaria, and other allergic reactions may occur, but are thought to be less common than with neomycin. Cross-sensitivity with polymyxin may occur. Thus, if a reaction occurs from use of a combination agent, this may not obviate future use of bacitracin alone.

Polymyxin, also produced from *B. subtilis,* is active primarily against gram-negative organisms, although its in vivo activity against *Pseudomonas* species may be limited. Polymyxin is generally available as a combined preparation with other topical antibiotics. It is thought to produce allergic reactions only rarely. but may cross-react with the related antibiotic bacitracin.

Neomycin is an aminoglycoside antibiotic, primarily active against gram-negative aerobic organisms, but with some activity against gram-positive cocci. It is generally believed to be more likely to produce contact dermatitis and other allergic reactions than other topical antibiotics, but this has been disputed. Because of its limited activity against common skin pathogens, it is generally available in combination with polymyxin or bacitracin (see above).

Some combination creams also contain topical corticosteroids (**Corticosporin**); these preparations should **not** be used on infected skin ulcers because they are likely to retard healing.

Gentamicin skin ointment is available but its use is discouraged because of the fear that the production of resistant strains will harm its importance as a systemic antibiotic. It is topically sensitizing and its antimicrobial spectrum is more or less comparable to that of neomycin.

Silver sulfadiazine (Silvadene) is a topical antibiotic of the sulfonamide family with a broad spectrum of activity against both gram-negative and gram-positive organisms, including *Staphylococcus aureus.* It causes adverse skin reactions uncommonly. It may be absorbed systemically if applied over a large area, but clinical consequences of this are most commonly observed in patients with extensive burns. The extent to which cross-sensitivity to other agents of the sulfonamide family occurs is not known, but patients with known allergy to sulfonamides should be considered to be at potential risk.

When Are Systemic Antibiotics Indicated?

Antibiotics are generally not required in the treatment of skin ulcers unless there is evidence of cellulitis, metastatic infection, sepsis, or deep infection, such as fasciitis or osteomyelitis. Stage-I decubitus ulcers require only that pressure, moisture, and friction be avoided, and they resolve spontaneously. Stage-II lesions are colonized by many organisms and may have purulent discharge, but if infection is mild and truly localized, local wound care usually suffices. Neither topical nor systemic antibiotics will necessarily speed healing further. Surrounding cellulitis should be treated with systemic antibiotics.

Stage-III lesions are more likely to produce systemic involvement; these ulcers not only are deeper but are often covered with eschar, which may harbor high concentrations of bacteria. Debridement of eschar commonly produces bacteremia, and systemic antibiotics should be considered as prophylaxis against infection of heart valves or prosthetic devices in susceptible patients (see below).

Stage-IV lesions are frequent sites of deep infection and are often associated with bacteremia. If osteomyelitis is present, the antibiotic must be one that penetrates bone.

Determining the Etiologic Organism

The decubitus ulcer is a polymicrobial lesion and local culture may produce more confusion than useful information. Anaerobic organisms may participate in those wound infections that occur in areas of compromised blood flow. In the event of a systemic infection, the etiologic organism will not be easily isolated from the ulcer itself, but may be recovered in a blood culture, which is less likely to be falsely positive. However, gram stain of infected skin ulcers may reveal the presence of one overwhelming organism, information that could be very helpful in interpreting culture results.

Cellulitis surrounding decubitus ulcers is thought to be produced by the same spectrum of organisms producing other forms of cellulitis (see below). However, when cellulitis complicates sacral or trochanteric decubitus ulcers, enteric pathogens are more likely to be involved.

Chronic osteomyelitis requires bone biopsy for identification of the etiologic organism.

VENOUS STASIS ULCERS

Decisions regarding antibiotic treatment of venous stasis ulcers are subject to the same considerations as other skin ulcers. Bacterial spectrum is roughly the same as that of decubitus ulcers, although contamination by fecal flora is less likely to occur. Diabetics and those who are immunosuppressed are more likely to have mixed gram-negative and anaerobic infections. Systemic antibiotics should be administered if there is associated cellulitis or if there are signs of systemic infection. Otherwise, strict wound care generally suffices (see Chap. 33). Use of topical antibiotics should be limited, as in the case of decubitus ulcers.

Selection of antibiotics is dependent on blood cultures, if positive, or on empiric considerations. Swabs may be misleading. Punch biopsy is often negative and should not be done at all in patients with compromised arterial circulation.

Arterial ischemic ulcers of the foot are colonized by the usual skin organisms. However, diabetic foot ulcers may also be infected with anaerobic organisms and gram-negative aerobes. Although arterial ulcers have a worse prognosis than venous stasis ulcers, systemic antibiotics may penetrate the ulcer poorly and should be used only if systemic infection threatens or is present. Topical antibiotics should be used sparingly.

CELLULITIS OF THE LOWER EXTREMITIES

Cellulitis is a common complication of severe venous stasis and of ulcers of the legs and feet. Antibiotics may be given orally in mild cases, or otherwise should be given parenterally. Cellulitis may be confused with stasis dermatitis, which does not require antibiotic treatment. In the former, there is more inflammation and pain, reflecting the deeper tissue infection. Topical antibiotics should be avoided because of the possibility that they will produce contact sensitivity.

Needle aspiration and punch biopsy have a low yield and are generally not recommended in uncomplicated cellulitis. In most cases, treatment should be empiric, directed against what are believed to be the most common etiologic organisms—beta-hemolytic streptococcus and *S. aureus*. This belief has been reinforced by the good response achieved by patients treated with penicillin or staphylocidal antibiotics. However, certain patients, particularly diabetics and those who are immunocompromised, may also be infected with gram-negative and anaerobic organisms. In other debilitated or functionally impaired elderly, the skin of the lower part of the body is often contaminated with fecal flora, and gram-negative infection may occur.

RECOMMENDED ANTIBIOTICS FOR CELLULITIS AND COMPLICATED SKIN ULCERS

In the absence of positive cultures of blood or unequivocal wound infection, the following antibiotics are recommended as empiric therapy. These antibiotic regimens always provide coverage of beta-hemolytic streptococcus and non-methicillin-resistant *S. aureus*. Specific choice of antibiotic hinges on whether additional coverage of gram-negative organisms or anaerobes is desired.

Oral

First-Line
Dicloxacillin
Amoxicillin-clavulanate

Alternative Agent
First-generation cephalosporin

Parenteral

First-Line
Oxacillin or nafcillin
Ampicillin-sulbactam

Alternative Agents
Cefazolin
Clindamycin
Cefoxitin
Clindamycin plus aztreonam or aminoglycoside

PNEUMONIA

Like many other infections, pneumonia frequently presents with minimal or nonspecific symptoms in elderly patients, especially if they are chronically ill or neurologically impaired. Cough may be absent or not prominent, while lethargy, altered mental status, or frank sepsis may be the first sign. Physical findings may be misleading—chronic rales are often heard because of other disorders or because chronic basilar atelectasis is frequently present in the nonambulatory patient. Chest X ray may be falsely positive or falsely negative.

The most common cause of community-acquired pneumonia in the elderly is *Streptococcus pneumoniae* (pneumococcus), and this pathogen is among the most common causes in the nursing home as well. Patients who have received pneumococcal vaccine may still develop pneumococcal infection. They may be infected with a strain not covered by the multivalent vaccine; in fact, many elderly were vaccinated with the earlier 14-valent preparation, not the more recently introduced 23-valent preparation. Even if vaccinated, debilitated elderly may remain unprotected (see Chap. 32).

Aspiration pneumonia is very common in patients who are neurologically impaired or who are taking medications that alter the level of consciousness, but it is rarely possible to distinguish aspiration pneumonia from other etiologies in such patients. The use of nasogastric feeding tubes increases rather than reduces the risk of aspiration because the tubes further impair the swallowing mechanism and reduce the competence of the lower esophageal sphincter. Nor are patients fed by gastrostomy or jejunostomy protected from aspiration, since these high-risk patients continue to aspirate oropharyngeal secretions, often have impaired lower esophageal sphincter tone, and may not be able to handle the volume of the feed that is instilled. Aspiration should be strongly considered as a cause of pneumonia in neurologically impaired patients regardless of how they are fed.

In institutionalized elderly, the etiologic organisms in aspiration pneumonia are generally a combination of anaerobic and aerobic gram-positive and gram-negative organisms. The latter are commonly involved because gram-negative colonization of the oropharynx is very common in such patients. This is partly related to institutional flora and partly related to host factors.

Legionella pneumophila is a relatively uncommon cause of pneumonia, but age is an independent risk factor for infection with this organism. Cigarette smoking increases the risk further. *Branhamella (Moraxella) catarrhalis*, chlamydia, and *Mycobacterium tuberculosis* are other pathogens that are more common causes of respiratory infections in the elderly.

Empiric Treatment of Respiratory Infections

Empiric treatment of pneumonia is often indicated in elderly patients. The diagnosis should be made clinically and liberally because of the unreliability of the chest X ray and the signs and symptoms. Sputum specimen may be extremely difficult to obtain in debilitated patients without resorting to inappropriately invasive methods. When obtained, sputum should be examined by gram and

AFB stain. Blood cultures should be done whenever possible. Pending appropriate cultures, the following antibiotics are recommended.

In Clinically Stable Patient with Bronchitis

First-Line
Amoxicillin-clavulanate
Trimethoprim-sulfamethoxazole

Alternative Agents
Cefaclor
Erythromycin

In Pneumonia

First-Line
Penicillin or ampicillin plus aminoglycoside
Penicillin or ampicillin plus aztreonam

Alternative Agents
Clindamycin plus aminoglycoside
Cefuroxime or cefoxitin
Ampicillin-sulbactam
Ticarcillin-clavulanate

ANTIBIOTIC PROPHYLAXIS

Endocarditis

Antibiotic prophylaxis should be given to elderly patients about to undergo procedures likely to produce bacteremia, according to the American Heart Association (AHA) criteria. Endocarditis is frequently misdiagnosed in elderly patients and mortality is high.

Although 80% of patients over the age of 80 have cardiac murmurs, most of these are hemodynamically insignificant, and it is not known whether all lesions producing these murmurs increase the risk of endocarditis. In addition, the likelihood of such patients developing endocarditis after routine procedures such as urethral catheterization is not known. Until the risk-benefit ratio of antibiotic prophylaxis is further elucidated, it is prudent to give routine prophylaxis as currently recommended by the AHA (see Table 31–1). The AHA criteria have been critically reviewed by Kaye (see Bibliography).

Dosage regimens that include an aminoglycoside call for a single dose. Since age-related toxicity of aminoglycosides depends on maintenance rather than loading dose, adjustments are not required. Aminoglycosides are discussed in further detail below.

Artificial Joint

Joint prostheses can be secondarily infected by blood-borne bacteria. The total joint arthroplasty appears to be vulnerable to such infection and when infected usually requires removal for the infection to be eradicated. There is no information regarding the risk of bacterial seeding of pins, nails, and hemiprostheses used to repair hip fractures.

Table 31-1. Regimens for Endocarditis Prophylaxis

Dental and Upper Respiratory Procedures	Gastrointestinal and Genitourinary Procedures
Oral	
Amoxicillin 3 g 1 hr before and 1.5 g 6 hr after	Same
Penicillin allergy: Erythromycin 1 g 2 hr before and 500 mg 6 hr after	See below
Parenteral*	
Ampicillin 2 g IM/IV 30 min before plus gentamicin 1.5 mg/kg IM/IV 30 min before	Same
Penicillin allergy: Vancomycin 1 g IV over 1 hr beginning 1 hr before procedure	Same plus gentamicin 1.5 mg/kg IM/IV 30 min before

*For patients with prosthetic heart valves or prior history of endocarditis.
Adapted from *Medical Letter* 31:112, 1989.

Although reported cases do suggest that pathogenic bacteria from distant foci such as the mouth, skin, gastrointestinal tract, and lung are capable of establishing serious infection in joint prostheses, the incidence of these occurrences is not known. It is likely that many cases go unreported.

Antibiotic prophylaxis prior to dental manipulation has been recommended by some physicians, but this practice is controversial. Most reported cases of late infection have been due to *S. aureus* and beta-hemolytic streptococcus, and only rarely *S. viridans* and other ordinary mouth organisms. Gram-negative organisms, which are frequently found in the mouth flora of elderly patients, are rarely implicated, and when found, have more often come from sites other than the mouth. It is possible that in some cases the organisms isolated in infected joint prostheses represent latent primary infection rather than secondary seeding, despite their temporal association with dental manipulation. Another possibility is that they do seed from distant sites, perhaps skin infections or the diseased mouth that might be infected with pathogens that are capable of infecting the joints.

This controversy notwithstanding, the infection of the prosthesis has disastrous consequences. For this reason, many orthopedic surgeons in clinical practice recommend that patients with hip prostheses receive antibiotic prophylaxis with cephalosporins prior to dental manipulations to guard against the spectrum of organisms that have been implicated in joint infections (see Jaspers & Little). This appears to be a sensible solution, although there is no scientific evidence that this approach is effective.

A complicating factor in elderly patients is the high prevalence of cardiac lesions. Those patients undergoing prophylaxis against seeding to joint prosthesis are frequently candidates for endocarditis prophylaxis as well, in which a different antibiotic regimen is indicated.

Recommendations

The efficacy of antibiotic prophylaxis in patients with artificial joint prostheses who are about to undergo dental procedures is not known. Consideration should be given to a regimen that includes a first-generation cephalosporin such as cephradine (Velosef), or amoxicillin-clavulanate (Augmentin). These would cover most organisms that have been implicated in late prosthetic joint infections. In preparation for a urological or lower gastrointestinal procedure, prophylaxis against enterococcus should be considered (see endocarditis recommendations).

Patients with joint prostheses should receive appropriate antibiotics when they have suspected or proved infections of the skin, lung, mouth, or other distant site, when the infection has the potential to seed the prosthesis hematogenously.

There is presently no data on which to recommend specific prophylaxis for patients with pacemakers, arterial grafts, or other implanted devices.

AGE-RELATED ASPECTS OF ANTIBIOTICS

Toxicity

Dose-related toxicity, which is potentially avoidable, is undoubtedly more common in older patients, particularly from those antibiotics eliminated primarily through the kidney. The risk of toxicity is probably also enhanced because of the increased vulnerability of certain end organs. Important pharmacodynamic toxicity that is likely to be more common in older patients includes ototoxicity, renal failure, seizures, hepatitis, gastrointestinal disturbances, and confusion.

This chapter does not address all side effects produced by antibiotics, but highlights those that are more likely to occur in elderly patients, so that precautionary measures can be taken.

Dosing

Most antibiotics are largely dependent on renal clearance for their elimination. As mentioned elsewhere in this book, older adults frequently have decreased renal function that is not reflected in an elevated serum creatinine. It is not always practical or possible to accurately assess glomerular filtration rate and predict the highest safe dose of renally eliminated antibiotics for a given patient, and it is important to administer an adequate dose in a life-threatening infection.

The loading dose of antibiotic does not have to be adjusted for age-related renal decline. However, it is crucial to adjust the **maintenance** dose of renally excreted **antibiotics with a narrow therapeutic index**, such as the aminoglycosides. When it is not practical or possible to obtain an accurate 24-hour urine for precise calculation of creatinine clearance, it is appropriate to estimate the creatinine clearance until more precise methods of assessing antibiotic dosage are available. A method of estimating creatinine clearance is discussed in Chap. 1.

It is not crucial to adjust the dosage of **antibiotics with a wide therapeutic index**, such as penicillin, unless extremely high doses are given. In serious infections, it is better to err on the side of giving a slightly higher dose of such an antibiotic than a lower one. For agents with a narrower margin of safety, therapeutic serum monitoring should be obtained when possible. For drugs that are highly bound to serum proteins (usually albumin), therapeutic monitoring may be inexact. Sick elderly patients frequently have hypoalbuminemia and increased free, active drug levels, which may not be reflected in serum drug levels if the laboratory reports only total (bound plus unbound) levels of the drug. Fortunately, most potentially toxic antibiotics, such as the aminoglycosides and vancomycin, are not highly protein-bound.

Elimination of agents not cleared by the kidney is less predictable. Recommendations are best based on adequate pharmacokinetic studies, which have not always been performed with the geriatric patient in mind. This is particularly true for older antibiotics, which came into use before appropriate assays were available for this purpose.

SPECIFIC AGENTS

The following section highlights aspects of antibiotics most relevant to the geriatric patient. **Dose recommendations assume normal serum creatinine, average age-related decline in creatinine clearance,** and **normal hepatic function.** Specific doses depend on the nature of the infection being treated. For a complete guide to antibiotic dosing, the reader is referred to the Bibliography readings (see Reese et al.).

Sulfonamides

Sulfonamides are active against a range of gram-positive and gram-negative aerobic organisms. The most commonly used agent of this group is sulfamethoxazole used in combination with the non-sulfonamide trimethoprim. Both components of **trimethoprim-sulfamethoxazole (TMP-SMZ) (cotrimoxazole, Bactrim, Septra)** are metabolized by the liver, with inactive metabolites and parent compounds being excreted in the urine. It is generally recommended that dose adjustments be made in patients with GFR less than 30 ml/min, a degree of renal dysfunction that is more severe than that in the average aged patient with normal serum creatinine. Fortunately, dose-related toxicity is unusual with ordinary oral use of this drug. Excessive doses of intravenous TMP-SMZ may produce acute tubular necrosis.

Sulfonamides may produce hemolysis in patients with glucose-6-phosphate deficiency, although elderly patients tend to have milder forms of this condition. Sulfonamides may produce other forms of anemia, however, particularly in patients with acquired immune deficiency syndrome.

Rash is a very common side effect of sulfonamides and a variety of other hypersensitivity reactions have been described.

Sulfisoxazole (Gantrisin) continues to be a very appropriate drug to use in patients having a first-time urinary tract infection but it is less practical than TMP-SMZ because it must be given more often than twice a day.

Important Drug Interactions

Sulfonamides are bound to serum proteins, some to a greater extent than others. All are potentially capable of enhancing the effect of certain highly bound drugs, such as warfarin, sulfonylureas, and phenytoin; it is unclear if this is due to displacement from protein binding sites or to inhibition of the metabolism of these drugs.

Dose Adjustment in Elderly

Oral use: Not required.
Intravenous use of TMP-SMZ: Adjust dose according to calculated creatinine clearance.

The Penicillins

Except for the high incidence of allergic reactions, the penicillins are rather safe antibiotics, with a wide therapeutic index. They are primarily eliminated by the kidney, however, so at high doses some dose-related toxic reactions can occur. The risk is greatest to patients with glomerular filtration rate under 60 ml/min, as seen in about 50% of patients over the age of 70. Autoimmune hemolytic anemia may occur after a week or more of high doses. Fortunately, this side effect is rare. Benign, reversible leukopenia may also occur at high doses.

Of the semisynthetic, antistaphylococcal penicillins in use, methicillin is the one most likely to cause interstitial nephritis. This is a hypersensitivity reaction and probably not age-associated.

Carbenicillin and **ticarcillin** contain substantial amounts of sodium compared to other penicillins. Dosage regimens of carbenicillin and ticarcillin can respectively deliver up to 140 mEq and 85 mEq of sodium per day. In some cases sodium overload and fluid retention can occur. This is unlikely to be clinically important in the elderly patient who is hemodynamically robust, because of age-related declines in renal sodium conservation. However, in the presence of congestive heart failure or other fluid-retaining states, the sodium burden could produce cardiac decompensation. Alternative agents exist, and are generally preferred in high-risk patients. Hypokalemia is another potential consequence of increased sodium delivery to the tubules. Since clinically important hypokalemia is more likely to occur when potassium-wasting diuretics are taken concurrently, diuretic administration should not be a routine means of preventing the sodium burden of these antibiotics.

High doses of carbenicillin and, to a lesser extent, ticarcillin may interfere with platelet aggregation. The risk of bleeding is enhanced when concurrent antiplatelet agents are administered, such as aspirin or nonsteroidal anti-inflammatory agents. Other mechanisms have also been implicated in the bleeding diathesis that can be produced by these drugs.

The related broad-spectrum penicillins **mezlocillin** and **piperacillin** contain less sodium and appear to have less of an effect on platelet function than carbenicillin or ticarcillin, and are preferable in patients for whom these considerations would be important.

Ampicillin commonly causes diarrhea due to a direct irritant effect in the colon. In addition, it is frequently implicated in pseudomembranous enterocolitis due to overgrowth of *Clostridium difficile*, a clinical entity that can be produced by a wide range of broad-spectrum antibiotics. There is some evidence that the elderly are at increased risk of developing antibiotic-associated diarrhea; in addition, they are more prone to dehydration and other more serious complications once diarrhea develops. *C. difficile* enterocolitis may occur and should be recognized and treated promptly (see Vancomycin and Metronidazole below). **Amoxicillin** is better absorbed orally than ampicillin, is less likely to produce diarrhea, and is preferred to oral ampicillin in most situations.

Certain penicillins are available in combination with beta-lactamase inhibitors, extending their spectrum of activity to organisms that are capable of inactivating beta-lactam antibiotics such as the penicillins via the enzyme beta-lactamase. Available agents include **amoxicillin-clavulanate** (Augmentin) for oral use and **ampicillin-sulbactam** (Unasyn) and **ticarcillin-clavulanate** (Timentin) for parenteral use. The beta-lactamase inhibitor does not alter the pharmacokinetics of the penicillin with which it is combined, but it may increase the incidence of gastrointestinal adverse effects.

Dose Adjustment in Elderly

Mild infections: Dose adjustments optional.
Serious infections: No adjustments; observe for anemia when high doses of intravenous penicillin are given; observe for fluid overload at high doses of ticarcillin or carbenicillin or use alternative agents.

Cephalosporins

Most members of this group of antibiotics depend entirely on the kidney for elimination. However, dose-related toxicity is uncommon. Cephalothin may produce dose-related acute tubular necrosis (ATN) but this is rare. There were fears that cephalothin and possibly other cephalosporin antibiotics produced a synergistic nephrotoxicity in conjunction with aminoglycoside antibiotics. Although this claim has not always held up under scrutiny, the aged patient would most likely be at higher-than-average risk, and the combination is increasingly being replaced by alternative antibiotics. Cephalosporins may produce Coombs positivity by altering the stickiness of the wall of blood cells, causing a nonimmune adherence of serum proteins; this phenomenon does not lead to hemolytic anemia.

In general, the **first-generation cephalosporins** have a favorable therapeutic index, and are quite safe for use in aged and debilitated patients. Among the parenteral antibiotics, the favored member of this group is cefazolin because it is relatively inexpensive, is very active against streptococci and staphylococci, and has a record of safety.

Second- and third-generation cephalosporins are more expensive and generally sacrifice gram-positive coverage for extended gram-negative coverage. Some (e.g., cefoxitin) also have potent activity against anaerobes, and individual agents provide specific additional coverage or tissue activity, making their applicability unique rather than all-encompassing. For detailed discussion of these agents, the reader should consult the Bibliography references (see Reese et al.).

In most ways, the newer cephalosporins are no more toxic than the first-generation agents. However, several of these drugs may produce a bleeding diathesis. Bleeding has been reported most often with **moxolactam**, a broad-spectrum cephalosporinlike agent, and with **cefamandole**, so that these agents are now seldom used. **Cefoperazone** and **cefotetan** may also affect coagulation but the incidence of clinical bleeding may be uncommon. The bleeding diathesis is vitamin-K-dependent, but, in the case of moxolactam and possibly cefoperazone, platelet function may also be affected. An additional problem that has occurred with some of these agents is a disulfiramlike reaction.

One third-generation agent, **ceftriaxone**, may have specialized use in geriatric practice for practical reasons. Unlike most other cephalosporins, it undergoes nonrenal elimination and has a very long half-life. It can be given once a day as an intramuscular injection. This may be useful in the home-bound dependent patient with certain infections, who can receive daily injection from a visiting nurse as an alternative to hospitalization. This must be done selectively, however, because ceftriaxone has less activity against streptococcal and staphylococcal organisms than first-generation cephalosporins.

Dose Adjustments in Elderly

Mild infections: Dose adjustment optional.
Serious infections: No adjustments; avoid cephalosporins that produce bleeding diathesis if possible.

Aminoglycosides

Systemic aminoglycosides include gentamicin, amikacin, tobramycin, and netilmicin. Neomycin is mainly used topically. Streptomycin is discussed below in connection with the treatment of tuberculosis.

The aminoglycosides have a narrow therapeutic index and their most important toxicity is dose-related. Since these agents are excreted primarily by the kidney, great caution must be observed when they are used in elderly patients. The drug concentrates in renal tissue itself and is retained for up to 3 weeks after being discontinued. There is some evidence that the elimination half-life of gentamicin increases progressively while the drug is being used. Because of this and because renal function is not static during nonrenal illness, therapeutic drug monitoring should be done throughout the course of treatment.

The most important and common toxicity from these agents is renal failure. Generally, aminoglycosides produce nonoliguric renal failure, which is reversible, but which places the patient in great jeopardy. If this is not recognized early and dose adjustments are not made, irreversible kidney damage may result. Age-related decline in renal function increases the risk of toxicity by reducing the clearance of these agents, but it is not known if this otherwise predisposes the kidney to damage. However, debility, dehydration, and use of potent loop diuretics increase the age-associated risk.

Fulminant renal failure occurs rarely; reported cases are thought to represent a hypersensitivity reaction for which age is not a major independent risk factor.

Ototoxicity also occurs in a dose-related fashion and may present as impaired hearing, tinnitus, or vertigo. The incidence of this effect is a subject of debate and the clinical importance has been questioned (see Brummett & Fox). Cautious dose adjustments for renal insufficiency may have reduced the risk in recent years. In at least 50% of cases, ototoxicity due to aminoglycosides is irreversible or only partly reversible. However, it is important that ototoxic symptoms not be wrongly attributed to the effects of aging.

Confusional states have been reported with aminoglycosides, but the mechanism is not known. Neuromuscular blockade with reversible paralysis has been reported rarely, and is probably more likely to occur in predisposed patients, such as those with myasthenia gravis.

Dosing Adjustments in Elderly

Loading dose: No adjustment.
Maintenance dose: Adjust dose according to calculated creatinine clearance until results of serum levels are available. Thereafter, serum levels should be rigorously monitored and dosage adjusted accordingly.

Vancomycin

Vancomycin is largely eliminated by the kidney and older individuals may develop toxic levels more readily than younger adults. The most important dose-related problem in older patients is ototoxicity, which can manifest as tinnitus or hearing loss. However, it is uncertain if ototoxicity occurs when vancomycin alone is used. The frequency of vancomycin-associated ototoxicity is not known but the risk is greater when other ototoxic agents, such as aminoglycosides and possibly furosemide, are taken concurrently.

In the past, nephrotoxicity was reported to occur with vancomycin, but current preparations do not contain the impurities implicated in those reactions.

Thrombophlebitis is a common complication of intravenous vancomycin.

Oral vancomycin is used primarily for the treatment of antibiotic-associated enterocolitis due to *C. difficile.* This form is poorly absorbed by the gastrointestinal tract so that clinically important concentrations are unlikely to be achieved.

Dose Adjustment in Elderly

ORAL. No adjustment.
INTRAVENOUS
Loading dose: No adjustment.
Maintenance dose: Adjust dosage according to calculated creatinine clearance until results of serum levels are obtained; thereafter follow serum levels if available.

Erythromycin

Erythromycin is metabolized by the liver with small amounts being excreted unchanged in the urine. The therapeutic index of this antibiotic is quite wide and serious toxicity is unusual. Gastrointestinal symptoms, which are partly dose-related, are generally mild, although pseudomembranous enterocolitis has been reported. High doses of parenteral erythromycin may produce reversible hearing loss in seriously ill patients. Hepatotoxicity has occurred but is unusual and occurs primarily with the estolate form of erythromycin. It is a hypersensitivity reaction that is not age-related.

Important Drug Interactions

Erythromycin reduces the activity of hepatic microsomal enzymes and may retard the metabolism of theophylline, anticonvulsants, warfarin, and corticosteroids, increasing their effect. Careful monitoring is required.

Erythromycin may also increase serum levels of digoxin in the minority of patients whose digoxin metabolism is dependent on gut bacteria (see Chap. 14); this phenomenon has been observed with certain other antibiotics.

Dose Adjustments in Elderly
Not required.

Tetracyclines

Tetracyclines differ in their mode of elimination, half-life, and spectrum of side effects. **Doxycycline** that has been absorbed reenters the intestine where it is deactivated by chelating cations and is eliminated largely in the feces. Other tetracyclines that reenter the gut are not deactivated and are largely dependent on the kidney for elimination. They are more likely to produce gastrointestinal symptoms than doxycycline and have occasionally been reported to produce pseudomembranous enterocolitis.

Tetracyclines inhibit protein synthesis and produce azotemia related to the nitrogenous wastes of amino acid metabolism. This problem is compounded in patients with renal insufficiency. If azotemia becomes significant, dehydration and other symptoms may occur. Tetracyclines should not be given to patients with renal insufficiency; doxycycline is considered safe, although it cannot be used for infections of the urinary tract because inadequate levels are attained in the urine in renal failure.

Fatty liver may also occur in the high dose range, but this is unusual.

Minocycline has a high tendency to produce dizziness and vertigo and should generally be avoided by older patients.

Dose Adjustments in Elderly

Oral use: Dose adjustments not required.
Note: Avoid tetracyclines (except doxycycline) in patients with elevated BUN or serum creatinine level.

Chloramphenicol

A highly useful antibiotic, chloramphenicol has been eclipsed by less-toxic alternative drugs for most indications. The best known adverse reaction is anemia, of which there are two distinct types. Dose-related bone marrow suppression associated with elevated serum iron occurs relatively commonly and does not appear to augur serious consequences, but the drug should be discontinued if counts decline significantly. There is no pharmacokinetic data for chloramphenicol in geriatric patients and it is not known if they are more susceptible to bone marrow suppression, which is more likely to occur when blood levels are supratherapeutic (i.e., greater than 25 μg/ml). It is the rare, idiopathic variety of aplastic anemia that has received the most publicity. This form of anemia is irreversible and may be produced by oral, intravenous, and even ocular administration. It does not appear to be an age-related phenomenon.

Other dose-related adverse effects include delirium, optic neuritis, stomatitis, and peripheral neuropathy.

Important Drug Interactions

Chloramphenicol inhibits hepatic microsomal enzymes and has been reported to increase the concentration of warfarin, phenytoin, and oral hypoglycemic agents. Acetaminophen may retard the hepatic clearance of chloramphenicol, increasing concentrations of the antibiotic.

Dose Adjustment in Elderly

No pharmacokinetic data. Adjustments probably not required, but hematocrit and serum drug levels should be monitored.

Clindamycin

Clindamycin is a well-tolerated drug that had the misfortune of being the first drug to be associated with pseudomembranous enterocolitis produced by *C. difficile*. This adverse effect occurs as commonly, if not more commonly, with other antibiotics, notably ampicillin and cephalosporins. It is more likely to occur with oral than with parenteral clindamycin. However, parenteral clindamycin can be recovered in the gut for up to 2 weeks, and diarrhea, including that produced by *C. difficile,* may occur with a delayed onset. Otherwise, serious side effects are rare.

The drug is metabolized by the liver and dose adjustments are required in liver disease.

Dose Adjustment in Elderly

Not required.

The Quinolones

The quinolones are a group of antibiotics that have recently regained popularity because of the development of new fluoride-containing compounds. These are structurally related to the original quinolone, nalidixic acid, which had not been widely used because it was often poorly tolerated and resistant strains developed readily. **Norfloxacin, ciprofloxacin,** and ofloxacin are the fluoroquinolones currently available in the United States.

The fluoroquinolones, which are taken orally, are more potent than nalidixic acid and have a much broader spectrum of activity. The antibiotic activity outlasts the relatively short serum half-life and they need be given only twice a day. Ciprofloxacin is even active against pseudomonas species and methicillin-resistant staphylococcus (but less effective against streptococcus), and it penetrates bone.

Elderly patients achieve higher blood levels of quinolones than do younger adults, an observation that has not been fully explained. Despite this, there is no evidence of age-related toxicity. Mild CNS symptoms have been reported, but in general these agents have a wide margin of safety.

Because of their useful spectrum of activity, ease of administration, and low toxicity, these drugs are widely used and it is tempting to overuse them in geriatric practice. However, experts caution that they must be prescribed judiciously because abuse may result in the production of resistant strains of microorganisms.

Important Drug Interactions

Absorption of quinolones is significantly inhibited by antacids and sucralfate. Concurrent administration should be avoided. Ciprofloxacin inhibits hepatic microsomal enzymes and can enhance the effect of theophylline and warfarin. An interaction with warfarin has also been reported with norfloxacin and ofloxacin.

Dose Adjustments in Elderly

Mild infections: Optional.
Serious infections: No adjustments.

Metronidazole

Metronidazole is used in geriatric practice primarily to treat gram-negative anaerobic infections and colitis due to *C. difficile.* The antibiotic is cleared by renal and nonrenal mechanisms; clearance is impaired in hepatic disease but in renal failure only when creatinine clearance is below 10 ml/min.

Adverse effects include gastrointestinal complaints and a metallic taste. Peripheral neuropathy has been reported but only with long-term use, such as when this agent is used in Crohn's disease. Seizures have been reported rarely.

An important aspect of metronidazole is its ability to participate in hepatically mediated drug interactions; an interaction with warfarin has been reported. A disulfiramlike reaction may occur when metronidazole is given together with alcohol, but this is unlikely to be seen in most clinical situations when metronidazole is used in geriatrics.

Dose Adjustments in Elderly

Not required.

Aztreonam

A member of the monobactam group of antibiotics, aztreonam is similar in structure and function to the cephalosporins and penicillins. Its antimicrobial spectrum overlaps with that of the aminoglycosides in that it is very effective against gram-negative aerobic organisms, including *Pseudomonas.* Because it does not produce ototoxicity and nephrotoxicity seen with the aminoglycosides, aztreonam is often touted as being a suitable alternative in the elderly. Aztreonam's spectrum of activity is narrower than that of the aminoglycosides, however, and it cannot be used in all situations calling for an aminoglycoside.

Aztreonam is renally excreted and dose recommendations are recommended in renal failure (creatinine clearance below 30 ml/min). However, to date, this drug has exhibited a very good therapeutic-to-toxic ratio, so that, in contrast to the aminoglycosides, it is not essential to ascertain creatinine clearance in elderly patients with normal serum creatinine.

As in the case of quinolones, experts caution that this drug should not be overused. It is presently more expensive than gentamicin. However, in certain situations it may serve as an alternative to aminoglycosides for frail elderly patients when therapeutic blood levels are not readily available.

Dose Adjustments in Elderly

This antibiotic should be reserved for use in serious infections. Assuming that this recommendation is followed, dose adjustments should not routinely be made for elderly patients with normal serum creatinine level.

Imipenem

Imipenem belongs to a new class of antibiotics, the carbapenems. It has a very broad spectrum of activity and penetrates well into all body tissues, including bone. For these reasons it has the potential to be overused.

Imipenem is renally excreted and may produce seizures at high doses. Seizures might not be grand mal in type and in someone with depressed consciousness, certain seizures, such as those of the myoclonic variety, might go unrecognized. The sick geriatric patient with a history of CNS disease, including remote stroke, would be at particularly high risk of developing seizures from this antibiotic. It should be reserved for serious infections resistant or not responding to other antibiotics.

Dose Adjustment in Elderly

Adjust dose according to creatinine clearance.

TUBERCULOSIS

As compared to younger adults, tuberculosis in the elderly is more often recrudescent than primary, and may present in an atypical fashion. Cough may be mild, fever may be absent, and the presentation may be one of depression, weight loss, or failure to thrive. The presentation may also be classic, with cough, fever, and night sweats. Primary tuberculous pneumonia may also occur, and epidemics have been reported in closed communities of elderly. The index case may be a patient who develops recrudescent tuberculosis, or a health care worker who becomes ill with a pulmonary form of the disease.

Prophylaxis for Positive Tuberculin Skin Test

A 6- to 12-month course of treatment with isoniazid markedly reduces the risk of developing active tuberculosis if a patient is skin-test positive. The prevalence of positive skin test among elderly Americans has declined markedly over the years, but is still estimated to be greater than 20%. In addition, many skin-test-negative individuals among the present geriatric population were skin-test positive in the distant past and may still harbor the organism. Most elderly, whether skin-test-positive or -negative, will never develop symptomatic tuberculosis and it is generally agreed that routine treatment is not justified because the risk of antimicrobial toxicity (namely isoniazid hepatitis) is greater than the risk of developing active tuberculosis. There is controversy over this argument, however, with some experts saying that the risk of isoniazid hepatitis has been overstated, that it is outweighed by the public health benefits that would accrue. The United States Public Health Service (USPHS) recommends treatment with antituberculosis medications on the basis of a positive skin test and suspected disease (i.e., an abnormal chest X ray). If there are no signs or symptoms, the decision is more complicated for an older individual. The person's living situation and proximity to high-risk individuals may influence the decision to treat. The risk of developing active disease is clearly greater for certain groups of skin-test-positive patients. Those with diabetes, cancer, gastrectomy, and various states of immunosuppression, including corticosteroid treatment, should be considered as a group separate from the robust elderly when calculating the risks and benefits of chemoprophylaxis.

Baseline testing in nursing homes is recommended for institutional health purposes, in order to avert an epidemic if one case were to develop. "New converters," who represent newly infected individuals, have a much higher risk of developing active clinical disease than do patients with remote history of skin test positivity or positive status of unknown duration, and should be treated with chemoprophylaxis regardless of age and immune status. The skin test should be performed twice, 1 week apart, to take into account the "booster phenomenon," in which true positivity becomes apparent only on retesting. The booster phenomenon occurs in about 6% of elderly people who initially test negative.

Some older individuals harbor subclinical infection but have a negative skin test. This is because age-related immune changes increase the tendency to develop skin anergy to *M. tuberculosis*. Since it is difficult to distinguish asymptomatic infected patients who are anergic from uninfected patients, antimicrobial treatment of skin-test negative elderly should be reserved for those in whom active tuberculosis is confirmed or strongly suspected.

Active Tuberculosis

Patients with confirmed or strongly suspected TB should be treated with isoniazid and rifampin (see below), unless culture and sensitivity testing dictate otherwise. The vast majority of American elderly with TB have strains of *M. tuberculosis* that are sensitive to these agents. However, recent immigrants from developing countries and those who acquire primary infection in a community harboring resistant strains may require other agents.

Antituberculosis Drugs

Isoniazid (INH)

Isoniazid (INH) is the first-line drug for tuberculosis and is effective in the vast majority of elderly Americans.

The absorption of isoniazid may be reduced by food. The drug is metabolized by acetylation in the liver to a group of compounds, some of which have been postulated to be more toxic than others. Two genetically distinct groups of patients metabolize isoniazid at different rates and are referred to as *fast* and *slow acetylators*. There does not appear to be any age-associated alteration in the metabolism among adults, with geriatric patients retaining their genetically determined rate of acetylation. Fast acetylation does not reduce clinical efficacy of the parent compound and slow acetylation is not thought to be important in overall toxicity. Thus, official recommendations do not include dose adjustments for age or acetylation status.

ADVERSE EFFECTS. The most important adverse effect of isoniazid is hepatitis, the risk of which increases with age. A significant minority of patients of all ages will develop mild, transient **elevations in serum transaminase enzymes,** but it is generally not recommended that treatment be discontinued unless levels are more than 3–5 times normal or if there are premonitory symptoms of **hepatitis.** If hepatitis develops, isoniazid should be discontinued. When hepatitis resolves, rifampin may be instituted with close monitoring for rifampin hepatotoxicity (see below).

By altering the metabolism of pyridoxine (vitamin B_6), isoniazid may produce a deficiency state manifested as **peripheral neuritis.** Some investigators recommend pyridoxine supplements only for high-risk patients, such as alcoholics, diabetics, and patients with poor nutrition. High-risk patients cannot always be identified and pyridoxine deficiency may be difficult to distinguish from other infirmities in sick elderly. Since many older patients with TB have marginal nutritional status and since low-dose pyridoxine is safe, routine supplementation is warranted in this group. The recommended daily dosage is approximately 10 mg for each 100 mg of isoniazid given. **Sideroblastic anemia** may also occur as a result of the isoniazid effect on pyridoxine metabolism. This is not necessarily accompanied by other signs of pyridoxine deficiency, but may be reversed by the administration of vitamin B_6.

Other adverse effects of isoniazid include **rash, fever, lupuslike syndrome,** and **central nervous system effects,** including confusional states, somnolence, sleep disorders, headache, and anxiety. Confusional states are more common in elderly patients than in younger adults, and toxic psychosis, euphoria, and memory loss have been reported. A possible explanation for this is that isoniazid, which enters the central nervous system readily, is thought to possess slight mono- and diamine oxidase inhibiting activity. This property has been implicated in rare isoniazid-food interactions (see below). Urinary retention has been reported with isoniazid, but the significance of these reports is not known and an explanation of the effect has not been offered.

DRUG AND NUTRIENT INTERACTIONS The absorption of isoniazid may be impaired by food and antacids. If possible, the drug should be taken on an empty stomach.

Isoniazid inhibits hepatic microsomal enzymes and may increase serum levels of warfarin, phenytoin, and carbamazepine. There is inconclusive evidence of similar interactions with benzodiazepines, corticosteroids, and antiarrhythmic agents. In general, it is wise to monitor for alterations in effect of the concurrently administered drug.

As mentioned earlier, isoniazid may possess mono- and diamine oxidase inhibiting activity in humans. This may potentiate the effects of tyramine and histamine found in high concentrations of certain foods, such as aged meat and cheese, fish, chianti, and sauerkraut. Symptoms such as headache and flushing have been reported but because of their apparent rarity and unpredictability, routine avoidance of these foods may be impractical.

DOSE ADJUSTMENT IN ELDERLY
None.

Rifampin

Rifampin is a well-tolerated, first-line drug used for the treatment of tuberculosis. It has activity against a broad spectrum of bacteria, including gram-positive and gram-negative organisms, but because resistant strains are rapidly produced, there are few applications of rifampin other than tuberculosis. They will not be considered here.

SIDE EFFECTS. Like isoniazid, rifampin may produce **hepatitis,** and the elderly are probably more susceptible to this effect. The exact frequency with which rifampin-induced hepatitis occurs is not known, since the drug is generally used in combination with isoniazid and other antituberculosis drugs with potential hepatotoxicity.

It has been suggested that rifampin may increase the risk of isoni-

azid hepatitis. However, if hepatitis occurs in elderly patients taking
the combination of isoniazid and rifampin, isoniazid is considered
the most likely drug to be producing this effect. Both drugs should
be stopped until hepatitis subsides. At that time, rifampin may be
reintroduced as part of a new drug regimen but the patient should be
monitored closely for reappearance of hepatotoxicity. There is some
evidence that the combination of isoniazid and rifampin produces
hepatotoxicity by an independent mechanism.

Other adverse effects of rifampin occur with a low frequency, but
may include rash, gastrointestinal disturbances, dizziness, and confusion. Pseudomembranous colitis has been reported. High doses
given in once-a-week regimens (no longer recommended) may produce a flulike or more severe immunologic reaction.

Rifampin confers an orange color to all body secretions, most obvious in urine and tears. Although this is a benign effect, it may produce alarm in the patient who is not forewarned.

IMPORTANT DRUG INTERACTIONS. The major disadvantage of
rifampin in the geriatric patient is its ability to participate in a large
number of drug-drug interactions. Rifampin is a potent stimulator
of the hepatic microsomal enzyme system and accelerates the metabolism of many drugs. Important interactions seen in the elderly
include that with warfarin, phenytoin, digitoxin, corticosteroids,
theophylline, verapamil, and oral hypoglycemic agents. In these
cases, metabolism of the coadministered drug is increased and its
effect is reduced. Although rifampin also increases the metabolism
of quinidine, active metabolites are produced and the effects of quinidine are maintained.

Rifampin is thought to increase the metabolism of exogenous estrogens. Based on observations of reduced effectiveness of oral contraceptives, it is possible that postmenopausal estrogens might also
be reduced in potency. Digoxin is subject to extrarenal metabolism
in a minority of patients and could be influenced by rifampin, manifesting as reduced digoxin efficacy.

Rifampin may also induce the metabolism of isoniazid to a hepatotoxin different from metabolites believed to produce isoniazid hepatitis, but the importance of an isoniazid-rifampin interaction is outweighed by the importance of the combination in antituberculous
therapy.

For a complete discussion of rifampin interactions, the reader is
referred to the Bibliography readings (see Baciewicz et al.).

DOSE ADJUSTMENT IN ELDERLY
None.

Pyrazinamide

This drug, which is structurally related to nicotinamide (see Chap.
17), is capable of producing hepatotoxicity. Unlike rifampin and isoniazid, pyrazinamide hepatotoxicity is dose-related. Pyrazinamide is
eliminated primarily by the kidney, making dose-related hepatotoxicity a potential risk for the elderly. This drug is generally added to
a regimen of INH and rifampin only if short-course (less than 9-
month) therapy is intended.

Pyrazinamide raises uric acid levels. A limited regimen of pyrazinamide is unlikely to produce clinical gout but is a potential risk in
patients with a history of gout or chronic hyperuricemia.

DOSE ADJUSTMENT IN ELDERLY. Adjust dose according to creatinine clearance. A dose of 25 mg/kg/day should generally not be exceeded.

Other Antituberculosis Agents

Ethambutol (Myambutol)

The major disadvantage of ethambutol is its ability to produce dose-related **optic neuritis,** which can result in decreased visual acuity, scotomata, and impaired color vision. Since this drug is primarily eliminated by the kidney, older patients may be at increased risk of toxicity. Early discontinuation of the drug halts progression of the visual disorder. Baseline and periodic ophthalmologic evaluation are useful but may fail to detect early changes. Patients who come to ethambutol therapy with visual disorders, and those unable to report visual changes, may elude early recognition and should receive other drugs if possible.

Like pyrazinamide, ethambutol may produce **hyperuricemia,** but clinical gout is unusual.

DOSE ADJUSTMENT IN ELDERLY. 15 mg/kg/day should generally not be exceeded.

Streptomycin

Until recently an important component of triple-drug regimens, streptomycin is less commonly used today. It is mentioned here because of its potential toxicity in older patients. Streptomycin is an aminoglycoside antibiotic with a narrow therapeutic-to-toxic ratio. It may produce **ototoxicity** and, less often, **nephrotoxicity.** Geriatric patients are particularly susceptible to vestibular and auditory VIII nerve damage and are more likely to develop toxic levels of this renally excreted drug. Although streptomycin is still useful in patients unable to take other drugs, it should generally be avoided in the elderly. A potential advantage of this agent is that it is given parenterally and can be given to patients unable to take drugs by mouth.

DOSE ADJUSTMENT IN ELDERLY
Maximum daily dose: 500 mg IM.

Other drugs used for tuberculosis are not commonly used in geriatric patients today and will not be discussed here. For a complete discussion of the remaining agents, the reader is referred to the Bibliography readings (see Pérez-Stable & Hopewell).

ANTITUBERCULOUS TREATMENT RECOMMENDATIONS FOR GERIATRIC PATIENTS

Chemoprophylaxis for Skin-Test Positive

Found by routine testing of healthy elderly (previous reactivity unknown): Treatment controversial (see text).
Found by routine testing of high-risk patients: Isoniazid 300 mg/day for 6–12 months.

Active tuberculosis (after Dutt et al.)

Isoniazid 300 mg (5 mg/kg) plus rifampin 600 mg (15 mg/kg) daily for 1 month,
then

Isoniazid 900 mg (10 mg/kg) plus rifampin 600 mg twice a week for 8 months.

Isoniazid treatment should be accompanied by daily administration of vitamin B_6 (pyridoxine).

Note: This regimen is recommended because it is at least as well tolerated by elderly patients as daily treatment and the twice-weekly regimen lends itself well to the home-bound patient who requires visiting nurse services. The 9-month regimen avoids the need to add a third potentially toxic drug, pyrazinamide, which is required when short-course treatment is given.

Recent USPHS data supporting short-course triple-drug therapy includes 8 weeks of pyrazinamide 30 mg/kg, a dose that might be excessive for many elderly patients (see Combs et al.). The patient population in that study may, furthermore, not be representative of the geriatric population. In short-course therapy using pyrazinamide, dose of that agent should be adjusted according to creatinine clearance.

Short-Course Regimen

Daily isoniazid 300 mg plus rifampin 600 mg plus pyrazinamide (dose adjusted for creatinine clearance) for 8 weeks,
then

Daily isoniazid 300 mg plus rifampin 600 mg for 16 weeks.

Short-course and other treatment regimens are discussed in the Bibliography readings (see American Thoracic Society).

ANTIVIRAL AGENTS

Two antiviral agents are commonly used in geriatric practice. **Acyclovir** is useful in the early treatment of shingles (herpes zoster) and is discussed in Chap. 33. **Amantadine** is used in the prevention and treatment of influenza A (see Chap. 32).

BIBLIOGRAPHY

Boscia, J. A., and Kaye, D. Asymptomatic bacteriuria in the elderly. *Clin. Geriatr. Med.* 4:57–70, 1988.

Breitenbucher, R. B. Bacterial changes in the urine samples of patients with long-term indwelling catheters. *Arch. Intern. Med.* 144:1585–1588, 1984.

Brummett, R. E., and Fox, K. E. Aminoglycoside-induced hearing loss in humans. *Antimicrob. Agents Chemother.* 33:791–800, 1989.

Hirschmann, J. V. Topical antibiotics in dermatology. *Arch. Dermatol.* 124:1691–1700, 1988.

Jaspers, M. T., and Little, J. W. Prophylactic antibiotic coverage in patients with total arthroplasty: current practice. *J. Am. Dent. Assoc.* 111:943–948, 1985.

Kaye, D. Prophylaxis for infective endocarditis: an update. *Ann. Intern. Med.* 104:419–423, 1986.

Lutomski, D. M., Trott, A. T., Runyon, J. M., et al. Microbiology of adult cellulitis. *J. Fam. Practice.* 26:45–48, 1988.

Micolle, L. E., McLeod, J., McIntyre, M., et al. Significance of pharyngeal colonization with aerobic gram-negative bacilli in elderly institutionalized men. *Age Ageing* 15:47–52, 1986.

Norman, D. C., Castle, S. C., and Cantrell, M. Infections in the nursing home (clinical conference). *J. Amer. Geriatr. Soc.* 35:796–805, 1987.

Pancoast, S. J. Aminoglycoside antibiotics in clinical use. *Med. Clin. N. Amer.* 72:581–612, 1988.

Reese, R. E., Sentochnik, D. E., Douglas, R. G., et al. *Handbook of Antibiotics.* Boston: Little, Brown, 1988.

Seiler, W. O., and Stahelin, H. B. Practical management of catheter-associated UTIs. *Geriatrics* 43(8):43–48, 1988.

Terpenning, M. S., Allada, R., and Kauffman, C. A. Intermittent urethral catheterization in the elderly. *J. Amer. Geriatr. Soc.* 37:411–416, 1989.

Valenti, W. M., Trudell, R. G., and Bentley, D. W. Factors predisposing to oropharyngeal colonization with gram-negative bacilli in the aged. *N. Engl. J. Med.* 298:1108–1111, 1978.

Warren, J. Catheters and catheter care. *Clin. Geriatr. Med.* 2:857–871, 1986.

Warren, J. W., Damron, D., Tenney, J. H., and Hoopes, J. M. Fever, bacteremia, and death as complications of bacteriuria in women with long-term urethral catheters. *J. Infect. Dis.* 155:1151–1158, 1987.

Zimmer, J. G., Bentley, D. W., Valenti, W. M., and Watson, N. M. Systemic antibiotic usage in nursing homes. A quality assessment. *J. Amer. Geriatr. Soc.* 34:703–710, 1986.

Tuberculosis

American Thoracic Society. Treatment of tuberculosis and tuberculosis infection in adults and children. *Amer. Rev. Resp. Dis.* 134:355–363, 1986.

Baciewicz, A. M., Self, T. H., and Bekemeyer, W. B. Update on rifampin drug interactions. *Arch. Intern. Med.* 147:565–568, 1987.

Combs, D. L., O'Brien, R. J., and Geiter, L. J. USPHS Tuberculosis short-course chemotherapy trial 21: Effectiveness, toxicity, and acceptability. *Ann. Intern. Med.* 112:397–406, 1990.

Comstock, G.W. Prevention of tuberculosis among tuberculin reactors: maximizing benefits, minimizing risks. *J.A.M.A.* 256:2729–2730, 1986.

Creditor, M. C., Smith, E. C., Gallai, J. B., Baumann, M., and Nelson, K. E. Tuberculosis, tuberculin reactivity, and delayed cutaneous hypersensitivity in nursing home residents. *J. Gerontol.* 43:M97–M100, 1988.

Dutt, A. K., Moers, D., and Stead, W. W. Short-course chemotherapy for tuberculosis with mainly twice-weekly isoniazid and rifampin. *Am. J. Med.* 77:233–242, 1984.

Nagami, P. H., and Yoshikawa, T. T. Tuberculosis in the elderly geriatric patient. *J. Am. Geriatr. Soc.* 31:356–363, 1983.

Pérez-Stable, E. J., and Hopewell, P. C. Current tuberculosis treatment regimens. *Clin. Chest Med.* 10:323–339, 1989.

Immunizations

INFLUENZA

Deaths from influenza and its complications occur mainly in people 65 and older. Although the majority of deaths that occur during influenza epidemics are actually due to noninfluenza viruses, influenza is the only respiratory virus for which an effective vaccine exists. Immunization reduces the risk of clinical infection, secondary pneumonia, and death in healthy elderly exposed to influenza virus.

Unfortunately, the vaccine may be less effective in reducing infection rates in chronically ill or debilitated elderly, who mount a less vigorous antibody response. However, vaccination has been demonstrated to reduce the rate of hospitalization, degree of illness, and mortality in such patients. In addition, population-based immunization programs promote the development of "herd immunity," namely the establishment of a high degree of population resistance, which protects poorly immunized and immunocompromised individuals.

Alternative approaches to immunizing the elderly are being studied, including the use of high-dose vaccine, inhaled vaccine, boosters, and adjuvants, but until these methods are shown to improve efficacy, ordinary adult doses and established methods should be used.

Influenza Vaccine

Influenza vaccines are preparations of virus strains prevalent in the previous influenza season, generally containing both A and B strains. Vaccines are prepared from inactivated virus grown in chicken eggs. Some are chemically treated (*split-virus* preparations) to reduce the likelihood of febrile reactions, a process more important in young children than adults.

Adverse Effects

Mild to moderate soreness around the vaccination site occurs in one third of recipients and may last up to 48 hours. A brief flulike illness, beginning 6 to 12 hours after vaccine is given, occurs in a very small proportion of vaccinees, lasts no longer than 48 hours, and seems to be less severe in elderly recipients. Rarely, allergic reactions occur in individuals with extreme sensitivity to egg protein and may manifest as hives, angioedema, asthma, or anaphylaxis.

Guillain-Barré syndrome has not been attributed to flu vaccine prepared with strains used since the 1976 swine flu vaccine debacle.

Interactions and Noninteractions

Interactions with influenza vaccine are probably less important than previously believed. The vaccine has been reported to interact with phenytoin, increasing seizure frequency, and with warfarin. However, these interactions have been disputed and the clinical significance is not known (see Chap. 29). Contrary to earlier belief, theophylline does not appear to interact with killed virus vaccine, the form given exclusively in recent years.

Influenza vaccine may be given in conjunction with pneumococcal vaccine (see below).

Contraindications and Precautions

Influenza vaccine is contraindicated in individuals with severe allergy to egg protein or with previous history of Guillain-Barré syndrome. Vaccine should not be given during acute febrile illness because certain microbial antigens can blunt the production of antibodies to influenza vaccine.

Recommendations

Influenza vaccine is recommended in all persons age 65 and over. In addition, doctors, nurses, and other personnel, regardless of age, who have close contact with patients at risk and are capable of infecting them, should receive vaccine.

Timing and Administration

One standard dose (0.5 ml) of vaccine is injected in the deltoid muscle. Many debilitated elderly have muscle atrophy. If atrophy precludes intramuscular injection into the deltoid, the preferred injection site is the thigh or upper outer quadrant of the buttock. This minimizes the risk of subcutaneous injection, which may result in local inflammatory reactions, including granuloma formation or necrosis.

The dose should be given in late fall at the beginning of flu season, early enough to permit immunity to develop but late enough for it to last the season. November is generally considered the ideal month in the Northern Hemisphere, but in locales where cases appear early vaccination programs may have to be instituted earlier. Vaccine may be given even after influenza outbreaks have occurred.

Influenza virus undergoes antigenic drift, with the result that natural or acquired immunity to a given strain does not guarantee immunity against a similar strain that may be prevalent in a subsequent year. Thus, immunization should be performed annually. Vaccine containing strains from a previous year may be ineffective and should be discarded.

The efficacy of influenza vaccine can be maximized in the nursing-home setting if institutionwide vaccination rate approaches 75%. Certain strategies may need to be employed in order to achieve this because patients, families, and health care workers are often poorly informed regarding the importance of vaccination, resist because of fear, or simply are not notified when vaccination time arrives.

Isolation of patients with influenza, and limitation of visitors or admissions during an epidemic, have **not** proved effective in limiting outbreaks and are measures that need not be routinely taken.

Chemoprophylaxis with amantadine should be considered as an adjunct to flu vaccine program for prevention of influenza A (see below).

Amantadine (Symmetrel)

Amantadine is an antiviral agent with activity against influenza A, which is sometimes given as an adjunct to or substitute for influenza vaccine. This agent interferes with the replication of influenza A virus, reduces the risk of infection when given to individuals exposed to influenza A, reduces viral shedding, and may reduce the severity of illness when given within the first 48 hours of active infection. Administration of amantadine does not reduce the antibody response to the virus. It has no activity against influenza B.

Amantadine also has dopaminergic action and is employed in the management of Parkinson's disease. A full discussion of this agent is found in Chap. 10.

Indications

Chemoprophylaxis with amantadine is indicated in high-risk patients unable or unwilling to take influenza vaccine, and those vaccinated late in the flu season when influenza has already occurred in the community. Amantadine may also be used during illness with influenza A.

Dosing

Usual dose: 100 mg bid.
Note: A lower dose, usually 100 mg daily, should be given to neurologically impaired or debilitated elderly, or to any patient who develops dizziness, confusion, or other central effects on a higher dose of amantadine.

Duration of Therapy

Unimmunized and immunosuppressed patients: Duration of the epidemic (6 to 12 weeks).
Late immunization: 2 weeks following immunization.
Treatment of influenza A: 5 to 7 days.

PNEUMOCOCCAL DISEASE

The incidence of pneumococcal disease increases dramatically with age, the elderly population experiencing more severe disease and greater mortality. These risks are substantially higher in chronically ill and institutionalized patients.

Pneumococcal Vaccine (Pneumovax)

Pneumococcal vaccine is a polyvalent preparation containing purified capsular polysaccharides from 23 serotypes of *Streptococcus pneumoniae*. This preparation has replaced the earlier vaccine, in which 14 serotypes were represented.

Antibody response to this vaccine seems to be satisfactory in healthy elderly recipients, and an efficacy of 60%–70% can be expected. Unfortunately, efficacy may be reduced in the chronically ill. This is due to impaired antibody response to the vaccine, and, since killing of pneumococcus requires opsonization as well, the dysfunction of white blood cells in infected elderly may further reduce the efficacy of immunization.

Adverse Effects

Local reactions consisting of discomfort, erythema, and induration occur commonly and last approximately 2 days. Less commonly, a transient **febrile reaction** occurs. More severe febrile reactions accompanied by myalgias, headache, and chills are extremely rare in elderly recipients of this vaccine when a one-time dose is given. Anaphylactoid reactions are likewise rare.

No drug interactions have been reported to occur with pneumococcal vaccine.

Recommendations

Pneumococcal vaccine should be given to all individuals 65 and over, for the prevention of pneumonia and other systemic illness caused by strains of *S. pneumoniae* represented in the vaccine. The current vaccine affords no protection against other capsular types.

Pneumococcal vaccine 0.5 ml is administered subcutaneously or intramuscularly as a one-time dose. It may be given at the same time as influenza vaccine, but a separate injection site should be used.

Although the duration of protection is not certain, booster doses do not increase efficacy, and the incidence of local and systemic adverse effects increases substantially with repeat doses. Therefore, pneumococcal vaccine should not be given more than once and recipients of the earlier 14-valent preparation should not receive the 23-valent preparation.

In order to ensure an adequate antibody response, the vaccine should be given at least 10 days prior to immunosuppressive therapy. It should not be given during acute febrile or respiratory illness.

TETANUS AND DIPHTHERIA

Tetanus is a severe, often fatal illness caused by the anaerobic, spore-forming bacterium *Clostridium tetani*. Although the disease is not communicable and is preventable by administration of tetanus toxoid, roughly 100 cases occur in the United States annually, and the majority of patients are under- or unimmunized elderly. Many cases are not caused by the classic puncture wound or laceration, but occur in conjunction with decubitus ulcers or gangrene, to which the elderly are particularly susceptible, as well as to burns and abrasions.

The current generation of elderly have not been exposed to school immunization programs, and in the case of most women, not even to military immunization programs. Although active immunization with tetanus toxoid usually produces adequate antibody response in elderly recipients, the average 10-year duration of protective titers may be somewhat shorter than the usual 10 years in a minority of elderly. These facts dictate that, unless a clear-cut immunization history dictates otherwise, a primary immunization series should be considered over a perfunctory booster shot when tetanus toxoid is given to an elderly patient. Boosters should be given at least every 10 years, as in younger individuals.

Diphtheria is a severe communicable disease caused by *Corynebacterium diphtheriae*. Although immunization programs have resulted in a dramatic decrease in incidence, sporadic outbreaks occur in the United States. The highest mortality among adults is seen in the elderly, and disease occurs primarily in this age group because of underimmunization.

Tetanus and Diphtheria Toxoids

Tetanus toxoid is an exotoxin that has been rendered nontoxic by treatment with formaldehyde but which retains its immunogenicity. It is available in aluminum salt adsorbed and nonadsorbed fluid forms, the former conferring antibody titers for a longer duration. It may be given alone or with **diphtheria toxoid** antigen as a combination preparation. The usual adult preparation (Td) should be given to elderly recipients. The abbreviation *Td*, to be distinguished from the pediatric preparation (DT), indicates the lower concentration of diphtheria antigen used to reduce the risk of adverse effects.

Adverse Effects

Local erythema and **swelling** may occur. Systemic reactions are uncommon, but severe **allergic reactions** have been reported. Neurological reactions, including encephalopathy and seizures, have been reported but are rare and their direct link to toxoid has not been firmly established.

Contraindications

Patients with known serious reactions to either toxoid should not receive them.

Recommendations

Physicians should consider giving tetanus and diphtheria toxoids electively to all elderly patients. If immunization history is unknown or is inadequate, tetanus toxoid is indicated at the time of puncture wound or laceration, or development of decubitus ulceration or gangrene. When wounds are incurred in a setting favoring infection with *C. tetani*, antitoxin should be given in addition to tetanus toxoid.

Individuals exposed to diphtheria should be given a booster even if they have been adequately immunized within 5 years.

Timing and Administration

Primary tetanus toxoid schedule consisting of 3 separate injections should be followed for elderly people who have not been immunized, who have not received tetanus or a booster within the previous 10 years, or whose immunization history is not known. Primary immunization consists of 0.5 ml single or combined toxoid given at least 4 weeks apart and a third smaller dose given 6 to 12 months later.

Booster injection is administered every 10 years. Although there is some evidence that protection may not last for 10 years in certain elderly, serious adverse reactions may be related to very high antibody levels. Thus, the ordinary adult recommendations of 10-year intervals between boosters apply to elderly individuals.

Patients with muscle atrophy should receive the intramuscular injection in the thigh muscle rather than the deltoid in order to avert potentially irritating subcutaneous administration.

Elective (but not emergency) immunization should be postponed

IMMUNIZATION SCHEDULE FOR PEOPLE 65 AND OLDER

Vaccine	Timing	Repeat
Influenza	Late fall	Annual
Pneumococcus	Optional	No
Tetanus	Primary series (see text)	Booster every 10 years
Diphtheria	Same as tetanus	Same as tetanus

in immunosuppressed states, which can foster an inadequate antibody response, and during acute febrile illness.

BIBLIOGRAPHY

Bentley, D. W., Immunizations in the elderly. *Bull. N.Y. Acad. Med.* 63:533, 1987.

Center for Disease Control. Diptheria, tetanus, and pertussis: Guidelines for vaccine prophylaxis and other preventive measures. *Ann. Intern. Med* 103 (6 pt. 1):896, 1985.

Center for Disease Control. Prevention and control of influenza: Recommendations of the Immunization Practices Advisory Committee. *Ann. Intern. Med.* 107:521, 1987.

Committee on Immunization. *Guide for Adult Immunization.* Philadelphia: American College of Physicians, 1990.

Degelau, J., Somani, S., Cooper, S. L., et al. Occurrence of adverse effects and high amantadine concentrations with influenza prophylaxis in the nursing home. *J. Amer. Geriatr. Soc.* 38:428–423, 1990.

Mostow, S. R. Influenza—a controllable disease? *J. Amer. Geriatr. Soc.* 36:281, 1988.

Simberkoff, M. S., Cross, A. P., Al-Ibrahim, M., et al. Efficacy of pneumococcal vaccine in high-risk patients: results of a Veterans Administration cooperative study. *N. Engl. J. Med.* 315:318–327, 1986.

Sims, R. V., Steinmann, W. C., McConville, J. H., et al. The clinical effectiveness of pneumococcal vaccine in the elderly. *Ann. Intern. Med.* 108:653–657, 1988.

Prescribing for Skin Problems

TREATMENT OF SKIN ULCERS

The most common forms of skin ulcers seen in the elderly are pressure (decubitus) ulcers, venous stasis ulcers, and arterial ulcers. Treatment principles are outlined below, with emphasis on specific agents and appliances now commercially available. Although commercial products represent a major advance in the treatment of ulcers, there is no real substitute for good medical and nursing care, and, above all, prevention.

DECUBITUS ULCER (PRESSURE SORE, BEDSORE)

Treatment of decubitus ulcers depends on the extent of the ulcer and whether or not complications are present. Several staging classifications exist. In general, decubitus ulcers are classified according to their depth. The following classification has been adopted by a national pressure ulcer advisory panel and will be referred to in this book.

NATIONAL PRESSURE ULCER ADVISORY PANEL CLASSIFICATION
OF DECUBITUS ULCERS

Stage 1: Non-blanchable erythema of intact skin; the heralding lesion of skin ulceration.

Stage 2: Partial thickness skin loss involving epidermis and/or dermis. The ulcer is superficial and presents clinically as an abrasion, blister, or shallow crater.

Stage 3: Full thickness skin loss involving damage or necrosis of subcutaneous tissue which may extend down to, but not through, underlying fascia. The ulcer presents clinically as a deep crater with or without undermining of adjacent tissue.

Stage 4: Full thickness skin loss with extensive destruction, tissue necrosis or damage to muscle, bone, or supporting structures (e.g., tendon, joint capsule, etc.).

—*From National Pressure Ulcer Advisory Panel, 1989.*

Decubitus ulcers develop as the result of pressure, friction, and moisture, and can occur in virtually any location on the body. The likelihood of developing a decubitus ulcer increases when pressure exceeds mean capillary pressure of 32 mm Hg, in which case blood flow is occluded and the stage is set for tissue death and skin breakdown. The most common sites are the sacrum, greater trochanter, ischial tuberosity, heel, and lateral malleolus. Areas of bony prominence are unusually susceptible because subcutaneous fat is sparse and pressure concentrating on that site easily exceeds capillary pressure. Patients with contractures and amputations may have ulcers in unexpected sites. In short, any area of the body that is exposed to unrelenting pressure or friction is at risk.

Risk Factors

Advanced age is an independent risk factor for decubiti because the skin thins with age, tends to abrade more readily, and heals more slowly. Loss of subcutaneous fat with age enhances the susceptibility to skin breakdown in areas of bony prominence. Healing may be further complicated by nutritional deficiencies that occur commonly in debilitated patients, protein, calorie, zinc, and vitamin-C deficiencies being those most likely to contribute to ulcer severity. Anything that reduces a patient's ability to move around while recumbent and shift pressure voluntarily or reflexly while asleep increases the risk. Thus, patients who are immobilized, physically restrained, paralyzed, oversedated, comatose, or who have impaired sensation to noxious stimuli are at particularly high risk. Dementia itself is a risk factor because it impairs a person's ability to follow instructions, and it may lead to nutritional deficiencies and, when agitation is present, to repeated skin trauma. The presence of diabetes adds additional risks, including reduced vascularity and increased susceptibility to infection.

Knowledge of risk factors helps the physician to identify patients at risk and to order precautionary measures **before** the ulcer forms. Ulcer cure is far more difficult and expensive to achieve than ulcer prevention. Stubborn ulcers can lead to pain, deformity, systemic infection, osteomyelitis, fasciitis, myositis, and death.

Prevention

The prevention of decubitus ulcers rests in reversing modifiable risk factors.

a. Avoid prolonged pressure or friction on one site.
b. Turn recumbent patients from side to side every 2 hours or more, 24 hours a day. Position and prop the patient using pillows. The patient's body should generally lie in the 30-degree lateral oblique position rather than directly on his or her side, avoiding pressure on areas of bony prominence.
c. Move patients by lifting, not sliding. Two or more workers may be needed to accomplish the task. A sling constructed from a sheet or other appliance may be employed.
d. Get chair-bound patients up regularly, or move them from chair to bed and back. Cushion chair with "egg crate" foam cushions, which distribute pressure, or sheepskin, which absorbs moisture.
e. Keep incontinent patients meticulously dry.
f. Maximize nutritional status. Correct deficiencies of protein, calories, vitamin C, and zinc. Correct anemia if possible.
g. Pad pressure sites such as heels, elbows, knees, or any other site that appears at risk of excessive pressure or friction in individual patients. Sheepskin rather than synthetic padding should be used.
h. Use only sheets that have a smooth, soft surface; they should be washed with mild detergent, rinsed thoroughly, and should not be bleached.
i. Maximize staffing.

Treatment

For all grades of ulcer, treatment must include the same measures used in a prevention program, as outlined above. Stage 1 lesions require only removal of pressure and they generally resolve without further treatment. For stage 4 ulcers, surgical or medical management is complex and surgical consultation is recommended. Stage 3 ulcers must also be carefully explored and evaluated before standard care is given, particularly when there is significant undermining of skin. The following discussion is primarily applicable to the treatment of ulcers of intermediate grade—stage 2, and occasionally stage 3.

Cleaning: Should Antiseptics Be Used?

Prior to dressing or debriding a wound, the skin should be cleaned with sterile water or saline and patted dry with clean gauze. The use of antiseptic agents is controversial. While they effectively reduce wound odor and are commonly prescribed in the widely held belief that they hasten wound healing, antiseptics are irritating and should be applied sparingly.

Hydrogen peroxide is very irritating to disrupted skin and may be counterproductive to the healing process. Its use should be reserved for debridement purposes (see below). **Povidone-iodine (Betadyne), sodium hypochlorite (Dakin's solution)**, and **acetic acid** are other antiseptic agents commonly used but equally or more harmful to normal tissue. All antiseptics are antibacterial, but the greater their antibacterial potency, the greater their toxicity to normal and regenerating tissue. This risk-benefit ratio must be taken into consideration before prescribing.

The specific antipseudomonal action of acetic acid does, however, give it a potential advantage. A low concentration (¼%) is felt to confer sufficient antibacterial activity while minimizing harm to normal tissue.

Debridement

Surgical debridement may be required in severely necrotic areas, if thick eschar is present, if the extent or severity of an ulcer below necrotic tissue is not known, or if the ulcer has produced substantial undermining of normal skin. Once the lesion is well defined or if lesser amounts of necrotic tissue are present, nonsurgical debridement may be undertaken.

Occlusive dressings (see below) may soften hard eschar if the layer is thin, promoting a sort of autodebridement. However, it is important to carefully inspect and explore the extent of the wound before applying the dressing.

The necrotic area may be scrubbed with **hydrogen peroxide,** applied directly with a cotton-tipped swab. Normal and regenerating tissue should be protected from this treatment, since it may retard healing and produce pain, and hydrogen peroxide should be rinsed immediately with sterile saline or water.

Wet-to-dry dressings (gauze soaked in saline, allowed to dry) are an effective debriding method but can be very painful to the patient.

Enzymatic debriding agents, such as fibrinolysin-desoxyribonuclease (Elase) are available commercially (see Table 33–1). Their purpose is to digest necrotic tissue, but, not surprisingly, they may damage underlying or surrounding normal tissue and should be used only as long as the ulcer itself is the source of necrotic tissue. They have limited effect on thick eschar, which should, in any case, be explored before enzymatic agents are applied. These agents should be applied only after the wound is cleaned. They should not be used in conjunction with other irritating agents, such as antiseptics or hy-

Table 33–1. Enzyme Debriding Agents

Elase (fibrinolysin-desoxyribonuclease)
Biozyme-C, Santyl (collagenase)
Travase (sutilains)
Granulex (trypsin)
Panafil (papain)

drogen peroxide, which may deactivate the enzyme, or which may themselves enhance disruption of normal tissue.

Enzymatic agents generally do not produce pain, but may be less effective than other debriding methods. Manufacturers recommend that enzymatic agents be applied up to 4 times a day. They often prove to be an expensive means of accomplishing what might be achieved with other measures.

Another enzyme, sutilains (Travase), is inactive until moistened. This may require around-the-clock changing of wet dressings, increasing the likelihood of maceration and increasing nursing time.

Enzymatic agents may lose potency with time, so product shelf life should be strictly heeded.

Managing Excessively Moist Ulcers

Skin ulcers frequently produce large amounts of purulent or serous exudate, especially in the early stages of healing. "Wound cleaning" substances are sometimes used in these situations in order to absorb this excessive moisture. **Dextran hydrophilic spherical beads (Debrisan, others)** are roughly 0.2 mm in diameter and are applied in a layer to the surface of such wounds. Not only is fluid absorbed, but proteins are trapped, which is said to retard the formation of eschar. A layer of beads is sprinkled loosely into the clean, debrided ulcer crater and a dressing is applied. Dressings are changed and the crater is cleaned 2 to 4 times a day or as needed. Hydrophilic beads do not remove hard eschar but do help to keep the wound clean and may speed healing of wet ulcers when compared to traditional methods. Use of these substances should be discontinued if discharge ceases or if granulation tissue forms. Debrisan is also available as a paste, which may be easier to apply.

Dextran beads have lost popularity since the introduction of hydrocolloid dressings and granules (see Dressings, below), which absorb fluid and produce a gel, resulting in less pain to the patient when the dressing is removed.

Dressings

GAUZE. **Wet-to-dry** dressings should only be used if debridement is required. Once sufficient debridement is accomplished, such dressings do little to speed healing but may disrupt normal tissue. Furthermore, it is currently held that healing progresses faster in a moist environment, since desiccation is believed to retard the healing process. **Saline-moistened** gauze may be used, but must be changed at very frequent intervals to avoid drying, at which point it becomes converted to a wet-to-dry dressing. With all moistened gauze dressings, care must be taken to avoid maceration of normal tissue. **Dry sterile** gauze and nonstick **Telfa** dressings are still popular, inexpensive, and simple, but are increasingly discouraged by the experts in favor of moist or occlusive dressings.

OCCLUSIVE DRESSINGS. Evidence suggests that healing of intermediate-stage ulcers is accelerated by the use of occlusive dressings, which keep the wound slightly moist. The moist environment prevents desiccation, and this preserves normal tissue and minimizes the pain and disruption of new tissue that occurs when a dry dressing is removed. The occlusive dressing retains in the wound healing substances produced by the wound itself. These substances prevent bacterial growth, autodigest necrotic tissue, and stimulate epithelialization. Occlusion also prevents exogenous bacterial contamination. Some commercially available occlusive dressings are designed to remain on for up to a week at a time. This allows epithelial cells and fibroblasts to migrate undisturbed, further speeding healing.

It is not known to what extent occlusion is ideal. A few cases of exuberant granulation tissue have been reported. In addition, occlusive dressings can theoretically increase the risk of anaerobic infection, although this is probably important only in deep ulcers, those related to vasculitis, and in patients with immunosuppression. Established infection (as opposed to bacterial colonization) should be eliminated before the occlusive dressing is applied. Stasis dermatitis associated with leg ulcers, and surrounding cellulitis of any ulcer should be treated prior to applying an occlusive dressing over the affected area.

The use of occlusive dressings in ischemic ulcers is controversial. It is prudent to avoid them in this setting because of the possibility that anaerobic organisms are present and because oxygenation of tissues is important. Patients with peripheral arterial insufficiency who have stasis ulcers that are clearly of venous origin can generally use occlusive dressings safely.

Commercially available occlusive dressings must be used in conjunction with a total decubitus care regimen because they are an adjunct to, and not a substitute for, good nursing. Finally, it should be emphasized that the reduction of nursing time that results may reduce the time in which the patient receives human contact, a factor of no small importance to the dependent or demented patient.

Several types of occlusive dressings exist.

A **hydrocolloid dressing (DuoDerm)** is opaque and composed of an inner hydrocolloid layer and an outer polyurethane layer. The inner layer that contacts the wound is permeable to moisture from the wound and vapor from normal skin. It absorbs wound fluid, creating a nonadherent gel over the surface of the wound, and absorbs skin moisture, creating an adhesive. The outer backing is water resistant and essentially impermeable to oxygen. While the dressing is in place, wound healing properties are maximized and the dressing can also be removed atraumatically. The dressing itself prevents the entry of exogenous bacteria, friction, and irritating substances, such as urine.

The dressing is applied to the clean wound of which surrounding skin has been thoroughly dried. The intact dressing may be cut down to size but this is not necessary and is only practical if the wound is small enough to allow an adequate margin to provide a seal with the remaining amount large enough to be used properly for the next application. Backing paper is removed from the hydrocolloid surface and the edges of the dressing smoothed to create a tight seal. Additional adhesive tape may be used if the wound is on a greatly curved surface, and may increase adherence during bathing. The dressing may remain in place for up to 7 days but should be removed if leakage occurs, as frequently happens in wet wounds in the early stages of healing. Once the dressing has been opened, it should be discarded and replaced with a fresh dressing.

This type of dressing has practical advantages. It is easy to apply, reduces nursing time significantly, and, in the long run, may reduce nursing cost. It is ideal for the geriatric outpatient with venous stasis ulcers who may lack the manual or cognitive ability to care for a wound. The dressing often adheres without the use of additional adhesive tape, and is thus useful in patients with contact sensitivity to tape. The intact dressing may also reduce pain.

A disadvantage of DuoDerm is that is may give a false sense of security to nursing staff and vigilance may be reduced. This is particularly important in institutionalized patients.

DuoDerm is available in granules and is intended for wounds with excess fluid and for those with some crater formation. In the latter case, the granules fill in the crater, improving application of the dressing itself. If the granules are applied to moist wounds prior to putting the dressing on, gel formation occurs and is said to reduce the frequency of dressing changes. There is no rationale for using the Debrisan-type granule under an impermeable dressing.

Maceration may occur if the dressing is left on too long or if the wound itself produces more moisture than the dressing can absorb. Leakage of fluid around the dressing should prompt inspection of the wound and a dressing change. The dressing should be changed as soon as leakage occurs, but frequent changes are otherwise discouraged because this will facilitate removal of normal, regenerating epidermis.

Exudative fluid in a shallow ulcer is not a contraindication to the use of this type of dressing. In fact, by dissolving fibrinous wound tissue, this type of dressing produces a fluid that looks like a purulent exudate and in the early stages of use the wound seems to become wetter. However, close inspection should be done to rule out deep infection, which may require further debridement or antibiotic treatment.

A **polyurethane dressing (OpSite)** is thin, transparent, and permeable to air and water vapor, but is impermeable to liquids. Thus, it protects the ulceration from contamination and irritation, but wound fluid is not absorbed into the dressing and must be evacuated. Contamination is somewhat more likely than with hydrocolloid dressings, and dressing changes may be required more frequently with certain wounds. Once healing begins, the adhesive may also produce dressing adherence to the wound itself, resulting in pain and tissue disruption when the dressing is removed. Maceration of surrounding normal skin may also occur. In addition, this type of dressing may not adhere as well to normal skin and may buckle. The dressing is capable of stretching to a greater width, a property that helps it to conform to greatly curved areas of the body; however, excessive stretching may produce undue pressure to critical areas. Although its transparent nature offers a potential, though minor, advantage, this dressing has more disadvantages than hydrocolloid dressings. It is theoretically safer in the presence of anaerobic infection because it is permeable to oxygen.

Plastic wraps (Saran Wrap, others) are uncommonly used today. They provide a transparent covering that is impermeable to air and liquid. The disadvantage of this type of dressing is that surrounding normal skin may easily become macerated, and the dressing may fall off easily. It requires adhesive tape, to which the patient may be sensitive. Since this type of dressing does not adhere to the wound, removal is painless. However, it is not known whether the hermetic nature of this dressing has other disadvantages.

Although commercially available dressings may increase healing in otherwise well cared for ulcers, they are an **adjunct to and not a substitute for** good nursing care. Decubitus ulcers require constant vigilance and preventive maneuvers as outlined above. **Pressure must be avoided regardless of the dressing used.** All skin ulcers must be tended carefully and require regular follow-up (see below).

A wide variety of techniques, appliances, and auxiliary methods are available. The reader is referred to the Bibliography readings for a complete discussion (see Fowler). **There is no strong evidence that any particular ulcer aid is superior to another in any general sense.** What is most important is good, regular nursing care. The physician and nursing staff generally provide maximal care when they adopt a particular regimen with which they have most experience and which they apply regularly.

Contraindications. Occlusive dressings should not be used in stage-4 pressure ulcers or similarly extensive venous stasis ulcer, or in the presence of frank infection. They should be used with extreme caution in ischemic arterial ulcers and should be not be used on ulcers produced by vasculitis or an infectious agent. They should not be used as a substitute for pressure removal on any type of pressure ulcer.

Pressure Relief Devices

Many devices, cushions, and beds are available commercially and may or may not contribute to wound healing.

CUSHIONS. The "donut" cushion has long been popular, used by thin, chair-bound patients to relieve sacral pressure. Experts generally discourage this because donuts are thought to reduce arterial flow to the very area at risk. Alternatively, experts recommend a "waffle" or "egg carton" cushion constructed from foam rubber, which distributes pressure more widely. Waffle cushions are designed to prevent ulceration, however, and if ulceration is already present, all pressure must be removed. Cushions should always be covered by a smooth, moisture-absorbing covering.

BEDS AND MATTRESSES. Specialized mattresses are frequently used but it is not known if they increase the likelihood of healing or reduce the risk of decubitus ulcers beyond standard preventive maneuvers and meticulous nursing care. The theoretical efficacy of these mattresses and beds depends on their ability to maintain extrinsic pressure on the skin at or below mean capillary pressure.

High density egg-carton foam mattresses are relatively inexpensive but difficult to keep clean.

Air mattresses are easier to keep clean and are available as simple, air-filled mattresses or more expensive and sophisticated air-cell mattresses with air flow or adjustable pressure systems. The latter are claimed to reduce the frequency with which patients must be turned. An advantage of some air mattresses is that they can be quickly deflated when cardiopulmonary resuscitation must be done.

Simple **water** mattresses are relatively inexpensive and can be cleaned but need to be relatively thick for pressure reduction to be attained. **Water beds** are more cumbersome and expensive, but are thicker and theoretically more effective because extrinsic pressure changes inherently and continually. In addition, some can be heated, which adds to comfort.

The **air-fluidized bed** (Clinitron, Skytron) is composed of silicon beads through which warm air flows under pressure. This system takes on the property of a fluid, mimicking a water bed. While this system is said to be bacteriostatic, it may be difficult to clean; moreover, the air flow may increase insensible fluid loss, the patient may be difficult to position, and the bed is very expensive. A recent study concluded that conventional treatment of patients using the air-fluidized bed was more effective than in patients on an alternating air-mattress system, and less frequent turning time was required (see Allman). However, the gains achieved by the air-fluidized system may not be great enough to justify the cost. Decubitus ulcers in debilitated elderly may heal very slowly and the number of patients who could avail themselves of each bed would be limited.

VENOUS STASIS ULCER

The principles of cleaning, debridement, dressing, and antibiotic treatment of the decubitus ulcer are applicable to the treatment of venous stasis ulcers. In addition, there are some specific aspects of treating these leg ulcers that bear discussion.

Whereas extrinsic pressure produces decubitus ulcer, intrinsic forces of decreased venous return initiate skin damage in stasis ulcer, and treatment must be directed towards checking this process. Significant pitting edema is usually present and must be corrected. Diuretics must often be used. If patients cannot tolerate adequate diuretic dosages, **graded elastic compression stockings** (Jobst, Sigvaris) should be employed, unless the patient has coexisting arterial compromise. These stockings are measured and custom-fit to the patient, unlike antiembolic (TED) stockings, which are ready-made and available only in a few sizes. **Ace wrap** does not provide the same type of reliable compression as graded elastic compression stockings but the fact that it is less tight may be advantageous for patients with significant pain. In addition, skeletal limitations prevent many geriatric patients from putting on graded elastic compression stockings but they may be able to apply the Ace wrap.

Leg elevation is useful but impractical, since edema rapidly returns when the legs are lowered. It is probably more useful to recommend an afternoon or evening "rest," in which the patient "stretches out" for an hour or so. The patient should avoid prolonged standing or sitting in one position. In severe ulceration, prolonged recumbency may be required. If bedrest is expected to be prolonged in these circumstances, leg exercises should be prescribed and prophylactic antithrombotic treatment considered.

Medications such as nifedipine and occasionally other vasodilators worsen venous insufficiency and may produce edema; these should be discontinued if possible.

Stasis dermatitis may be confused with cellulitis. Both lesions are erythematous and scaly. However, stasis dermatitis is an eczematous eruption that is not painful and that occurs in the setting of chronic stasis changes, including edema and pigmentation. Topical corticosteroids are generally recommended. Antibiotics should be given if there is accompanying cellulitis.

Compression Boots

The **Unna boot** is a zinc oxide, glycerine, and gelatine bandage, which is molded to the foot and kept on for approximately a week. It promotes healing by keeping the wound clean, preventing trauma, and absorbing exudate. Because the boot is a pressure dressing, it is able to mechanically counteract increased venous pressure, reducing edema. The boot can remain on for up to a week or more, although it generally loses its strength and effectiveness after a week. Early on in wound healing the duration of effectiveness depends on the amount of wound weepage. Compression boots have lost popularity to commercial occlusive dressings that are easier to apply.

A compression boot should not be used in patients with significant arterial insufficiency.

HERPES ZOSTER (SHINGLES)

Shingles is a painful cutaneous eruption believed to be due to reactivation of latent varicella zoster virus (herpes zoster, VZV) in a dermatomal distribution. Among immunocompetent individuals, it is most commonly seen in late life. In most cases, the appearance of shingles does not require a workup for an underlying malignancy or immune deficiency.

Management of shingles consists of local care to prevent superinfection, analgesics, and instituting measures to prevent postherpetic neuralgia. Timely use of the antiviral agent acyclovir may shorten the duration of acute zoster.

Acyclovir (Zovirax)

Pharmacologic Considerations

MECHANISM OF ACTION. Acyclovir (Zovirax) is a nucleoside analogue that inhibits DNA replication of herpes viruses. It is presently used clinically against herpes simplex viruses (HSV) 1 and 2, as well as VZV. Acyclovir inactivates HSV at relatively low concentrations but concentrations nearly 30 times higher are required to inactivate VZV. Cellular DNA is not affected until much higher, suprapharmacologic concentrations are reached.

Oral acyclovir speeds the rate of healing of vesicles and reduces the degree and duration of acute pain in acute herpes zoster infection. It is possible that acyclovir reduces the incidence of long-term complications of ophthalmic zoster. It has not yet been proved to reduce the incidence of postherpetic neuralgia. Its apparent lack of effect in this regard may be due to the fact that the drug would have to be instituted very early in the course of treatment of this condition, which almost always occurs only once in the lifetime of an immunocompetent patient, and individuals may not seek treatment until the inflammatory reaction has set in. The goal of using acyclovir in herpes zoster is thus to shorten the duration of pain and rash of acute zoster.

PHARMACOKINETICS. Oral acyclovir is slowly and incompletely absorbed. On the average, peak plasma concentrations are not reached for 2 hours or more, but the percentage of absorption may decrease further with increasing dosage, due to poor solubility or to saturable absorption of the drug. Approximately 75% of the drug is excreted unchanged in the urine after intravenous administration, but the proportion is only 14% after oral administration. Acyclovir is only about 15% bound to serum proteins, and it distributes widely, with concentrations in infected vesicle fluid approximating the concentration in plasma. However, assuming normal renal function, mean steady state plasma concentrations capable of inactivating VZV require oral doses that are considerably higher than those required in the treatment of genital herpes simplex. Clinical experience supports this observation. Concentrations in aqueous humor are only 40% that in plasma.

The plasma elimination half-life of intravenous acyclovir is 2–3 hours in adults with normal creatinine clearance. A small proportion of oral acyclovir is metabolized, the rest being eliminated by the kidney. Plasma half-life correlates with creatinine clearance, so that plasma half-life can be expected to increase with age.

Adverse Effects

Oral acyclovir is very well tolerated. Nonspecific complaints such as nausea, dizziness, and headache have been reported, but are no greater than those reported with placebo.

Adverse effects do occur with intravenous administration. The concentration of acyclovir is 10 times greater in the kidney than in plasma and at high doses it crystallizes in the tubules and collecting system, causing potentially reversible renal failure. This danger can be minimized by increasing urine flow rates with adequate hydration, giving each dose over 1 hour, with each gram of drug given matched with a liter of fluid. Gastrointestinal disturbances, rash, and phlebitis at the intravenous site, and mild elevations of serum transaminases have also been reported.

Indications

Oral acyclovir is indicated for the treatment of acute cutaneous herpes zoster infection of less than 72-hours' duration. Antiviral activity occurs only when there is actual viral shedding, so the drug must be given as early as possible in the acute infection, and clinical efficacy cannot be ensured if the drug is begun after roughly 1 week. Acyclovir cannot be relied upon to prevent postherpetic neuralgia and other measures should be taken (see below).

The ophthalmic division of the trigeminal nerve is a commonly affected dermatome in herpes zoster infection, but good results have not been consistently obtained with oral acyclovir in preventing ocular complications. This observation has not been fully explained. It has been suggested that viral shedding in ophthalmic zoster is of shorter duration and may be on the wane when the drug is instituted.

Intravenous acyclovir is not indicated in uncomplicated VZV infection. Topical acyclovir has no therapeutic effect and should not be used.

Other Uses

Oral acyclovir is effective in reducing the recurrence of genital HSV. Primary genital infection with HSV is uncommon in the elderly. Those few who have been infected in the past generally have only rare recurrences, in accordance with the natural history of this infection. Recurrences of herpes labialis are even less common over time. Topical acyclovir only modestly reduces pain and increases healing rate in genital HSV infections and has no clinical effect in labial infection.

Dosing in Cutaneous Zoster

Recommended dose: 800 mg PO every 4 hr while awake (5 doses) for 7 days.

Although dose adjustments are generally recommended in the elderly for renally excreted drugs such as acyclovir, this dosage has been found safe and effective in elderly patients. The drug has a very wide therapeutic index when given orally, and clinical experience in the treatment of shingles with oral acyclovir in immunocompetent adults is based primarily on patients over 60. Since shingles is an extremely debilitating and painful affliction, full doses should be given. However, in frank renal insufficiency, dosage adjustments should be made by changing the dosage interval (800 mg every 8 hr for creatinine clearance < 30 ml/min and every 12 hr for creatinine clearance < 10 ml/min).

As a practical matter, patients who require supervision to comply with a multidose regimen may do well on less-frequent dosages if their home situation demands this type of dosing. Lower doses in elderly patients have not been studied, but because renal function may be impaired in the face of normal serum creatinine, therapeutic levels may well be achieved in many elderly.

POSTHERPETIC NEURALGIA

Postherpetic neuralgia is defined as pain that persists beyond the duration of the rash. However, the natural history of zoster pain is such that the majority of patients are pain-free within a few months, and it is not easy to know where the syndrome of persistent acute pain ends and a chronic entity begins. Postherpetic neuralgia may last for a year or more.

The discomfort may include lancinating or shooting pain, itching, or tingling. The symptoms may be disabling and result in depression, social withdrawal, and disordered behavior.

The incidence of postherpetic neuralgia increases dramatically with age, and disabling symptoms are most common in the elderly. Thus, aggressive measures are justified to prevent this affliction in the patient over 60.

Prevention of Postherpetic Neuralgia

The apparent inability of acyclovir to prevent postherpetic neuralgia may be due to the fact that patients come to therapy too late in the course of the infection. It has been suggested that acyclovir would be successful if it were instituted in the prodromal phase of the infection, but this is therapeutically unrealistic in a syndrome that almost always occurs only once in the lifetime of a patient.

The likelihood of developing postherpetic neuralgia may decrease when systemic corticosteroids are given in the early stages of infection. The rationale for this treatment is that inflammation of the acute infection is responsible for damaging the affected nerves, sometimes permanently. Although the use of corticosteroids is not universally recommended, there is some evidence that elderly patients are more likely to benefit than other groups. This may well be because they are at greater risk of developing postherpetic neuralgia.

Fears have been expressed that corticosteroids might precipitate disseminated zoster, but this rarely if ever occurs in immunocompetent patients. However, systemic corticosteroids should not be given to the immunocompromised patient, or to the patient who develops shingles as the result of corticosteroid use.

The use of corticosteroids in the elderly is discussed in Chap. 3. Short-term use suggested here is much better tolerated than long-term use.

Dosing

Prednisone 40–60 mg daily for 1 week, then taper rapidly to complete a 2-week course.

Treatment of Postherpetic Neuralgia

Capsaicin Cream (Zostrix)

MECHANISM OF ACTION. Capsaicin is derived from capsicum, the pepper plant. It is the ingredient thought to mediate the well-known irritative effects of hot peppers on the skin and mucous membranes. Applied to the skin surface, capsaicin produces erythema, pain, and inflammation.

Recent suggestions as to its therapeutic efficacy in reducing pain of postherpetic neuralgia are explained by the observation that topical capsaicin depletes peripheral nerves of substance P, a substance thought to be important in transmission of pain impulses to the central nervous system. Substance P is chemically related to the kinins and other vasoactive peptides, and shares some of their properties.

Limited study of capsaicin for the treatment of postherpetic neuralgia has been promising. Anecdotal reports and open studies must be interpreted in light of the fact that postherpetic neuralgia usually does subside with time. Clinical experience with capsaicin has thus far been somewhat disappointing, clinicians reporting that their patients may not tolerate capsaicin well enough to use it continuously. Scientific trials have studied patients with intractable symptoms. These patients might be more highly motivated, might have clinical pain that outweighs local irritant effects, and might have a neurohormonal environment in their peripheral nerves that is particularly susceptible to the beneficial effects of capsaicin.

ADVERSE EFFECTS. Topical capsaicin often produces **erythema** and a **burning sensation** at the site of application. Painful symptoms due to postherpetic neuralgia may be temporarily increased and this frequently limits compliance. These adverse effects may subside with time.

PRECAUTIONS. To avoid eye irritation, the patient must wash the hands carefully after applying the ointment, or should apply the ointment while wearing gloves.

INDICATIONS. Capsaicin cream is indicated in the treatment of postherpetic neuralgia. It is not indicated for treatment of pain due to painful herpetic rash.

DOSING

Usual dose: 0.025% cream applied to painful dermatome in a thin layer tid to qid. The cream should not be used until after herpetic vesicles have healed.

Note: If burning from the cream is intolerable or limits compliance, the patient may apply lidocaine cream prior to applying capsaicin.

Other Treatments for Postherpetic Neuralgia

A number of agents and treatment modalities have been studied. Although none have been shown to be widely effective, anecdotal reports and scattered evidence from some clinical trials have supported their use. These are summarized on Table 33–2.

Systemic agents, such as tricyclic antidepressants (TCAs), may be poorly tolerated in the elderly. However, TCAs may be effective in neuropathic pain at much lower doses (10–25 mg of amitriptyline) than prescribed for depression and therefore may be better tolerated in this setting. TCAs are discussed more fully in Chap. 8.

TREATMENT OF PHOTOAGING

Photoaging is a group of pathological alterations in the skin that occur as a result of sunlight exposure. The term *extrinsic aging* is sometimes used because some of the changes may be due to toxic factors other than sunlight. These changes differ from normal age changes that occur in the skin, both grossly and histologically. Chronic sunlight exposure produces skin that is finely and coarsely wrinkled, has a yellowish hue and rough to leathery texture, and contains benign hyperpigmented freckles and lentigoes, and premalignant actinic keratoses. These changes are most pronounced in light-skinned individuals. Sunlight, not normal aging, is the main factor that promotes wrinkling, as evidenced by the lack of wrinkles on skin that has not been exposed to the sun and other harsh factors in the environment (e.g., abdomen, lower back).

In normal aging, the skin becomes thin, loses elasticity and sags, and there is deepening of normal expression lines.

Tretinoin (Retin-A)

Tretinoin (Retin-A) is a naturally occurring retinoid, all-*trans* retinoic acid, which has incomplete vitamin A activity, but which, like its isomer isotretinoin (Accutane), influences epidermal proliferation and differentiation in a variety of ways. Tretinoin, however, has a low therapeutic index, being too toxic to be taken systemically, and is available for topical use only.

Table 33–2. Some Suggested Treatments for Postherpetic Neuralgia

Tricyclic antidepressant

Capsaicin cream

Transcutaneous electrical nerve stimulation (TENS)

Ethyl chloride coolant spray; may be followed by rubbing affected area

Topical lidocaine

Nerve blockade

Acupuncture

Intralesional corticosteroids

Other less commonly advocated approaches:
    Amantadine
    Levodopa-carbidopa (Sinemet)

Tricyclic antidepressant plus anticonvulsant (carbamazepine, phenytoin, valproic acid, or clonazepam)

Mechanism of Action

Topical application of tretinoin stimulates dermal collagen synthesis, alters the production of other skin proteins, and stimulates growth of epithelial cells and superficial vessels. It is systemically absorbed and undergoes local and systemic conversion to isotretinoin. Systemic absorption is not felt to be clinically important.

Tretinoin has been most widely prescribed for treatment of acne, but is being increasingly prescribed for prevention and reversal of symptoms of photoaging (dermatoheliosis), although it has not yet been approved for this use. When applied daily for several months, tretinoin reverses fine wrinkling, and confers a pinkish hue to the skin that may be pleasing to users but which represents a low-grade irritant dermatitis. These changes occur as early as 2 to 12 weeks of regular use. Coarse wrinkling and tactile roughness also improve with treatment, but less rapidly. Benign lesions such as freckles and senile lentigos seem to become depigmented with time. Further research will be needed to know whether tretinoin is an effective topical agent for actinic keratoses.

Presently, there is no evidence that tretinoin or any other agent prevents or reverses the changes that occur in the skin as a result of normal aging. Furthermore, at least one investigator feels that tretinoin is less effective for photoaging in patients over the age of 70, who tend to have more advanced skin changes. However, further study of these questions is required.

It is not known how long tretinoin needs to be used for therapeutic efficacy, and presumably it would have to be used indefinitely or repeatedly, provided sunlight exposure were to continue. Avoidance of excessive sunlight exposure and use of potent sunscreens (solar protection factor 15 or higher) are the best way to prevent photoaging.

Adverse Effects

Dermatitis occurs in almost all patients who use tretinoin for dermatoheliosis. Erythema, scaling, localized swelling, pruritus, and burning sensations may occur. This dermatitis resolves when the product is discontinued or when frequency of application is reduced, and is alleviated by topical corticosteroid creams. It may resolve spontaneously only to recur in a "second phase," which may herald the reduction in dermatoheliosis. In most cases, the problem becomes less apparent with time because with treatment, the skin undergoes "hardening," a thickening of the epidermis, which renders it less sensitive to the irritating effects of tretinoin. The dermatitis itself may actually be less severe the older the patient because aged skin mounts a reduced inflammatory response.

At present, there is no evidence that topical tretinoin has long-term adverse systemic or topical effects. Topical tretinoin has been used safely since the 1970s for acne and most likely systemic effects are limited by the small quantity that is applied. However, the treatment of extrinsic aging may well require indefinite use, and the long-term effects on the skin of older individuals are not known.

Retin-A is available in liquid, gel, and cream form; .025%, .05%, and 0.1% strength. Published studies have used creams at varying strengths in 1 thin application at bedtime. Dermatologists generally recommend that patients apply the substance on sites of fine wrinkling or at specific sites that the patient is most concerned about.

Recommendations

It is not known if topical tretinoin is effective in advanced photoaging in patients over the age of 70. It may be used in geriatric patients, but the patient should recognize that the results might not be satisfactory.

Actinic keratoses and other suspicious skin lesions should be treated with established methods.

Pending further research, topical tretinoin should not be touted as a cure for intrinsic skin aging.

Topical 5-Fluorouracil (Efudex, Fluroplex) for Actinic Keratoses

5-fluorouracil is an antineoplastic antimetabolite that is used topically for the removal of actinic keratoses, which affect a large proportion of light-skinned elderly individuals. These are premalignant lesions that occur in sun-exposed areas and that patients often consider unsightly. Topical 5-fluorouracil is a highly effective treatment but it is extremely irritating and should be prescribed by the dermatologist who has experience in its use. It is available in 1% and 5% concentrations.

BIBLIOGRAPHY

Skin Ulcers

Agate, J. N. Aging and the skin—pressure sores. In J. C. Brocklehurst (ed.), *Textbook of Geriatric Medicine and Gerontology* (3rd ed.). Edinburgh: Churchill Livingstone, 1985. Pp. 915–934.

Allman, R. M. Pressure ulcers among the elderly. *N. Engl. J. Med.* 320:850–853, 1989.

Allman, R. M., Walker, J. M., Hart, M. K., et al. Air-fluidized beds or conventional therapy for patients with pressure sores. *Ann. Intern. Med.* 107:641–648, 1987.

Fowler, E. M. Equipment and products used in management and treatment of pressure ulcers. *Nurs. Clin. N. Amer.* 22:449–461, 1987.

National Pressure Ulcer Advisory Panel. Pressure ulcers. Prevalence, cost and risk assessment: Consensus Development Conference statement. *Decubitus* 2:24–28, 1989.

Witkowski, J.A., and Parish, L.C. Cutaneous ulcer therapy. *Int. J. Dermatol.* 25:420, 1986.

Herpes Zoster (Shingles)

Bernstein, J. E. Capsaicin in the treatment of dermatologic disease. *Cutis* 39:352–353, 1987.

Bernstein, J. E., Korman, N. J., Bickers, D. R., et al. Topical capsaicin treatment of chronic postherpetic neuralgia. *J. Amer. Acad. Dermatol.* 21:265–270, 1989.

McKendrick, M. W., McGill, J.I ., White, J. E., et al. Oral acyclovir in acute herpes zoster. *Brit. Med. J.* 293:1529, 1986.

Post, B. T., and Philbrick, J. T. Do corticosteroids prevent postherpetic neuralgia? A review of the evidence. *J. Amer. Acad. Derm.* 18:605–610, 1988.

Watson, C. P. N. Postherpetic neuralgia. *Neurol. Clin.* 7:231–248, 1989.

Watson, C. P., Evans, R. G., and Watt, V. R. Post-herpetic neuralgia and topical capsaicin. *Pain* 33:333–340, 1988.

Ophthalmic Agents

Most geriatric patients are being treated by ophthalmologists for one or more disorders of the eye. Unfortunately, information about what medication they are getting, and why, is not always shared with the primary care physician. Ophthalmic agents, both oral and topical, can produce important systemic effects and can participate in drug-drug interactions. It is important for the primary care physician to do a complete drug history that inquires about eye medications, both on the initial visit and whenever a patient develops a new symptom.

SYSTEMIC EFFECTS OF EYE DROPS

Agents instilled into the eye may be systemically absorbed. If the punctum is not occluded during instillation, the ophthalmic solution may enter the nasolacrimal duct, gain access to the nasopharynx, and be swallowed. However, ingested medication can be removed by the liver on first pass, reducing the bioavailability of this small amount of drug. A more important means of access for ophthalmic agents is via direct absorption through the nasopharyngeal mucosa and the conjunctival and other ocular vessels. These modes of entry avoid first-pass hepatic metabolism, so that active drug enters the circulation directly, producing a more rapid onset of action. For certain medications, this process is analagous to the sublingual route of administration. Systemic absorption may be further enhanced by local factors, such as inflammation, "dry eye," lid laxity, and recent eye surgery.

Ophthalmic agents can also cause local symptoms such as burning, irritation, eye pain, allergic reactions, and, occasionally, more serious ocular problems. Vision can be reversibly impaired by eye drops if they produce miosis or cycloplegia. It has also been suggested that certain agents may accelerate the formation of cataracts, although this is somewhat controversial.

PROPER INSTILLATION OF EYE DROPS

Ideally, the patient should tip the head back slightly and gaze upward while instilling eye drops. Immediately after instillation, the eye should be closed and the punctum should be occluded with the finger for a full minute. This will minimize leakage of the drop out of the eye and will prevent drainage into the nasolacrimal duct.

Unfortunately, many elderly patients have anatomical problems mitigating against proper instillation of drops. Musculoskeletal and arthritic problems of the neck often limit range of neck motion, preventing proper positioning of the head. Diminished ability to gaze upward is another age change that can impede instillation. If the patient has impaired manual dexterity or a tremor, it becomes extremely difficult to operate small dispensers properly. Ectropion, an eversion of the lower eyelid due to age-related skin laxity, is very common and promotes spillage of the drops out of the eye. However, lid laxity may increase the reservoir capacity of the eyelid and systemic absorption of the agent will increase. Lax eyelids also tend to become inflamed, producing local vasodilation, which further enhances systemic absorption of medication.

If eye drops fall out of the eye, or have missed the eye, the patient may try again, so that it will be impossible to judge what the actual dose was. The physician should observe the patient instilling eye drops to ensure that this is being done properly.

The incidence of systemic side effects from topical ophthalmics is not known. Over 60% of adverse effects reported to the National Registry of Ocular Drug Induced Side Effects are systemic ones. Although the direct link of these side effects to the eye drop is not always firmly established, it is less important to know the precise incidence than to be aware that such effects may occur. It is entirely possible that many effects have not been reported in the literature or to the registry because they go unrecognized. Vigilance is required, particularly by the nonophthalmologist, who may be the person contacted by the patient when systemic symptoms develop, but may have less experience in recognizing these problems.

GLAUCOMA DROPS

Beta Blockers

Mechanism of Action

Topical beta blockers are currently the most widely prescribed glaucoma drops. These agents reduce the production of aqueous humor by an unknown mechanism. They are used therapeutically for the treatment of glaucoma and intraocular hypertension. Beta blockers have surpassed other topical agents in popularity because they do not produce pupillary constriction and are therefore less likely to impair vision than older agents, such as pilocarpine. Unfortunately, when sufficient concentrations reach the systemic circulation, they are capable of producing all of the systemic effects seen with the oral beta blockers. There is some evidence that betaxolol, which selectively blocks $beta_1$ receptors, is less likely to produce bronchospasm in susceptible individuals, but, as with oral $beta_1$ selective agents, this is not an entirely reliable property and bronchospasm has been reported. Four agents now in use are listed in Table 34-1.

Systemic effects of ophthalmic beta blockers probably occur much less often than with oral agents, so that many patients who do not tolerate the oral agents may be able to tolerate eye drops. Proper instillation will further reduce the likelihood of systemic effects.

Pharmacologic aspects of ophthalmic beta blockers are similar to those of other beta blockers (see Chap. 12).

Table 34-1. Ophthalmic Beta Blockers

Available Agents (Brand)	Duration of Effect (hr)
Nonselective	
Timolol (Timoptic)	12–24
Levobunolol (Betagan)	12–24
Metipranolol (OptiPranolol)	12–24
Beta₁ selective	
Betaxolol (Betoptic)	12

Adverse Effects

The side-effect profile of beta blockers is discussed fully in Chap. 12. In general, if a systemic effect of beta blockade occurs, the ophthalmic agent should be assumed responsible until proved otherwise. A very large number of **systemic effects** have been reported with these ophthalmic agents since their introduction. These have included approximately 400 cases of cardiorespiratory collapse and many cases of neuropsychiatric syndromes, such as confusion, dementia, and depression. Exacerbation of myasthenia gravis has also been reported.

Although most patients tolerate ophthalmic beta blockers well, it is important to emphasize the systemic problems so that they are not misdiagnosed.

Local effects consist of **stinging** and, with prolonged use, **corneal anesthesia**.

Interactions with Systemic Drugs

Ophthalmic agents may participate in drug-drug interactions. The most important interactions are those involving cardiac medications, and other drugs known to affect cardiac conduction and contractility (see Chap. 12).

Pilocarpine (IsoptoCarpine, Others)

Mechanism of Action

Pilocarpine is a parasympathomimetic agent that acts directly on the muscarinic receptors in the eye to produce pupillary constriction and contraction of the ciliary muscle. This facilitates drainage of aqueous humor and reduces intraocular pressure. Other local effects may be operating as well to reduce aqueous humor production or facilitate outflow. Pilocarpine is used in the treatment of chronic open angle, as well as acute angle closure, glaucoma.

Adverse Effects

By producing miosis, pilocarpine may reduce the visual field and **impair visual acuity**. This may be particularly problematic in older patients with cataracts or macular degeneration, who have a reduced capacity to use the central field of vision. Stimulation of the ciliary muscle produces overactive accommodation in younger people, but in the elderly, impaired ability to accommodate may prevent this effect; however, spasm of the ciliary muscle can occur, producing **eye or brow pain,** problems that may subside with continued therapy.

Of particular importance to the examining physician is the fact that pilocarpine produces a **pinpoint pupil,** confounding the physical examination; if the eye drop is used only in one eye, the pupils will be strikingly unequal. The duration of miosis may be prolonged and the pupillary inequality may be mistaken for an acute neurologic sign in patients presenting to emergency rooms for other reasons.

Systemic effects of pilocarpine are less common than with beta blockers. Systemic toxicity is more likely to be seen with high doses used in acute angle closure glaucoma than with low-dose chronic use. Sufficient systemic concentrations of pilocarpine may produce **gastrointestinal symptoms, hypersalivation, lacrimation, increased bronchial and gastric secretions, bronchospasm, hypotension,** and **bradyarrhythmias. Confusional states, hallucinations,** and **urinary disturbances** have occurred in elderly patients.

Carbachol (IsoptoCarbachol)

Carbachol is a parasympathomimetic agent, similar to pilocarpine in its mechanism of action. Unlike pilocarpine, it has intrinsic anticholinesterase activity and is therefore very long acting. It is somewhat more likely than pilocarpine to produce systemic effects, and these would tend to be of a longer duration.

Echothiophate Iodide (Phospholine Iodide)

Echothiophate iodide acts by irreversibly inhibiting acetylcholinesterase, the enzyme that degrades acetylcholine. Thus, it is a potent cholinomimetic agent, with a mechanism of action and spectrum of effects similar to pilocarpine, but with a very long duration of action. It is only infrequently used today in the treatment of glaucoma.

Systemic effects from echothiophate may present in a delayed fashion, presumably because of gradual accumulation of the drug. A particularly important aspect of echothiophate use is that it can prevent the breakdown of succinylcholine, which is used in conjunction with electroshock treatment and as a muscle relaxant in surgery. In these settings prolonged apnea can occur. It is very important that patients discontinue use of echothiophate for 6 weeks prior to exposure to succinylcholine.

Epinephrine and Other Sympathomimetics

Sympathomimetic agents are used for a variety of purposes. In open angle glaucoma, they act by complex mechanisms to reduce the production of aqueous humor and to increase outflow. These agents are also useful as mydriatic agents to facilitate fundoscopic examinations. The mydriatic effect is sometimes used in chronic glaucoma management to counteract the miotic effect of cholinergic agents.

Epinephrine preparations (Epifrin, Epinal, others) are potent activators of alpha- and beta-adrenergic receptors.

One epinephrine congener, dipivefrin (Propine), is a pro-drug, which is much more lipophilic than epinephrine and penetrates ocular structures more readily. It is converted to epinephrine in the eye, and for this reason it is thought to have a lower incidence of systemic effects.

Epinephrine and its congener should not be used in the aphakic (postcataract) eye because they can produce cystoid macular edema with decreased visual acuity.

Phenylephrine is a sympathomimetic agent with a relatively short duration of action. It is used primarily as a diagnostic mydriatic agent and for its local vasoconstrictor action to reduce redness. Unlike epinephrine, phenylephrine has predominantly alpha-stimulating properties (see Important Drug Interactions, below). Older patients are particularly susceptible to the mydriatic effects of phenylephrine, so that high concentrations (10%) are not commonly used in this age group. Low concentrations (0.12%) are available without prescription.

Some sympathomimetic agents are listed in Table 34–2.

Systemic Effects

The most common systemic effects produced by sympathomimetic agents are cardiovascular. In addition to being a potent vasopressor, epinephrine has a direct effect on the heart; epinephrine preparations can elevate blood pressure, produce tachyarrhythmias, and

Table 34-2. Some Sympathomimetics

Agent (Brand)	Use
Epinephrine (Epinal, others)	Open angle glaucoma
Dipivefrin (Propine)	Open angle glaucoma
Phenylephrine (Neo-Synephrine, others)	
10%	Pupil dilatation, diagnostic use
2.5%	Pupil dilatation; diagnostic use
0.12%	Decongestant

precipitate cardiac ischemia. Tremor may also occur. Metabolic effects of ocular epinephrine have not been studied.

As a pure alpha agonist, phenylephrine is a vasoconstrictor with little direct effect on the heart, and is more likely to elevate blood pressure than produce cardiac arrhythmias, although reflex bradycardia may occur. Adverse effects from low concentrations of phenylephrine are probably rare, but caution should be observed in elderly patients with cardiovascular problems because they are particularly sensitive to adverse effects of these drugs.

By producing mydriasis, these agents may precipitate **angle closure glaucoma** in susceptible patients.

Important Drug Interactions

Adrenergic properties of epinephrine can be potentiated by concurrent administration of monoamine oxidase inhibitors. Various agents that affect the sympathetic nervous system, such as reserpine, guanethidine, tricyclic antidepressants, and beta blockers, may enhance sensitivity to sympathetic stimulation. Alpha-adrenergic agents in particular, such as phenylephrine, may produce large increases in blood pressure when given to patients on these medications or to those who have severe autonomic neuropathies. Elderly patients develop even a higher pressor response to these interactions than do younger patients. Sympathomimetic eye drops should be avoided in patients with cardiovascular disease and those taking any drug that modulates cardiovascular response or neurotransmitters. The same rule applies for nasal or oral decongestants that contain these chemicals.

Anticholinergic Agents (Cycloplegics)

Anticholinergic (atropinelike, parasympatholytic) ophthalmics are used primarily, though not exclusively, for diagnostic purposes. They act by competitively inhibiting the action of acetylcholine at muscarinic sites in various organ systems, including the brain, heart, bladder, and bowel. In the eye, they produce mydriasis and paralysis of accommodation (cycloplegia). Chief among their ophthalmologic uses are pupillary dilatation and cycloplegia for purposes of refraction and retinal examination. Strong cycloplegics are rarely required in elderly patients because the ability to accommodate to close vision is severely impaired. In late life, a sympathomimetic mydriatic, such as phenylephrine, is often used for this purpose instead.

Ocular anticholinergic agents are capable of producing the same effects as systemic agents possessing these properties. As mentioned elsewhere in this book, the elderly are particularly susceptible to anticholinergic side effects, such as dry mouth, urinary retention, constipation, and confusional states, including psychosis. Since most ophthalmic parasympatholytic agents are used on the short-term, **acute reactions,** such as acute **confusional states** and **cardiac arrhythmias,** are probably observed more often than chronic systemic effects. The ophthalmic and systemic effects of the longer-acting ocular agents may last several days.

Central nervous system effects occur more commonly with **cyclopentolate** (Cyclogyl) than with other topical anticholinergic agents, perhaps because a portion of the molecule is similar in structure to certain hallucinogens. **Psychosis, hallucinations, and other serious confusional states** have been reported more in older than in younger adults.

Since cycloplegics and mydriatics are frequently used only in one eye, a unilateral, fixed, and dilated pupil may mislead the physician who happens to be examining the patient for unrelated medical problems. This can be particularly troublesome in medical or neurologic emergencies. A commonly used ocular anticholinergic agent is tropicamide (Mydriacyl). Its duration of effect is relatively brief, making it practical for office evaluation.

CARBONIC ANHYDRASE INHIBITORS

Carbonic anhydrase inhibitors are oral agents with diuretic properties. The two most commonly used agents are acetazolamide (Diamox) and methazolamide (Neptazane). Although they are not particularly useful as diuretics for nonophthalmologic disease, they reduce the production of aqueous humor by inhibiting carbonic anhydrase, and are used in the treatment of glaucoma. In chronic open angle glaucoma, they are generally used as adjunctive therapy in patients who do not have an adequate response to topical ophthalmics.

Agents of this class inhibit carbonic anhydrase, the enzyme that catalyzes the reversible conversion of carbon dioxide and water to carbonic acid. Carbonic anhydrase promotes the generation of bicarbonate ion, which initiates a series of events that increases the tonicity of aqueous humor. Carbonic anhydrase inhibitors alter this process so that less aqueous humor is formed. Since carbonic anhydrase is present in the cells of many tissues, these agents may produce systemic effects.

Carbonic anhydrase inhibitors are excreted virtually unchanged in the kidney and their duration of action is probably prolonged in the elderly. With age, an increased uptake or prolonged binding of acetazolamide by various cells of the body has been noted. This could partly explain the higher incidence of side effects produced by these drugs in older patients.

Adverse Effects

Adverse systemic effects occur in a large proportion of patients and are particularly common in the elderly.

The most important electrolyte disturbance seen is **systemic acidosis,** which may be severe. **Hypokalemia** tends to be mild and transitory. However, potassium depletion may be profound when these agents are taken concurrently with potassium-wasting diuretics.

As diuretics, carbonic anhydrase inhibitors may produce **disturbances in micturition**. Although their diuretic action is weak, geriatric patients with underlying bladder dysfunction may find the effect significant.

Constitutional effects include **confusion, depression, paresthesias** of the extremities, and **decreased appetite**. It is unclear if these symptoms are related to systemic acidosis or are due to a direct action in the nervous system.

Some carbonic anhydrase inhibitors have been noted to promote **urolithiasis**. The mechanism may be related to alkalinization of urine and decreased renal excretion of citrate and magnesium, factors that reduce the solubility of urinary calcium. Stones have been reported more often with acetazolamide than other agents, but this may reflect higher use of the former.

Carbonic anhydrase inhibitors, which contain a sulfonamide moiety, are capable of producing **allergic reactions**.

Other side effects include **nausea, diarrhea,** and **malaise**. Carbonic anhydrase inhibitors are virtually devoid of ocular adverse effects.

Important Drug Interactions

As mentioned above, concurrent administration of potassium-wasting diuretics may result in severe hypokalemia. This is especially likely to occur with thiazides, which have weak carbonic anhydrase inhibiting properties. Since systemic hypertension and intraocular hypertension are epidemiologically (though not necessarily etiologically) related, and since these two conditions are usually treated by separate physicians, this drug combination occurs often and may go unnoted by the prescribers.

Hypokalemia may also occur when these agents are used in conjunction with corticosteroids. In addition, by alkalinizing the urine, carbonic anhydrase inhibitors can reduce renal clearance of certain drugs, including lithium and quinidine.

ARTIFICIAL TEARS

"Dry eye" is a relatively benign form of xerophthalmia that, though not confined to the elderly, affects primarily older individuals. Patients complain of irritative symptoms, such as itching, "sandy" feeling, burning, excessive tearing, redness, and inflammation. Impaired tear production reduces the delivery of endogenous antimicrobial substances to the eye and increases the likelihood of infectious conjunctivitis. Accompanying epithelial damage may enhance the systemic absorption of ophthalmic agents. Unlike other causes of xerophthalmia, such as vitamin-A deficiency, dry eye rarely impairs visual acuity to a significant degree. However, ocular epithelial damage is commonly present and visual acuity may be affected.

Dry eye may be subclinical, becoming symptomatic only because of environmental or climatic conditions, contact lens wearing, or drugs that impair tear formation, such as agents with anticholinergic effects, antihistamines, and some cardiovascular drugs.

The cause of dry eye is somehow related to decreased or erratic production of normal tears or production of tears with altered chemical composition. Normal tears are composed of an outer lipid layer, a water layer, and an inner mucoid layer, each with specific properties and functions. In dry eye, it has been suggested that one or more of these layers may be affected. In addition, a spectrum of ocular surface abnormalities may be present. It is not known if or when these are primary or secondary features of the condition. Keratoconjunctivitis sicca is a severe form of dry eye that is associated with autoimmune diseases, such as Sjogren's syndrome; it is probably responsible for only a small proportion of cases.

Xerophthalmia is best evaluated by an ophthalmologist, since ocular surface epithelial damage and other disorders may exist. Treatment consists of attempting to avoid external irritants, treating accompanying allergy or infection, such as blepharitis, ruling out autoimmune or other systemic disease, discontinuing drugs known to produce diminished tearing, avoiding vitamin-A deficiency, and, when indicated, instillation of artificial tears. Artificial tears may provide relief of irritative symptoms, improve visual acuity, and minimize damage to surface epithelium. However, their effect is palliative and of unpredictable benefit. Because their residence time in the eye is limited, they must be instilled throughout the day.

About two dozen preparations are currently on the market, and all bottled preparations are available without prescription. Artificial tears consist of a polymeric ingredient and a preservative with weak antimicrobial properties. Preservative-free brands are available for use in patients with hypersensitivity reactions to that component. The purpose of the polymer is to increase tear viscosity, prolonging their residence time in the eye. Since the physiology and composition of tears are complex, the constituents of artificial tears do not necessarily duplicate the natural environment. Furthermore, dry eye may be due to or associated with a number of factors, such as decreased tear production, decreased or abnormal mucin or lipid in the tear, decreased blinking, or ocular disease. Thus, the prescriber cannot predict the extent to which the various components of the preparation will ameliorate the problems in each individual case. Nor are artificial tears particularly helpful in patients with decreased blinking, such as those with Parkinson's disease, since blinking is important in tear renewal as well as protection of the eye surface.

The **preservative component** of artificial tears may pose problems for certain patients. One preservative, thimerosal, is an allergen that produces **hypersensitivity reactions**, including keratopathies and a stubborn condition known as giant papillary conjunctivitis. Though less sensitizing than thimerosal, benzalkonium chloride may also produce irritating symptoms in susceptible patients.

An **artificial tear insert** (Lacrisert) is available by prescription only. This preparation is a tiny hydroxypropyl cellulose stick, 3.5 mm long, which is inserted into the inferior cul de sac once or twice a day. The cellulose polymer is very viscous and **may blur the vision** or produce **crusting of the lids and lashes**. More expensive than bottled tears, Lacrisert is intended for use in patients with relatively refractory symptoms, but it may be appropriate for selected patients living at home, who have limited access to care providers but who are unable to instill tears themselves. A trained visiting nurse or family member could insert the preparation once a day or less often, as indicated. However, this viscous material should be dispensed only by a physician experienced in its use.

Artificial tears have not been reported to produce systemic symptoms.

CORTICOSTEROIDS

Topical corticosteroid preparations of prednisolone or dexamethasone play an important role in a variety of inflammatory and immunologic diseases of the eye, among them uveitis, allergic keratoconjunctivitis, and postoperative inflammation. These agents have the potential of producing **important local side effects**, including increased intraocular pressure, cataract formation, decreased wound or defect healing, and potentiation of herpes simplex keratitis. For this reason, they should only be used for important indications and dispensed by physicians experienced in their use, namely ophthalmologists.

Perhaps unfortunately, corticosteroids are available in combination with topical antibiotics (Cortisporin, Blephamide, TobraDex, others) and are liberally prescribed by nonophthalmologists who may be unfamiliar with the risks. In general, it is inadvisable to prescribe these combinations when the antibiotic alone would suffice.

ANTIBIOTICS

Ophthalmic antibiotics are more likely to produce local irritative and allergic symptoms than systemic ones. However, systemic absorption occurs. Idiosyncratic aplastic anemia has been reported with ocular chloramphenicol. This dreaded form of anemia is rare and not age-related.

Although the aminoglycosides, gentamicin, tobramycin, and neomycin, are potentially ototoxic and nephrotoxic, these are dose-related problems that are unlikely to occur at the blood levels achieved from ocular preparations.

Nonophthalmic forms of chloramphenicol, sulfonamides, and ciprofloxacin (recently available as an ophthalmic agent) participate in important drug interactions, as discussed elsewhere in this handbook. It is not known whether ocular antibiotics interact significantly with systemic drugs.

OCULAR ANTIHISTAMINE-DECONGESTANTS

Several ocular preparations are available and are used primarily for allergic conjunctivitis. They are available in combination with weak sympathomimetic agents to produce a decongestant effect. Both the antihistamine and the sympathomimetic agent are capable of producing mydriasis. There are no reports of systemic effects related to the antihistamine in these specific combination agents, but certainly they are theoretically possible. The adverse effects of antihistamines are discussed fully in Chap. 30. Precautions regarding sympathomimetic agents are discussed above.

PRESCRIBING NONOPHTHALMIC DRUGS FOR THE GLAUCOMA PATIENT

Approximately 95% of elderly patients treated for glaucoma have chronic open angle glaucoma or intraocular hypertension. Although the prevalence of the narrow anterior chamber angle increases with age, only a small minority of elderly patients have narrow angle glaucoma. It is important for the physician to be aware of the specific diagnosis when prescribing medications for the glaucoma patient.

A number of medications that dilate the pupil may precipitate an acute attack of glaucoma in susceptible individuals, namely those

Table 34-3. Drugs That Can Cause Acute Angle Closure Glaucoma

Drugs with Anticholinergic Action
  Antihistamines
  Antipsychotic drugs
  Gastrointestinal antispasmodics
  Urinary antispasmodics
  Some antiparkinson drugs
  Tricyclic antidepressants
  Topical mydriatics and cycloplegics

Adrenergic agents
  Bronchodilators
  Decongestants (oral, ocular, nasal)
  Central stimulants

---

with a narrow anterior chamber angle or a history of acute angle closure glaucoma. The susceptibility to this effect is increased with age proportional to the increased prevalence of the narrow angle, but it is difficult to predict risk in individual patients. The risk is greater from topical than systemic agents. Key medications are listed in Table 34-3.

The agents in the table are not, however, contraindicated in chronic open angle glaucoma or intraocular hypertension, which are unrelated to the size of the anterior chamber angle. This mistake is made frequently, with the consequence that useful medications may be withheld unnecessarily. However, corticosteroids, particularly those instilled in the eye, may raise intraocular pressure significantly. Although the institution of systemic steroids may not precipitate an acute emergency in the patient with open angle glaucoma, patients requiring systemic steroids should be referred immediately to their ophthalmologist for close consultation. Ocular steroids should generally be prescribed only by an ophthalmologist experienced in their use and indications.

BIBLIOGRAPHY

Holly, F. J. Aqueous tear substitutes. In D. W. Lamberts and D. E. Potter (eds.), *Clinical Ophthalmic Pharmacology*. Boston: Little, Brown, 1987. Pp. 497-518.

Pavan-Langston, D., and Dunkel, E. C. *Handbook of Ocular Drug Therapy and Ocular Side Effects of Systemic Drugs*. Boston: Little, Brown, 1991.

Selvin, B. L. Systemic effects of topical ophthalmic medications. *South. Med. J.* 76:349-358, 1983.

Zimmerman, T. J., Kooner, K. S., Kandarakis, A. S., and Ziegler, L. P. Improving the therapeutic index of topically applied ocular drugs. *Arch. Ophthalmol.* 102:551-553, 1984.

Index